D1714694

The Changing Nervous System

THE
CHANGING
NERVOUS
SYSTEM

Neurobehavioral Consequences
of Early Brain Disorders

Edited by

Sarah H. Broman

Jack M. Fletcher

New York   Oxford

OXFORD UNIVERSITY PRESS

1999

Oxford University Press

Oxford   New York
Athens   Auckland   Bangkok   Bogotá   Buenos Aires   Calcutta
Cape Town   Chennai   Dar es Salaam   Delhi   Florence   Hong Kong   Istanbul
Karachi   Kuala Lumpur   Madrid   Melbourne   Mexico City   Mumbai
Nairobi   Paris   São Paulo   Singapore   Taipei   Tokyo   Toronto   Warsaw

and associated companies in
Berlin   Ibadan

Copyright © 1999 by Oxford University Press, Inc.

Published by Oxford University Press, Inc.
198 Madison Avenue, New York, New York 10016
http://www.oup-usa.org

Library of Congress Cataloging-in-Publication Data
The changing nervous system :
neurobehavioral consequences of early brain disorders /
edited by Sarah H. Broman, Jack M. Fletcher.
p.   cm.   Includes bibliographical references and index.
ISBN 0-19-512193-7
1. Pediatric neurology.   2. Developmental neurobiology.
3. Developmental disabilities.   4. Neuroplasticity.
5. Nervous system—Growth.
I. Broman, Sarah H.   II. Fletcher, Jack, 1952–.
[DNLM: 1. Brain Diseases—in infancy & childhood.
2. Brain Diseases—complications.
3. Brain Injuries—in infancy & childhood.
4. Brain Injuries—complications.   5. Cognition Disorders—etiology.
6. Developmental Disabilities—etiology.
WS 340 C456 1999]   RJ486.C43   1999   618.92'8—dc21
DNLM/DLC   for Library of Congress   98-45750

2 4 6 8 9 7 5 3 1
Printed in the United States of America
on acid-free paper

*Thanks to F. J. Brinley, Jr.,
Stephen Groft and Rita Taylor
for their much appreciated support
and encouragement*

Foreword

This volume is a collection of valuable contributions on varied aspects of neuroscience, from basic to clinical, united around three important ideas. The first is that the nervous system is plastic rather that static. The second is that early brain disorders condition brain plasticity in a particular way. The third is that those plastic changes can now be better understood and that their understanding may lead to better treatment and care of the individuals affected by those disorders.

The volume starts out in the most auspicious manner, by calling the reader's attention to the word "changing" in the title. It is certainly true that the idea that the brain is changeable, rather than rigid, is not a new idea. That does not mean, however, that the idea does not need to be defended and supported with fresh evidence. The reason why such support is still needed is that, although not novel, it is an idea that is often forgotten. Old habits die hard, and one of the oldest habits when it comes to thinking about the brain is that, somehow, between the genome and early development, the brain acquires a steady state that only diseases or old age manage to modify. The idea of brain stability has been inculcated in the public's mind, and, unfortunately, in the minds of so many physicians and scientists that sometimes even substantial amounts of counter evidence have little effect in the prevailing attitude. There is no doubt, of course, that regeneration is hardly the distinctive feature of the human nervous system. There is little doubt also that neuron division will not turn out to be a principle. Also unquestionably, substantial damage to the nervous system is more likely to cause irreparable defects than functional improvements. And yet, the evidence is equally clear that the nervous system, and in that I include the human nervous system, can respond to injury in a most adaptive fashion. It is also evident that, because of the fundamentally plastic, changeable nature of the system, it is possible to direct modifications in a way that encourages compensation for the deficits incurred through brain damage. Perhaps most important, in relation to the material covered in this volume it is apparent that the age at which disorders have their onset is a critical factor in the profile of changes that subsequently occur in the damaged nervous system. Moreover, a number of other cofactors influence the ultimate outcome of damage and condition the prospects of therapeutically directed recovery.

The volume edited by Sarah Broman and Jack Fletcher brings together many scientists and practitioners dedicated, in one way or another, to the study of early brain damage. They are also concerned, in most diverse manners, with the direction taken by either the natural or the directed plastic changes of those affected brains. Since brain plasticity is now a central theme for investigators and clinicians working on different levels of the nervous system, on different species, and with different approaches, it is useful to have, under the same cover, a set of contributions that focuses on one particular problem: the neurobehavioral consequences of early brain disorders. The interested reader, especially the reader who may be just discovering the crossroads between plasticity and brain disease, will find those contributions grouped under logical partitions: three chapters on the basics of synaptic circuit development and on the effects of differential experience on those circuits; three chapters on mechanisms of reorganization of brain circuitry; seven chapters describing the course of neurobehavioral changes in a variety of early brain disorders; and two chapters on the matter of therapeutic intervention, one outlining fundamental issues in the design of effective treatments, and another reporting on some exciting new results which suggest that improvements of performance are indeed possible.

The editors should be commended on their choice of authors, most of whom are familiar names in the large family of neuroscience, and for showcasing their contributions in a way that will be both pleasant and useful to the large number of readers interested in this topic.

Antonio R. Damasio
M. W. Van Allen Professor and Head
Department of Neurology
University of Iowa College of Medicine

Preface

Beginning in the pre-Socratic era, philosophers and scientists have approached the prospect of acquiring new knowledge in about the same way. At first, the opportunities for exploration are only barely perceived. Then, as Aristotle commented, the emotion of wonder takes over, and the primary question is not merely "what do we know?" but "how do we know?" and "what evidence do we have to corroborate the explanation offered?"—all surprisingly modern questions. Thales and the other early Greek philosophers sought knowledge, evidence, and application for the sake of understanding, not for the sake of utility, although in other environments these ends have coexisted. We have sought understanding of changes in the central nervous system that take place during maturation and learning and after injury to the brain. The changes can occur within the cell or at the synapse, across a neural network, or in connections among networks. By examining changes in the central nervous system—in this instance in relation to early brain disorders—we increase our knowledge of the processes occurring in the developing, learning, and recovering brain. By following the gathering of evidence from its infancy to what is, perhaps, its adolescence, we share in the wonder of this scientific exploration.

Neural reorganization and plasticity are areas rich in discovery, new findings, and new insights. These discoveries and insights occur across several levels of analysis—at the cell and synapse, in animals and humans, and across multiple domains of behavior. Nowhere is this richness more apparent than in research on disorders of early brain development. Here neural plasticity issues are played out in multiple variations of maturational stages, amount of recovery after injury, and development in the injured brain—again, at both neural and behavioral levels of analysis. There are important interactions between the organism and the environment that can inhibit or facilitate central nervous system reorganization. At this time, few attempts have been made to evaluate findings from research on early brain disorders across levels of analysis, in neural and behavioral domains, and in animal and human models.

The objectives of this volume are to increase communication among the scientific disciplines engaged in research on neural plasticity, to encourage collaborative efforts, and to provide a current source of clinical and experimental findings in this critical area. The impetus for this book was a conference called The Role of Neuroplasticity in Rare Developmental Disorders sponsored by the National Institute of Neurological Disorders and Stroke and the Office of Rare Diseases, National Institutes of Health, in February 1997. The book has 15 chapters divided into four sections and a final chapter that integrates findings from a range of animal and human studies and discusses their implications for future research, remediation, and a better understanding of the development of the central nervous system.

Part I consists of three chapters that address how the central nervous system is shaped—first by the neurobiological processes of elimination of synapses and second by learning. Based on an elegant model system, the first chapter summarizes research on synapse elimination at the neuromuscular junction. This research suggests that chronic electrical stimulation initiates the process of synaptic elimination, leading to a cascade of chemically mediated events involving the actions of protein kinase C. How specificity of chemically mediated elimination of synapses is achieved is currently under investigation. In the second chapter, a series of pioneering studies providing the first evidence that enrichment of the environment could lead to changes in cognitive behavior and structural changes in the brain are described along with the theoretical and empirical background of this research. More recent work using a similar paradigm is presented in the third chapter. This research indicates that cerebellar cortex from rats raised in environmentally complex conditions shows increases in the number of synapses, capillary volume, and glia in the brain. The changes are related to learning as well as to increases in motor activity. This research has been extended to include the etiologies of selected developmental disorders. Together, these three chapters provide a rich summary of brain–environment interactions, initially from laboratory models but with clear application to human studies.

Part II is devoted to mechanisms of reorganization in the central nervous system and has three chapters. In the first of these, Chapter 4, structural changes underlying long-term memory are examined using the gill and siphon withdrawal reflex of the marine mollusc *Aplysia californica*. This reflex can be modified by sensitization and habituation, two types of nonassociative learning. Long-term memory was found to be accompanied by structural modifications of the synapse, specifically in focal regions of membrane specialization and in the total number of presynaptic varicosities per sensory neuron. These changes can also be effected by cAMP activated by serotonin. At the molecular level, synaptic reorganization involves cell adhesion molecules. Membrane remodeling at the synapse may represent the first morphological step underlying long-term facilitation. In Chapter 5, development and plasticity of local circuits in the motor cortex are discussed. Intrinsic connections may account for as many as 70% of synapses present in particular cortical regions in the rat motor cortex. Lesions, such as clipping the whiskers, introduced after patterns of intrinsic connections between representation zones are mapped, are shown to have modified these excitatory and inhibitory connections. In the final chapter in this section, the rewiring and behavioral sparing that follow lesions of the immature visual cortex are presented. Although the repercussions of these lesions are widespread and found throughout the neural circuitry of the visual system, emphasis is placed on the plastic capacities of the immature brain that permit it to overcome major challenges to its normal development. Again, these three chapters represent laboratory models of basic processes that can be extrapolated to studies of normal and abnormal development in humans.

Part III is devoted to the neurodevelopmental course of several early brain disorders and is the largest section in the book with seven chapters. The authors of these primarily empirical chapters have interwoven reviews of the areas covered with results of their own research and implications for theories of recovery of function. The disorders discussed include congenital malformations (Chapters 7 and 8), surgically induced focal lesions for treatment of epilepsy or tumors (Chapter 9), infant unilateral brain lesions (Chapters 10 and 11), and autism (Chapters 12 and 13). Each of these areas represents different issues for evaluating reorganization of the central nervous system after brain injury—usually in the first 5 years—and highlights principles clearly identified in the earlier laboratory-based experimental chapters. Chapter 7, the first in this part, investigates the corpus callosum as a model for brain plasticity in children with early hydrocephalus of different origins. Neurobehavioral assessments together with quantitative magnetic resonance imaging morphometry allow the effects of the congenital malformations to be disassociated from the more diffuse effects of hydocephalus. This research is integrated with broader views of the structure and function of the corpus collosum derived from experimental animal and human research in normal development and studies of other populations characterized by congenital abnormalities of the corpus collosum.

Chapter 8 addresses the effects of brain malformations in children on the acquisition and development of behaviors that include coordinated movement, visuospatial analysis, linguistic discourse, mathematical computation, and reading comprehension. Congenital malformations of the cerebellum and midbrain are described using magnetic resonance imaging. The contemporary view of the cerebellum is that it has a major role not only in the coordination of movement but also in the temporal integration of discrete cognitive and motor responses. In Chapter 8, a major goal is to link the findings for neural structure with those for behavioral dysfunction so that a coherent set of relations that describe the reorganization of cerebellar functions and its long-term impact on motor and cognitive skills can be developed.

Chapter 9 deals with the recovery of cognitive functions after surgery for intractable epilepsy. In a before and after intervention design, recovery of acquired reading and naming impairments following focal cerebral resection is discussed. A significant degree of spontaneous recovery of function was found, suggesting that stage of premorbid skill development is strongly associated with recovery of very specific cognitive functions. Extrapolating to a developmental disorder (autism), the authors suggest that very targeted training may be more effective than currently available therapies.

Developmental course and recovery of function following early unilateral brain injury is discussed in Chapters 10 and 11. In the first series of studies, focal lesions occurred prior to 6 months of age and in the second at an average age of about 4 years of age. The populations differ in their exclusions, but both reveal a fairly optimistic picture. In Chapter 10, findings include left temporal specialization for lexical and grammatic production. In Chapter 11, mild deficits in spoken syntax and comprehension were identified in left-lesioned subjects, while right-lesioned children were often characterized by attentional deficits. Most children operated in the normal range on most measures. Relatively rare subcortical lesions were found to be associated with the worst outcomes.

The last two chapters in this part on disorders discuss the serious developmental disability of autism. In Chapter 12, longitudinal findings show that a significant proportion of autistic children (approximately one-third) had increases in IQ scores from below to above 70 over a follow-up period, while comparison groups of Down syndrome and developmentally delayed children showed no such improvement over time. The authors suggest that targeting behaviors that appear to be disrupted in autism—coordinated joint attention, play, and responsiveness to other people—is a rational approach to treatment. They also suggest that it is probably time to consider the effects of environmental factors on the development of autistic children, including parenting. Chapter 13 discusses biological and behavioral heterogeneity in autism and its implications for etiology and for the biological and behavioral consequences of this disorder.

Part IV, the final part, deals with intervention, the corollary of plasticity. In an overview of issues in developing effective intervention strategies, the author of Chapter 14 cites data from interventions with very-low-birth-weight babies at risk for developing disorders affecting attention, motor function, and language, and from research on autistic children. The following general principles for designing effective interventions are proposed: testing with experimental designs that incorporate relatively large sample sizes, longitudinal follow ups, careful definition of diagnostic criteria, and selection of outcomes that assess a broad range of skills. To be successful, such programs should also take into consideration family and community factors, which may be vital environmental agents of intervention. In the second and final chapter of Part IV, what is envisioned as a nationwide intervention program for language-impaired children is described. There are important aspects of the design as well as the content in this training program. Based on a theory that language impairment stems from an inability to process auditory information rapidly enough and therefore a difficulty in processing phonemes so that speech can be easily understood, the authors have developed a computer-based therapy that is an animated video game for training language-impaired children. An intervention with children who have pervasive developmental disorders is reported in this chapter. The researchers are able to alter the amplitude and duration of recorded sounds, the core of the intervention, and the children, who undergo a period of intense training, are exposed to progressively more difficult or closely timed sound discriminations as their performance on the video game improves. The children are rewarded for their correct responses, and their progress on the computer tasks is displayed. Learning theorists and experimental psychologists will recognize many of the principles incorporated into this design. Both Chapters

14 and 15 emphasize a process of theory development, empirical evaluation of hypotheses from theory, and subsequent application in intervention studies.

The final chapter presents a summery and recommendations, and discusses the interrelations among the concepts of development, learning, and neuroplasticity, where we are now, and where we can expect to go.

Bethesda, Md.   S.H.B.
Houston, Tex.   J.M.F.

Contents

Contents

Contributors

DOROTHY M. ARAM
Division of Communications Disorders
Emerson College
Boston, Massachusetts

CRAIG H. BAILEY
New York State Psychiatric Institute
Columbia University
New York, New York

MARCIA A. BARNES
Department of Psychology
The Hospital for Sick Children
Toronto, Ontario, Canada

ELIZABETH BATES
Center for Research in Language
University of California at San Diego
La Jolla, California

KATHY E. BATES
Beckman Institute
University of Illinois at Urbana-
    Champaign
Urbana, Illinois

JAMES E. BLACK
Beckman Institute
University of Illinois at Urbana-Champaign
Urbana, Illinois

DANA BOATMAN
Department of Neurology
The Johns Hopkins University
Baltimore, Maryland

MICHAEL E. BRANDT
Department of Psychiatry and Behavioral
    Sciences
University of Texas-Houston Medical
    School
Houston, Texas

SARAH H. BROMAN
Division of Fundamental Neuroscience
    and Developmental Disorders
National Institute of Neurological
    Disorders and Stroke
Bethesda, Maryland

ERIC COURCHESNE
Department of Neurosciences
University of California at San Diego
La Jolla, California

RACHEL YEUNG COURCHESNE
Laboratory for Research on the
    Neuroscience of Autism
Children's Hospital Research Center
La Jolla, California

ROGER DAVENPORT
Laboratory of Developmental Neurobiology
National Institute of Child Health and
    Human Development
Bethesda, Maryland

MAUREEN DENNIS
Department of Psychology
The Hospital for Sick Children
Toronto, Ontario, Canada

JACK M. FLETCHER
Department of Pediatrics
University of Texas-Houston Medical
 School
Houston, Texas

BARRY GORDON
Department of Neurology
The Zanvyl Krieger Mind/Brain Institute
The Johns Hopkins University
Baltimore, Maryland

WILLIAM T. GREENOUGH
Beckman Institute
University of Illinois at Urbana-Champaign
Urbana, Illinois

H. JULIA HANNAY
Department of Psychology
University of Houston
Houston, Texas

JOHN HART
Department of Neurology
The Zanvyl Krieger Mind/Brain Institute
The Johns Hopkins University
Baltimore, Maryland

C. ROSS HETHERINGTON
Department of Psychology
The Hospital for Sick Children
Toronto, Ontario, Canada

WILLIAM M. JENKINS
Keck Center for Integrative Neurosciences
University of California at San Francisco
San Francisco, California

ASAF KELLER
Department of Anatomy
University of Maryland
Baltimore, Maryland

NORMAN KIM
Neuropsychiatric Institute
University of California at Los Angeles
Los Angeles, California

ANNA KLINTSOVA
Beckman Institute
University of Illinois at Urbana-
 Champaign
Urbana, Illinois

SUSAN H. LANDRY
Department of Psychology
University of Texas Medical School
Houston, Texas

RONALD P. LESSER
Department of Neurosurgery
The Zanvyl Krieger Mind/Brain Institute
The Johns Hopkins University
Baltimore, Maryland

MICHAEL M. MERZENICH
Keck Center for Integrative Neurosciences
University of California at San Francisco
San Francisco, California

STEVEN MILLER
Scientific Learning Corporation
Berkeley, California

PHILLIP G. NELSON
Laboratory of Developmental
 Neurobiology
National Institute of Child Health and
 Human Development
Bethesda, Maryland

BERTRAM R. PAYNE
Department of Anatomy and
 Neurobiology
Boston University School of Medicine
Boston, Massachusetts

BRET PETERSON
Scientific Learning Corporation
Berkeley, California

KAREN PIERCE
Children's Hospital Research Center and
 University of California at San Diego
La Jolla, California

MARK R. ROSENZWEIG
Department of Psychology
University of California
Berkeley, California

GABRIELLE SAUNDERS
Scientific Learning Corporation
Berkeley, California

BENNETT A. SHAYWITZ
Departments of Pediatrics and Neurology
Yale University Medical School
New Haven, Connecticut

MARIAN SIGMAN
Neuropsychiatric Institute
University of California
Los Angeles, California

BRENDA J. SPIEGLER
Department of Psychology
The Hospital for Sick Children
Toronto, Ontario, Canada

PAULA TALLAL
Center for Molecular and Behavioral
    Neuroscience
Rutgers University
Newark, New Jersey

IVAN JEANNE WEILER
Beckman Institute
University of Illinois at Urbana-
    Champaign
Urbana, Illinois

I

SHAPING THE CENTRAL NERVOUS SYSTEM

1

Wiring the Brain: Activity-Dependent and Activity-Independent Development of Synaptic Circuits

PHILLIP G. NELSON AND ROGER DAVENPORT

The fundamental dogma of neuroscience holds that the function of the brain is mediated by circuits formed via synaptic connections between neurons. The operation of these circuits may well be modulated in profound ways by various aspects of glial function. Moreover, some neuronal interactions may not require synaptic connections. However, the basic computational algorithms responsible for mental life are executed by appropriately wired neuronal assemblies. The questions of how these neural circuits form, how they are modified by experience, and what mechanisms mediate the plasticity of learning and memory are central to neuroscience. It seems eminently plausible that abnormalities in any of the stages of synaptic circuit development and function could result in pathological behavior of the brain. We do not attempt any specific pathogenetic interpretations, however, but rather summarize certain aspects of the current status of developmental neuroscience concerning the genesis of appropriate, functional synaptic circuitry of the brain and neuromuscular system.

Initial Activity-Independent Formation of Synaptic Connections

Early in development, after neuronal cells have divided, completed their genetic differentiation, and migrated to their final location, neurons are still faced with a task that is unmatched by any other cell in the organism. Neurons must extend processes that ultimately form the critical interconnections that enable our every thought and movement. This task is significantly complicated because these interconnections are dispersed across the large dimensions of the nervous system and across the entire organism. This crucial task requires that processes navigate through the young environment, find their appropriate target region and specific target zone within that region, form synapses, and begin a process of competition that leads eventually to the refined, stereotypic circuitry that enables the organism to function. Electrical activity and synaptic function serve a minimal role during axonal outgrowth and guidance, yet subsequently are essential for the functional circuit to form. This portion of the chapter outlines in broad terms the process of axon guidance and specifically describes some of the key findings regulating growth cone navigation. As a result of many recent discoveries concerning the surface and intracellular molecular control of growth cones, this necessarily remains an overview only touching on concepts involved and selected examples from the literature.

Guidance Cues

One of the most important concepts to realize is that growth cones do not lead their trailing axons through the embryonic environments by predestined paths regulated exclusively by the genetic code. Instead, growth cones respond actively to their environment, almost constantly contacting surfaces and redirecting accordingly. Guidance cues direct the growth cone by attracting them toward favorable directions, repelling them from unfavorable areas, and simply preventing their unregulated extension. Guidance cues are distributed within the nucleus of origin, along the path to the target nucleus, and within the target itself. Generally, these cues are distributed in one of two ways, either as guidepost cells or as distributed concentration gradients. Molecular and cellular characterizations of many guidance cues have appeared in recent literature. Some of these are briefly described separately according to their distribution in the developing nervous system.

Guidepost Cells

Guidepost cells have been discovered and may commonly function in the development of invertebrate nervous systems (Fig. 1-1A). One notable series of guidepost cells directs the axons from pioneer neurons across the developing limb bud into the central nervous system (CNS) in the grasshopper (Bentley and Keshishian, 1982a,b). The pair of Ti1 pioneer neurons are the first afferent neurons to extend axons in the limb buds, and they establish a pathway essential for normal development of the peripheral nervous system. As the Ti1 growth cones migrate across the limb bud, they cross multiple limb segment boundaries. The growth cones orient toward and contact guidepost cells, which are necessary for the pioneer axons to reach the CNS (Caudy and Bentley, 1986; Condic et al., 1989; Guthrie et al., 1989; Keshishian and Bentley, 1983; O'Connor et al., 1990).

Development of large nervous systems requires the mapping of millions of axons from one afferent nucleus to single or multiple target nuclei. Single identifiable guidepost cells may not be sufficient to orchestrate such large-scale mappings, although it is clear that vertebrate growth cones can redirect to guidepost distri-

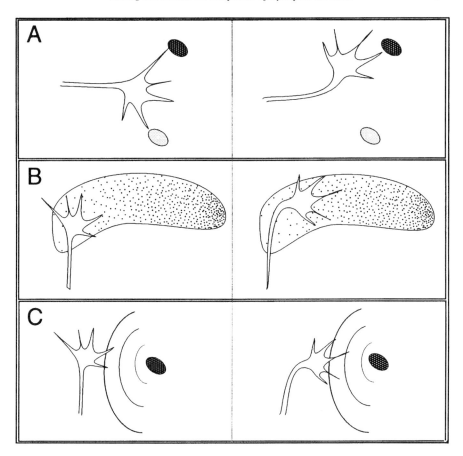

Figure 1-1. Neuronal growth cones encounter multiple cues in their environment that redirect their outgrowth. Guidance cues may be distributed as guideposts *(A)*, surface-bound concentration gradients *(B)*, or diffusible gradients *(C)*.

butions of both attractive and repellent cues (Fan and Raper, 1995; Kuhn et al., 1995; Raper et al., 1991). For example, a series of coated latex beads presented sequentially to dorsal root ganglion (DRG) growth cones can direct their outgrowth (Kuhn et al., 1995). Several molecules may exhibit guidepost distributions in the vertebrate (see discussion in Kuhn et al., 1995). However, guidance cues in the developing vertebrate nervous system are generally more widely distributed and affect many axons.

Distributed Contact-Dependent Cues

Contact-dependent guidance likely does serve a major role in the development of the nervous system by excluding axons from certain regions and by providing tracks of permissive or attractive components. For example, laminin is one of the most favorable substrates for retinal axon outgrowth. High levels of laminin are expressed along the optic nerve during development as retinal ganglion axons are extending from the retinae toward their multiple distant targets (Cohen et al., 1987). After the period of axonal extension, laminin expression is down-regulated (Cohen et al., 1986), and molecules inhibitory to neuronal outgrowth are up-regulated across the entire CNS (Schwab, 1996a,b; Schwab and Bandtlow, 1994). Particular regions can also express high levels of repellent molecules as well. Presumably high expression of collapsin molecules can prevent axons from entering certain regions and instead extend into neighboring regions (Luo and Raper, 1994; Luo et al., 1995; Shepherd et al., 1996, 1997). In each of these examples, regions of high expression are localized to particular locations and serve locally to restrict or permit extension of many afferent fibers. Thus, in many respects these examples are simple extensions of the guidepost guidance exhibited in invertebrates. To direct axons over the large dimensions of the vertebrate nervous system, however, guidance cues must be distributed over a wide area as well as affect local guidance events.

Sperry (1963) suggested that there were too few genes to encode the precise coordinates for mapping the entire vertebrate nervous system and suggested that limited numbers of cues may be distributed in concentration gradients that are read by the advancing growth cone. Sperry was specifically discussing the precise mapping of retinal axons across their target nuclei, which is discussed in a following section. Concentration gradients, however, may serve to direct outgrowth in many areas within the nervous system (Fig. 1-1B). Indeed this area of research presently receives considerable attention in developmental neurobiology. The molecular constituents comprising developmental gradients may be either diffusible or bound to the surface.

Diffusible Cues

Diffusible cues can attract or repel axonal outgrowth over large distances (Fig. 1-1C). Diffusible cues have been identified relatively recently (i.e., in the 1990s), whereas Ramon y Cajal (1890, 1937) had suggested their existence over 100 years ago. As Ramon y Cajal had suggested, molecules that are released from a given source diffuse across long distances and attract axons toward the source. One example of such interaction is observed in the developing spinal cord. Commissural axons extend toward the midline in part by being attracted toward the source there of diffusible molecules known as the *netrins* (Kennedy et al., 1994; Serafini et al., 1994, 1996; Shirasaki et al., 1996). These molecules are produced by midline cells and diffuse within the spinal cord such that a gradient of protein is observed, with highest levels at the midline, the primary destination of commissural axons. In culture, commissural growth cones turn toward a source of netrins (Kennedy et al., 1994). Similarly, axons can be repelled in culture by tissues that axons normally grow away from (Colamarino and Tessier-Lavigne, 1995; Guthrie and Pini, 1995; Keynes et al., 1997; Pini, 1993; Tessier-Lavigne, 1994). For example, olfactory bulb axons extend in all directions except toward a piece of co-cultured septum (Pini, 1993). Thus, axons can be directed by diffusible cues that guide their outgrowth either toward or away from the gradient source.

These examples are but a few of the likely numerous examples of long-range diffusible action of guidance cues on the direction of axon extension. Their effect is profound when one considers the number of axons that can be affected by essentially point sources of expression. Clearly, general outgrowth direction can be manipulated, and such a mechanism may partially underlie numerous developmental systems. Throughout the entire projection, a combination of multiple cues distributed along tracks, in discrete locations or diffused widely, can direct the elongating axons.

What happens once axons arrive at their target? In some systems, target areas are large relative to the size of individual growth cones, and therefore guidance mechanisms again must be relied on to coordinate axonal projections. The following example illustrates some of the fundamental studies that have recently led to the first molecular definition of Sperry's original hypothesis of retinotectal map formation. Here, graded distributions of contact-dependent cues may serve to separate and guide afferent axons to their final target zones.

An Example: Establishment of Retinotectal Maps

The mapping of retinal ganglion axons across their target nuclei in the brain serves as an exemplar system to study processes regulating precise mapping of afferent populations. The retinae are a two-dimensional sheet of cells containing only one efferent cell type, the retinal ganglion cells (RGC). RGC axons project to their targets and synapse across a two-dimensional layer of target cells. In each target, this two-dimensional set of connections matches the original cellular orientation within the retinae, preserving both nearest neighbor relationships and polarity orientation. A great deal of study has been focused on the processes that govern retinotopic maps because they are easily accessible and are established on relatively large nuclei during development and because the same cellular sequence of events is likely to be played out in many other areas of the nervous system. Retinal fibers lose orientation in the optic nerve (Chien and Harris, 1994; Harris, 1986; Rager, 1979, 1980, 1983) and therefore must sort out as they extend across their targets. Sperry (1963) predicted that gradients of guidance molecules exist on target cells that direct RGC axons to their correct target zones. This hypothesis has been supported by numerous studies in the intervening years. After arriving at their target zones, synapses develop and activity-dependent processes provide the final refinement of the retinotopic map.

Aimed toward a cellular and molecular definition of Sperry's original hypothesis, a number of studies have provided a great deal of insight into the processes regulating topographic development. It was shown that axons can correct for reorientation of the embryonic tecta (Harris, 1986; Sperry, 1963), suggesting that critical guidance information must be present within the tecta, the major target of RGC axons in birds and mammals. Several assays in culture demonstrated that indeed there was a repellent guidance activity present, that it was distributed in a gradient with highest concentrations in posterior tecta, and that it affected axons from temporal regions of the retinae, which do not project to the posterior tecta (Baier and Bonhoeffer, 1992; Bonhoeffer and Gierer, 1984; Bonhoeffer and Huf, 1982, 1985; Cox et al., 1990; Davenport et al., 1994; Karlstrom et al., 1997; Logan et al., 1996; Müller et al., 1990; Trowe et al., 1996; Walter et al., 1987a,b). Similar gradients of repellent material have now been shown to exist in birds, fish (Bastmeyer and Stuermer, 1993; Stuermer, 1990; Vielmetter and Stuermer, 1989; Vielmetter et al., 1991), and mammals (Godement and Bonhoeffer, 1989; Wizenmann et al., 1993).

These data clearly supported the hypothesis put forward by Sperry. Cellular and molecular characteristics, however, remained elusive until recently. Specific molecules (both receptors and ligands) that could account for these behaviors were recently cloned (Brennan et al., 1997; Cheng and Flanagan, 1994; Cheng et al., 1995; Drescher et al., 1995, 1997; Nakamoto et al., 1996; Winslow et al., 1995) and are part of the Eph family of receptor tyrosine kinases (Friedman and O'Leary, 1996; Orike and Pini, 1996; Orioli and Klein, 1997; Tessier-Lavigne, 1995; Tuzi and Gullick, 1994). The receptor EphA3 is distributed in a gradient across the retinae, with highest levels in temporal retinae, and the ligands ephrin-2A and -5A are distributed across the tecta, with highest levels in posterior tecta. A great deal of work remains before all of the events that underlie the formation of retinotopic maps are understood; however, the cloning of these molecules greatly aids in our understanding. Time-lapse observations of RGC growth cones as they encounter individual dissociated tectal cells revealed that the repellent guidance cues were present on tectal neurons (Davenport et al., 1996b). Interestingly, a separate guidance cue was suggested by these experiments, namely, a cue that essentially stopped outgrowth but did not repel it. Such attenuating or adhesive cues may serve essential roles in the development of retinotectal maps in birds (Davenport, 1997) and may help to explain differences in retinotopic map development across species. The data to date strongly suggest that there are various stages of axonal guidance regulated by separate environments that direct axons moment by moment to their final destinations.

Second Messengers

Especially through experimentation in cell culture it has been possible to characterize the effect of a number of factors on neuronal outgrowth. Exogenous factors applied to neuronal growth cones can cause a variety of changes, such as growth cone collapse, stall, and turn, but also more subtle changes such as increased filopodial length or number. Tissue culture studies that began with Harrison (1910) serve an important role in our increasing understanding of the mechanisms that regulate the individual growth cone's response to its environment. A great deal has been learned, and clearly very much still remains to be discovered concerning the transduction of external cues to internal changes in cytoskeletal motility. Central to this transduction process are the second-messenger systems, discussed in the following sections, that can relay information across the spatial dimensions of the growth cone and to the many different structural proteins involved in controlling growth cone motility.

Calcium

One of the clearest cases for a second messenger serving an important role in neuronal growth cone motility can be made for intracellular calcium. Large rises in calcium can cause rapid growth cone collapse. For some cell types, large rises in calcium alone may not be sufficient to induce growth cone collapse (Ivins et al., 1991), but in many cell types large rises in calcium change the cytoskeleton (Lankford and Letourneau, 1989, 1991) and induce growth cone collapse and retraction (Kater and Mills, 1991; Kater et al., 1988). These changes in intracellular calcium can be elicited by membrane depolarization due to direct manipulation or excitatory neurotransmitters (Kater and Mills, 1991; Kater et al., 1988) and by release from intracellular stores in response to particular cell surface antigens (Bandtlow et al., 1993). In the latter study, NI-35, which is an inhibitory molecule present on oligodendrocytes, caused rapid collapse of DRG growth cones. The rise in calcium in response to NI-35 exposure was necessary and sufficient to induce growth cone collapse.

More subtle growth cone behaviors have been shown to be under the regulation of calcium and other second messengers. For example, depolarization induces both elongation of filopodia and a subsequent decrease in filopodial number that are highly correlated with the induced rise in calcium (Kater and Rehder, 1995; Rehder and Kater, 1992). Local rises in calcium can have more local effects as well. For example, hot spots of calcium in motile growth cones have been correlated with local extensions of lamellipodia (Silver et al., 1990). Also, gradients of calcium induced across growth cones cause filopodia to lengthen and to increase in number and growth cones to turn (Bedlack et al., 1992; Davenport and Kater, 1992; Zheng et al., 1996). In part this filopodial response may be extremely local, resulting from local changes in calcium in individual filopodia (Davenport et al., 1993, 1996a). Even the shaft of neurites is susceptible to rises in calcium and can emit new lateral extensions when given sufficiently large depolarization-induced changes in calcium (Williams et al., 1995). Clearly this second messenger is very important to the navigation and survival of growth cones.

cAMP

Calcium is clearly not the only second messenger in growth cones or the only second messenger affecting changes in growth cone motility. For example, graded distributions of cAMP can cause growth cones to turn in culture (Lohof et al., 1992; Zheng et al., 1994). More interesting perhaps is that it appears that cAMP levels can interact with the effects of other guidance cues, causing them to exert either attractive or repellent forces on the growth cone (Song et al., 1997). Thus, multiple environmental signals interact with multiple second-messenger signals that exert multiple growth cone responses, from attractive to repellent.

Multiple Factors Affect Neuronal Outgrowth

These data only serve to remind us how much remains to be discovered concerning the relationship between the developing and regenerating axons and the complex environment *in vivo* through which they must traverse. Multiple factors are present simultaneously and throughout the many stages of outgrowth as growth cones first extend away from the cell body and then find their way to and across their target nuclei. Even when one considers an individual growth cone, multiple factors are able to simultaneously affect its varied and complex behavior. The express intent of this overview was not to define all of the factors that are known to affect growth cone motility and axon guidance but instead to make clear that a great many factors must be understood at many different levels of resolution to fully understand how a growth cone navigates during early development and regeneration. A great deal of work lies ahead.

Neural Plasticity

A conceptual framework was formulated for plasticity phenomena in cellular terms but from a psychological perspective by D. O. Hebb in 1949 that has had a remarkable and persistent influence in the field of neural plasticity. A "Hebb synapse" has the property that if activity in a presynaptic fiber succeeds in bringing a postsynaptic cell to threshold so that it fires an action potential, that synapse is strengthened. Conversely, it can be supposed that if a presynaptic fiber is *un*successful it will be weakened (Stent, 1973). These rather general postulates were given considerable strength in 1973 when Lomo and Bliss discovered the phenomenon of long-term potentiation (LTP) (see Bliss and Collingridge, 1993, for review.) Rather brief, high-frequency activation of synapses in the hippocampus was shown to be followed by a prolonged interval (up to several days) of increased synaptic responsiveness. A variety of experiments showed that this potentiation was dependent on a substantial depolarizing response of the postsynaptic cell during the conditioning stimulus. The basis for the contingency upon postsynaptic responsiveness has been greatly clarified by studies on properties of central excitatory neurotransmitter receptors. One of the glutamate receptors, the N-methyl-D-aspartate (NMDA) receptor, has been shown by Mayer and Westbrook (1987) and by Asher and Nowack (1988) to require both the presence of the agonist (glutamate or NMDA) and depolarization of the postsynaptic neuronal membrane to be activated. Thus, the responsiveness of the receptor is both voltage and agonist dependent. This has been shown to be due to a voltage-dependent block of the channel by magnesium ions, but in any event it confers a Hebb-like property to this receptor molecule. In a number of synaptic connections (but not all) LTP has been shown to be dependent on the function of NMDA receptors so that some synaptic circuits and even behavioral properties can be related fairly convincingly to properties of a molecule involved in those circuits. On the other hand, not all synapses depend for their plasticity on NMDA activation, and plasticity at different synapses may involve changes in presynaptic transmitter output or changed postsynaptic responsiveness or possibly both. The dependence of presynaptic transmitter output on postsynaptic responses implies some retrograde messenger moving from the postsynaptic to the presynaptic element. A model for the transduction pathways and mechanisms involved in LTP is shown in Figure 1-2 (see Bliss and Collingridge, 1993, for extensive discussion of LTP and other plasticity processing).

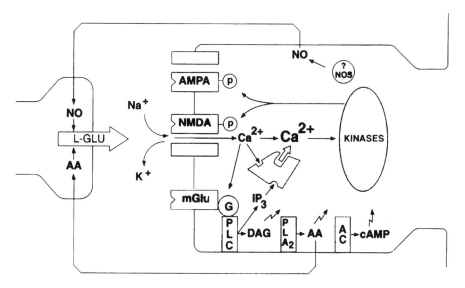

Figure 1-2. Pathways and mechanisms involved in LTP. The initial induction signal is a Ca^{2+} transient that permeates NMDA channels. This signal is then amplified by the release of CA^{2+} from Ca^{2+}/InsP3-sensitive intracellular stores. A parallel pathway that may be important for the induction of LTP is provided by mGluRs. These receptors can couple, through G proteins, to the phosphoinositide-specific phospholipase C (PLC), phospholipase A2 (PLA2), and adenylate cyclase (AC) to produce diacylglycerol (DAG) and arachidonic acid (AA) and to regulate the levels of cAMP, respectively. Note that the initial NMDA receptor-mediated Ca^{2+} transient may be necessary for the activation of the mGluR cascades by L-glutamate. The amplified Ca^{2+} signal, in association with the other activators of protein kinases (zig-zag arrows), then leads to the phosphorylation of substrate proteins, including, probably, AMPA and NMDA receptors. Other enzymes, such as nitric oxide synthase (NOS), if present, may also be activated by the Ca^{2+} transient. Biochemical changes in the presynaptic terminal may be initiated by the action of retrograde messengers, such as AA, nitric oxide (NO), and K^+, perhaps in conjunction with the action of L-glutamate on presynaptic mGluRs. (From Bliss and Collingridge, 1993.)

A reciprocal response to neural network activation, namely, a decrease in synaptic efficacy, has recently been demonstrated (Dudek and Bear, 1992). With low-frequency stimulation phosphatases are activated, and a consequent dephosphorylation (in contrast to kinase-mediated phosphorylation) of certain proteins is produced. The analysis of this form of synaptic plasticity (long-term depression [LTD]) is less advanced than for the sensitization or LTP models discussed above, but the discovery of LTD is of great theoretical significance (Bear, 1996).

The molecular mechanisms coupling neural activation to changes in neural gene expression that may be involved in memory storage have understandably received a great deal of study. In *Aplysia*, a marine mollusc, sensitization of a defensive reflex can be divided into short- and long-term phases. The sensitization is initiated by serotonin release, which produces an increase in cAMP and activation of protein kinase A (PKA). This second-messenger system in turn phosphorylates certain cAMP response element binding (CREB) proteins that are transcription factors and that activate synthesis of cAMP-inducible genes. This picture is complicated by the fact that long-term facilitation is dependent on the reciprocal regulation of two CREB proteins (for further discussion, see Bailey et al., 1996; and Bailey, Chapter 4).

In the hippocampus, the late LTP appears to involve cAMP and PKA-mediated synthesis of mRNA and protein. The use of transgenic and site- and stage-specific gene knockout mice represents a potentially extremely powerful approach to the investigation of memory storage mechanisms (Wilson and Tonegawa, 1997).

Developmental Plasticity of the Brain

A great deal of evidence has accumulated showing that stimulation of the developing organism by input from the environment can drastically affect nervous system development. The classic studies of Wiesel and Hubel (1963) on the visual systems of cats and monkeys showed the functional and structural consequences of altered visual stimulation (monocular occlusion or induced strabismus) that strikingly changed the ocular dominance of inputs to the cells in the visual cortex. Many subsequent studies by Stryker, Shatz, Singer, and others (see Shatz, 1990, for review) demonstrated both the strength and the subtlety of these influences. Further approaches of a more general behavioral sort are described by Rosenzweig (Chapter 2) and Greenough et al. (Chapter 3).

A generalization from the experiments on the visual system is that an initial rather diffuse afferent innervation of the visual cortex with poorly defined ocular dominance patterns in the newborn becomes more sharply and functionally specific with appropriate stimulation during the early postnatal weeks. Importantly, this involves a loss of many functionally inappropriate connections. A general pattern for the changes in cortical synapse number involves a massive increase in synapses early in the postnatal period, with a subsequent reduction of some 40% that occurs during the first few years of postnatal life in the primate (Bourgeois and Rakic, 1993; Huttenlocher, 1979). This massive process of synapse elimination or "pruning" probably plays a crucial role in the development of an optimally functional brain, and further understanding of the mechanisms involved seemed to us to be worthy of pursuit.

While many valuable mechanistic studies of synapse elimination have been done in the CNS, a simplified, more experimentally accessible system offered many advantages. It should be noted that the process of synapse elimination is only one side of a double process, and neuronal growth results from the action of a number of highly potent biomolecules, including the neurotrophins. These may be elaborated as a result of neural activity, and their powerful effects are exemplified by the action of brain-derived neurotrophic factor (BDNF). In the visual system, when BDNF is perfused into the developing cat visual cortex, the processes of synapse elimination and ocular dominance column formation are completely blocked (Cabelli et al., 1997). It may be that more local release of BDNF during the normal process of ocular dominance development is involved in some selective maintenance of appropriate connections.

The Neuromuscular Junction and Synapse Elimination

Redfern (1970) showed that, during the first 3 weeks of postnatal life in the rodent, the innervation of skeletal muscle cells went through a dramatic change. At birth, essentially every muscle fiber was innervated by two or more motor axons, but by 3–4 weeks of age each fiber was innervated by one, and only one, axon. This drastic reduction in polyneuronal innervation was substantially dependent on activity in the nerve and muscle in that paralysis by either a sodium channel blocker (tetrodotoxin) or acetylcholine receptor (AChR) blockers (curare or α-bungarotoxin [α-BGTX]) delayed or prevented the elimination. Furthermore, if one axon innervating a multiply innervated muscle fiber were stimulated, there was some selective loss of other axonal inputs to that muscle (for review, see Thompson, 1985; VanEssen et al., 1990). In apparent contradiction of this pattern of activity-dependent elimination of inactive muscle inputs were experiments by Callaway and colleagues (1987), who found that tetrodotoxin block of activity of a nerve innervating a limb muscle in the rabbit resulted in an enlargement of the motor units connected to this *inactive* nerve.

Experiments on synapse elimination at the neuromuscular junction have been vigorously pursued by Lichtman and colleagues (see Balice-Gordon and Lichtman, 1993; Nguyen and Lichtman, 1996). They labeled the nerve and the muscle AChR with fluorescent dyes *in vivo* and followed individual junctions over time with confocal microscopy. This showed that in many cases there appeared to be a loss of the postsynaptic receptors prior to a retraction and the loss of the overlying neurites during the elimination process. Furthermore, if they produced a local block of AChR function by a restricted application of α-BGTX, these blocked receptors disappeared and did so before the overlying neurite was lost. No loss of connections occurred in junctions where all receptors were blocked by a general application of α-BGTX (Balice-Gordon and Lichtman, 1994). These observations suggested that the elimination process was focused with extreme precision on inactive terminals, that postsynaptic receptor activity was crucial to initiate the elimination process, and that active nerve–muscle structures initiated some local process that sustained or protected these structures from the elimination process.

As in the case of the visual system, neurotrophins have been invoked as a positive mechanism for generating selective motoneuron and neuromuscular synapse survival (Oppenheim, 1989). A large number of molecules have been identified that influence neuromuscular developments, neurotrophin 3 and BDNF being examples. For none of them, however, does blockade completely or permanently prevent synapse elimination at the neuromuscular junction (Greensmith and Vrbova, 1996).

We have developed a tissue culture preparation designed to analyze activity-dependent synapse reduction (ADSR) (Nelson, et al., 1993). We wished to capture two aspects of the process, namely, the activity dependence and the competitive aspect whereby active inputs might be favored over inactive inputs (or conceivably the opposite could be true). To this end, we have used a three-compartment chamber in which two populations of cholinergic neurons project axons to converge on and innervate a common target population of skeletal muscle fibers. In some cases a given muscle fiber will receive innervation from at least one fiber from both populations of nerve cells, thus setting up a potential competitive interaction. A set of stimulating electrodes can be devised such that different patterns of electrical stimuli can be delivered independently to the axons of the two neuronal populations for extended periods (days or weeks). Synaptic efficacy can be monitored by counting the muscle fibers that twitch in response to stimulation of the afferent axons or by recording intracellularly from the muscle fibers and measuring synaptic potentials or currents directly. We have used both the superior cervical ganglion and the ventral spinal cord as sources for our innervating cholinergic neurons.

When axons from one side chamber are stimulated for about 20 hours (<1 day), there is a selective loss of inputs from the unstimulated side, indicating a Hebb-like behavior of this synapse. If more prolonged stimulation (2–3 days) is carried out, however, this stimulus selectivity is largely lost. It appears that the synapse-preserving effect of activation can be overcome by sufficiently prolonged, intense stimulation. There is a reliable, robust degree of expression of the ADSR, however, and we wished to exploit this system to test hypotheses as to mechanisms underlying the ADSR.

Proteases and the ADSR

Vrbova and colleagues during the late 1970s and early 1980s had proposed that proteolytic action might be involved in the ADSR process at the neuromuscular junction *in vivo* and provided a variety of experimental observations supporting this proposal (see O'Brien et al., 1978; Connold et al., 1986). Our initial mechanistic experiment involved the use of a broad-spectrum protease inhibitor, leupeptin, to see if blockade of proteolytic activity generally would interfere with the ADSR. We found that indeed the ADSR was completely blocked by the leupeptin (Liu et al., 1994b). There are several broad classes of proteases with inhibitors that specifically block each of the classes. When we tried to block the ADSR with different inhibitors for serine, thiol, and calcium-activated proteases (the calpains), we were unsuccessful (Fig. 1-3). One member of the serine protease family was notable in not being affected by the widely used serine protease inhibitor aprotinin, which in fact was the inhibitor that we had used for this class of proteases. The protease in question, thrombin, does have a highly specific and potent inhibitor, hirudin, derived from the leech. We found that hirudin, in nanomolar concentrations, completely blocked the ADSR, strongly suggesting that thrombin was involved in this process (Liu et al., 1994a; Fig. 1-4). *In vivo,* synapse elimination is delayed but not completely blocked by hirudin perfusion of the neuromuscular

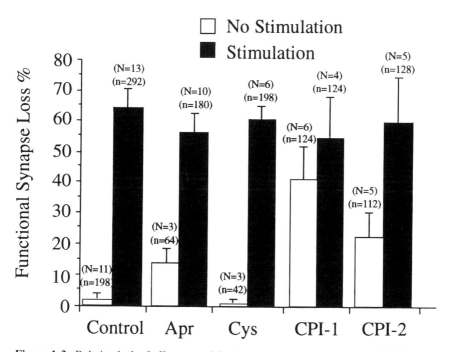

Figure 1-3. Relative lack of effect on activity-dependent synapse reduction (ADSR) by a variety of protease inhibitors. Apr is the serine protease inhibitor aprotinin; Cys is the cysteine protease inhibitor cystatin, and CPI-1 and CPI-2 are the calpain inhibitors 1 and 2. N indicates the number of individual cultures and n the number of synaptic connections that were analyzed for each condition. The open bars are synapse loss in the absence of stimulation, and filled bars represent synapse loss in the presence of electrical stimulation. Both are in the presence of the indicated inhibitors. With all of these inhibitors, synapse loss with stimulation is the same as in the case of stimulated controls without the inhibitors. Note that with calpain-1 inhibitor there is some loss in the absence of stimulation. (Modified from Liu et al., 1994a.)

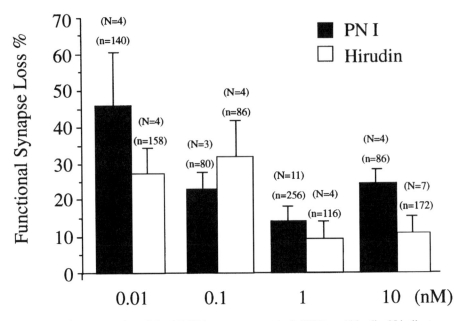

Figure 1-4. Suppression of the ADSR by protease nexin-1 (PN I) and hirudin. N indicates the number of individual cultures and n the number of synaptic connections that were analyzed for each condition. In all cases the preparations were being stimulated electrically so that synapse loss of controls was about 50%. Significant block of the elimination process is produced by both PN I and hirudin at concentrations of 1 nM or greater. (Modified from Liu et al., 1994a.)

junction (Zoubine et al., 1996). Thus, thrombin is probably involved, but other molecules also may mediate the elimination *in vivo*. If regulation of thrombin action is important for control of synapse effectiveness, it might be expected that some endogenous inhibitor would be produced. Protease nexin 1 is such an endogenous inhibitor of serine proteases in general and of thrombin in particular, and we found it also to be a potent blocker at subnanomolar concentrations of the ADSR (Liu et al., 1994a; Fig. 1-4).

Thrombin's essential role in the ADSR suggested that its synthesis or elaboration by muscle cells might be affected by activation of the muscle. To test this possibility in muscle cells grown in culture in the absence of nerve, we manipulated the state of activation of the muscle with tetrodotoxin (to block spontaneous spike activity) and veratridine (to activate the sodium spike mechanism) and with cholinergic stimulation (Glazner et al., 1997). We then measured the amount of thrombin activity released from the muscle cells into the culture medium and the levels of prothrombin mRNA synthesized by the myotubes. We found that elaboration of thrombin activity was increased by either electrical or cholinergic stimulation, and prothrombin mRNA synthesis was also increased by cholinergic (Glazner et al., 1997) or electrical activation (Kim et al., unpublished data). Developmental and denervation studies also indicate a high degree of regulation of prothrombin, protease nexin 1, and the thrombin receptor present on muscle cells (Kim et al., 1998). The involvement of a balance between thrombin and its inhibitor, PN-1, has been shown for a variety of neurobiological phenomena such as neurite extension and glial shape changes. The possible contribution of thrombin to some neuropathological processes is suggested by recent work showing that thrombin receptor activation can induce apoptosis in neurons (Donovan et al., 1997). Figure 1-5 shows a conceptual framework in which mechanisms involving thrombin action would generate the behavior of a Hebb synapse.

We have touched only briefly on some of the current work on plasticity in the nervous system with emphasis on the molecular and cellular mechanisms underlying neuroplasticity (see Nelson et al., 1995, for further review). Understanding of both functional plasticity in the mature nervous system (learning and memory) and environmental modification of brain development has increased dramatically in the past decade. The relationship between memory and developmental plasticity is unclear, but some common molecular mechanisms may be emerging. As noted at the beginning of this chapter, it is a generally accepted view that brain

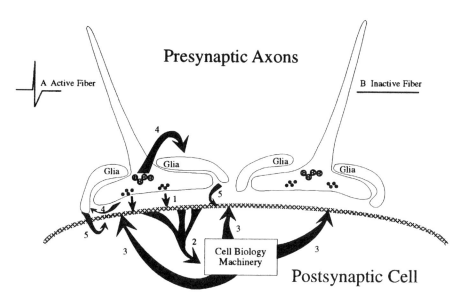

Figure 1-5. Schematic diagram for possible mechanisms underlying the Hebb synapse. 1, Classic transmitter (e.g., glutamate, acetylcholine) released by active axons and synapses. 2, Activation of postsynaptic cell couples into cell biology machinery (e.g., kinases, phosphates). 3, Proteases are released intra- or extracellulary over postsynaptic cell to eliminate synapses. 4, Co-transmitters (e.g., CGRP, VIP, or other peptides) released locally by presynaptic activity. 5, Protease inhibitors or trophic factors released locally by glia, near active synapses only, neutralize proteases or other synapse elimination factors.

function must be, at least in large part, determined by activity in appropriately connected synaptic circuits. Both an initially genetically programmed phase and a subsequent experientially modified process are crucial for the development of these circuits. A great deal of knowledge at the cellular and molecular levels is now available regarding both of these stages, although much more remains to be discovered. The application of the available knowledge toward an understanding of pathological development is still in a relatively primitive state, and it remains largely for the future to demonstrate the degree to which the plasticity-related mechanisms may play a role in such nervous system disorders as autism and dyslexia or some of the degenerative or destructive processes such as cerebral palsy. The molecular interactions involved in nervous system development are enormously complex, and sorting out the ways in which these interactions may produce abnormalities of development is correspondingly challenging. It seems eminently plausible that it is to this area that considerable effort might profitably be expended.

References

Ascher, P., and Nowack, L. (1988). The role of divalent cations in the N-methyl-D-aspartate responses of mouse central neurones in culture. *J. Physiol., 399,* 247–266.

Baier, H., and Bonhoeffer, F. (1992). Axon guidance by gradients of a target-derived component. *Science, 255,* 472–475.

Bailey, C. H., Bartsch, D., and Kandel, E. R. (1996). Toward a molecular definition of long-term memory storage. *Proc. Natl. Acad. Sci. U.S.A., 93,* 13445–13452.

Balice-Gordon, R. J., and Lichtman, J. W. (1993). *In vivo* observations of pre- and postsynaptic changes during the transition from multiple to single innervation at developing neuromuscular junctions. *J. Neurosci., 13,* 834–855.

Balice-Gordon, R. J., and Lichtman, J. W. (1994). Long-term synapse loss induced by focal blockade of postsynaptic receptors. *Nature, 372,* 519–524.

Bandtlow, C. E., Schmidt, M. F., Hassinger, T. D., Schwab, M. E., and Kater, S. B. (1993). Intracellular calcium mediates growth cone collapse evoked by the CNS myelin-associated neurite growth inhibitor NI-35. *Science, 259,* 80–83.

Bastmeyer, M., and Stuermer, C. A. (1993). Behavior of fish retinal growth cones encountering chick caudal tectal membranes: A time-lapse study on growth cone collapse. *J. Neurobiol., 24,* 37–50.

Bear, M. F. (1996). A synaptic basis for memory storage in the cerebral cortex. *Proc. Natl. Acad. Sci. U.S.A., 93,* 13453–13459.

Bedlack, R. S., Jr., Wei, M.-D., and Loew, L. M. (1992). Localized membrane depolarizations and localized calcium influx during electric field-guided neurite growth. *Neuron, 9,* 398–404.

Bentley, D., and Keshishian, H. (1982a). Pathfinding by peripheral pioneer neurons in grasshopper. *Science, 218,* 1082–1088.

Bentley, D., and Keshishian, H. (1982b). Pioneer neurons and pathways in insect appendages. *Trends Neurosci., 5,* 364–367.

Bliss, T. V. P., and Collingridge, G. L. (1993). A synaptic model of memory: Long-term potentiation in the hippocampus. *Nature, 361,* 31–39.

Bonhoeffer, F., and Gierer, A. (1984). How do retinal axons find their targets on the tectum? *TINS, 7,* 378–381.

Bonhoeffer, F., and Huf, J. (1982). *In vitro* experiments on axon guidance demonstrating an anterior–posterior gradient on the tectum. *EMBO J., 1,* 427–431.

Bonhoeffer, F., and Huf, J. (1985). Position-dependent properties of retinal axons and their growth cones. *Nature, 315,* 409–410.

Bourgeois, J.-P., and Rakic, P. (1993). Change of synaptic density in the primary visual cortex of the macaque monkey from fetal to adult stage. *J. Neurosci., 13,* 2801–2820.

Brennan, C., Monschau, B., Lindberg, R., Guthrie, B., Drescher, U., Bonhoeffer, F., and Holder, N. (1997). Two Eph receptor tyrosine kinase ligands control axon growth and may be involved in the creation of the retinotectal map in the zebrafish. *Development, 124,* 655–664.

Cabelli, R. J., Shelton, D. L., Segal, R. A., and Shatz, C. J. (1997). Blockade of endogenous ligands of TrkB inhibits formation of ocular dominance columns. *Neuron, 19,* 63–76.

Callaway, E. M., Soha, J. M., and VanEssen, D. C. (1987). Competition favoring inactive over active motor neurons during synapses elimination. *Nature, 328,* 422–426.

Caudy, M., and Bentley, D. (1986). Pioneer growth cone steering along a series of neuronal and non-neuronal cues of different affinities. *J. Neurosci., 6,* 1781–1795.

Cheng, H. J., and Flanagan, J. G. (1994). Identification and cloning of ELF-1, a developmentally expressed ligand for the Mek4 and Sek receptor tyrosine kinases. *Cell, 79,* 157–168.

Cheng, H. J., Nakamoto, M., Bergemann, A. D., and Flanagan, J. G. (1995). Complementary gradients in expression and binding of ELF-1 and Mek4 in development of the topographic retinotectal projection map. *Cell, 82,* 371–381.

Chien, C. B., and Harris, W. A. (1994). Axonal guidance from retina to tectum in embryonic *Xenopus. Curr. Top. Dev. Biol., 29,* 135–169.

Cohen, J., Burne, J. F., McKinlay, C., and Winter, J. (1987). The role of laminin and the laminin/fibronectin receptor complex in the outgrowth of retinal ganglion cell axons. *Dev. Biol., 122,* 407–418.

Cohen, J., Burne, J. F., Winter, J., and Barlett, P. (1986). Retinal cells lose response to laminin with maturation. *Nature, 322,* 465–467.

Colamarino, S. A., and Tessier-Lavigne, M. (1995). The axonal chemoattractant netrin-1 is also a chemorepellent for trochlear motor axons. *Cell, 81,* 621–629.

Condic, M. L., Lefcort, F., and Bentley, D. (1989). Selective recognition between embryonic afferent neurons of grasshopper appendages in vitro. *Dev. Biol., 135,* 221–230.

Connold, A. L., Evers, J. V., and Vrbova, G. (1986). Effects of low calcium and protease inhibitors on synapse elimination during postnatal development in the rat soleus muscle. *Dev. Brain Res., 28,* 99–107.

Cox, E. C., Muller, B., and Bonhoeffer, F. (1990). Axonal guidance in the chick visual system: Posterior tectal membranes induce collapse of growth cones from the temporal retina. *Neuron, 4,* 31–37.

Davenport, R. W. (1997). Functional guidance components and their cellular distribution in retinotectal co-cultures. *Cell Tissue Res., 290,* 201–208.

Davenport, R. W., Dou, P., Mills, L. R., and Kater, S. B. (1996a). Distinct calcium signaling within neuronal growth cones and filopodia. *J. Neurobiol., 31,* 1–15.

Davenport, R. W., Dou, P., Rehder, V., and Kater, S. B. (1993). A sensory role for neuronal growth cone filopodia. *Nature, 361,* 721–724.

Davenport, R. W., and Kater, S. B. (1992). Local increases in intracellular calcium elicit local filopodial responses in *Helisoma* neuronal growth cones. *Neuron, 9,* 405–416.

Davenport, R. W., Löschinger, J., Huf, J., Jung, J., and Bonhoeffer, F. (1994). Retinal axons suddenly stop elongating after significant extension onto gradients of posterior tectal material. *Soc. Neurosci. Abstr., 20,* 1065.

Davenport, R. W., Thies, E., and Nelson, P. G. (1996b). Cellular localization of guidance cues in the establishment of retinotectal topography. *J. Neurosci., 16,* 2074–2085.

Donovan, F. M., Pike, C. J., Cotman, C. W., and Cunningham, D. D. (1997). Thrombin induces apoptosis in cultured neurons and astrocytes *via* a pathway requiring tyrosine kinase and RhoA activities. *J. Neurosci., 17,* 5316–5326.

Drescher, U., Bonhoeffer, F., and Muller, B. K. (1997). The Eph family in retinal axon guidance. *Curr. Opin. Neurobiol., 7,* 75–80.

Drescher, U., Kremoser, C., Handwerker, C., Loschinger, J., Noda, M., and Bonhoeffer, F. (1995). *In vitro* guidance of retinal ganglion cell axons by RAGS, a 25 kDa tectal protein related to ligands for Eph receptor tyrosine kinases. *Cell, 82,* 359–370.

Dudek, S. M., and Bear, M. (1992). Homosynaptic long-term depression in area CA1 of hippocampus and effects of N-methyl-D aspartate receptor blockade. *Proc. Natl. Acad. Sci. U.S.A., 89,* 4363–4367.

Fan, J., and Raper, J. A. (1995). Localized collapsing cues can steer growth cones without inducing their full collapse. *Neuron, 14,* 263–274.

Friedman, G. C., and O'Leary, D. D. (1996). Eph receptor tyrosine kinases and their ligands in neural development. *Curr. Opin. Neurobiol., 6,* 127–133.

Glazner, G. W., Yadav, K., Fitzgerald, S., Coven, E., Brenneman, D. E., and Nelson, P. G. (1997). Cholinergic stimulation increases thrombin activity and gene expression in cultured mouse muscle. *Dev. Brain Res., 99,* 148–154.

Godement, P., and Bonhoeffer, F. (1989). Cross-species recognition of tectal cues by retinal fibers *in vitro. Development, 106,* 313–320.

Greensmith, L., and Vrbova, G. (1996). Motoneurons survival: A functional approach. *Trends Neurosci., 19,* 450–455.

Guthrie, P. B., Kater, S. B., and Bentley, D. (1989). Guidepost cells act as calcium sinks for pioneer growth cones *in vivo. Soc. Neurosci. Abstr., 15,* 1261.

Guthrie, S., and Pini, A. (1995). Chemorepulsion of developing motor axons by the floor plate. *Neuron, 14,* 1117–1130.

Harris, W. A. (1986). Homing behaviour of axons in the embryonic vertebrate brain. *Nature, 320,* 266–269.

Harrison, R. G. (1910). The outgrowth of the nerve fiber as a mode of protoplasmic movement. *J. Exp. Zool., 9,* 787–848.

Hebb, D. O. (1949). *The Organization of Behavior.* New York: John Wiley & Sons.

Huttenlocher, P. R. (1979). Synaptic density in human frontal cortex, developmental changes and effects of aging. *Brain Res., 163,* 195–205.

Ivins, J., Raper, J., and Pittman, R. (1991). Intracellular calcium levels do not change during contact-mediated collapse of chick DRG growth cone structure. *J. Neurosci., 11,* 1597–1608.

Karlstrom, R. O., Trowe, T., and Bonhoeffer, F. (1997). Genetic analysis of axon guidance and mapping in the zebrafish. *Trends Neurosci., 20,* 3–8.

Kater, S. B., Mattson, M. P., Cohan, C. S., and Conner, J. (1988). Calcium regulation of the neuronal growth cone. *TINS, 11,* 315–321.

Kater, S., and Mills, L. (1991). Regulation of growth cone behavior by calcium. *J. Neurosci., 11,* 891–899.

Kater, S. B., and Rehder, V. (1995). The sensory-motor role of growth cone filopodia. *Curr. Opin. Neurobiol., 5,* 68–74.

Kennedy, T. E., Serafini, T., de la Torre, J. R., Tessier, L. M. (1994). Netrins are diffusible chemotropic factors for commissural axons in the embryonic spinal cord. *Cell, 78,* 425–435.

Keshishian, H., and Bentley, D. (1983). Embryogenesis of peripheral nerve pathways in grasshopper legs. I. The initial nerve pathway to the CNS. *Dev. Biol., 96,* 89–102.

Keynes, R., Tannahill, D., Morgenstern, D. A., Johnson, A. R., Cook, G. M., and Pini, A. (1997). Surround repulsion of spinal sensory axons in higher vertebrate embryos. *Neuron, 18,* 889–897.

Kim, S., Buonanno, A., and Nelson, P. G. (1998). Regulation of prothrombin, thrombin receptor and protease nexin-1 during development and after denervation in muscle. *J. Neurosci. Res., 53,* 304–311.

Kuhn, T. B., Schmidt, M. F., and Kater, S. B. (1995). Laminin and fibronectin guideposts signal sustained but opposite effects to passing growth cones. *Neuron, 14,* 275–285.

Lankford, K. L., and Letourneau, P. C. (1989). Evidence that calcium may control neurite outgrowth by regulating the stability of actin filaments. *J. Cell. Biol., 109,* 1229–1243.

Lankford, K. L., and Letourneau, P. C. (1991). Roles of actin filaments and three second-messenger systems in short-term regulation of chick dorsal root ganglion neurite outgrowth. *Cell Motil. Cytoskel., 20,* 7–29.

Liu, Y., Fields, R. D., Festoff, B. W., and Nelson, P. G. (1994a). Proteolytic action of thrombin is required for electrical activity-dependent synapse reduction. *Proc. Natl. Acad. Sci. U.S.A., 91,* 10300–10304.

Liu, Y., Fields, R. D., Fitzgerald, S., Festoff, B. W., and Nelson, P. G. (1994b). Proteolytic activity, synapse elimination and the Hebb synapse. *J. Neurobiol., 25,* 325–335.

Logan, C., Wizenmann, A., Drescher, U., Monschau, B., Bonhoeffer, F., and Lumsden, A. (1996). Rostral optic tectum acquires caudal characteristics following ectopic engrailed expression. *Curr. Biol., 6,* 1006–1014.

Lohof, A. M., Quillan, M., Dan, Y., and Poo, M.-M. (1992). Asymmetric modulation of cytosolic cAMP activity induces growth cone turning. *J. Neurosci., 12,* 1253–1261.

Luo, Y., and Raper, J. A. (1994). Inhibitory factors controlling growth cone motility and guidance. *Curr. Opin. Neurobiol., 4,* 648–654.

Luo, Y., Shepherd, I., Li, J., Renzi, M. J., Chang, S., and Raper, J. A. (1995). A family of molecules related to collapsin in the embryonic chick nervous system [published erratum appears in *Neuron,* 1995, *15*(5), following p. 1218]. *Neuron, 14,* 1131–1140.

Mayer, M. L., and Westbrook, G. L. (1987). The physiology of excitatory amino acids in the vertebrate nervous system. *Prog. Neurobiol., 28,* 197–276.

Müller, B., Stahl, B., and Bonhoeffer, F. (1990). *In vitro* experiments on axonal guidance and growth-cone collapse. *J. Exp. Biol., 153,* 29–46.

Nakamoto, M., Cheng, H. J., Friedman, G. C., McLaughlin, T., Hansen, M. J., Yoon, C. H., O'Leary, D. D., and Flanagan, J. G. (1996). Topographically specific effects of ELF-1 on retinal axon guidance *in vitro* and retinal axon mapping *in vivo*. *Cell, 86,* 755–766.

Nelson, P. G., Fields, R. D., and Liu, Y. (1995). Neuroactivity, neuron–glia relationships and synapse development. *Perspect. Dev. Neurobiol., 2,* 399–407.

Nelson, P. G., Fields, R. D., Yu, C., and Liu, Y. (1993). Synapse elimination from the mouse neuromuscular junction *in vitro:* A non-Hebbian activity-dependent process. *J. Neurobiol., 24,* 1517–1530.

Nguyen, Q. T., and Lichtman, J. W. (1996). Mechanism of synapse disassembly at the developing neuromuscular junction. *Curr. Opin. Neurobiol., 6,* 104–112.

O'Brien, R. A. D., Osteberg, A. J. C., and Vrbova, G. (1978). Observation on the elimination of polyneuronal innervation in developing mammalian skeletal muscle. *J. Physiol.* (Lond.), *282,* 571–582.

O'Connor, T. P., Duerr, J. S., and Bentley, D. (1990). Pioneer growth cone steering decisions mediated by single filopodial contacts *in situ. J. Neurosci., 10,* 3935–3946.

Oppenheim, R. W. (1989). The neurotrophic theory and naturally occurring motoneuron death. *Trends Neurosci., 12,* 252–255.

Orike, N., and Pini, A. (1996). Axon guidance: Following the Eph plan. *Curr. Biol., 6,* 108–110.

Orioli, D., and Klein, R. (1997). The Eph receptor family: Axonal guidance by contact repulsion. *Trends Genet, 13,* 354–359.

Pini, A. (1993). Chemorepulsion of axons in the developing mammalian central nervous system. *Science, 261,* 95–98.

Rager, G. (1979). Arrangement and distribution of fibres in the developing optic nerve of the chicken [Proceedings]. *J. Physiol. (Lond.), 292,* 54 pp.

Rager, G. (1980). Retinotopy and order in the visual pathway of the chick embryo during development. *Folia Morphol (Praha), 28,* 72–75.

Rager, G. (1983). Structural analysis of fiber organization during development. *Prog. Brain Res., 58,* 313–319.

Ramon y Cajal, S. (1890). A quelle epoque apparaissent les expansions des cellules nerveuses de la moelle epiniere du poulet. *Anat. Anz., 5,* 609–613, 631–639.

Ramon y Cajal, S. (1937). *Recollections of My Life.* Cambridge: M.I.T. Press.

Raper, J. A., Chang, S., and Raible, D. W. (1991). Interactions between growth cones and axons: Selectively distributed extension-promoting and extension-inhibiting components. In P. C. Letourneau, S. B. Kater, and E. R. Macagno (eds.): *The Nerve Growth Cone.* New York: Raven Press, pp. 207–218.

Redfern, P. A. (1970). Neuromuscular transmission in newborn rats. *J. Physiol. (Lond.), 209,* 701–709.

Rehder, V., and Kater, S. (1992). Regulation of neuronal growth cone filopodia by intracellular calcium. *J. Neurosci., 12,* 3175–3186.

Schwab, M. E. (1996a). Molecules inhibiting neurite growth: A minireview. *Neurochem. Res., 21,* 755–761.

Schwab, M. E. (1996b). Structural plasticity of the adult CNS. Negative control by neurite growth inhibitory signals. *Int. J. Dev. Neurosci., 14,* 379–385.

Schwab, M. E., and Bandtlow, C. E. (1994). Neurobiology. Inhibitory influences [News]. *Nature, 371,* 658–659.

Serafini, T., Colamarino, S. A., Leonardo, E. D., Wang, H., Beddington, R., Skarnes, W. C., and Tessier, L. M. (1996). Netrin-1 is required for commissural axon guidance in the developing vertebrate nervous system. *Cell, 87,* 1001–1014.

Serafini, T., Kennedy, T. E., Galko, M. J., Mirzayan, C., Jessell, T. M., and Tessier, L. M. (1994). The netrins define a family of axon outgrowth-promoting proteins homologous to *C. elegans* UNC-6. *Cell, 78,* 409–424.

Shatz, C. J. (1990). Impulse activity and the patterning of connections during CNS development. *Neuron, 5,* 745–756.

Shepherd, I. T., Luo, Y., Lefcort, F., Reichardt, L. F., and Raper, J. A. (1997). A sensory axon repellent secreted from ventral spinal cord explants is neutralized by antibodies raised against collapsin-1. *Development, 124,* 1377–1385.

Shepherd, I., Luo, Y., Raper, J. A., and Chang, S. (1996). The distribution of collapsin-1 mRNA in the developing chick nervous system. *Dev. Biol., 173,* 185–199.

Shirasaki, R., Mirzayan, C., Tessier, L. M., and Murakami, F. (1996). Guidance of circumferentially growing axons by netrin-dependent and -independent floor plate chemotropism in the vertebrate brain. *Neuron, 17,* 1079–1088.

Silver, R. A., Lamb, A. G., and Bolsover, S. R. (1990). Calcium hotspots caused by L-channel clustering promote morphological changes in neuronal growth cones. *Nature, 343,* 751–754.

Song, H. J., Ming, G. L., and Poo, M. M. (1997). cAMP-induced switching in turning direction of nerve growth cones. *Nature, 388,* 275–279.

Sperry, R. W. (1963). Chemoaffinity in the orderly growth of nerve fiber patterns and connections. *Proc. Natl. Acad. Sci. U.S.A., 50,* 703–710.

Stent, G. (1973). A physiological mechanism for Hebb's postulate of learning. *Proc. Natl. Acad. Sci. U.S.A., 70,* 997–1001.

Stuermer, C. A. (1990). Target recognition and dynamics of axonal growth in the retinotectal system of fish. *Neurosci. Res. Suppl., 13,* s1–10.

Tessier-Lavigne, M. (1994). Axon guidance by diffusible repellents and attractants. *Curr. Opin. Genet. Dev., 4,* 596–601.

Tessier-Lavigne, M. (1995). Eph receptor tyrosine kinases, axon repulsion, and the development of topographic maps. *Cell, 82,* 345–348.

Thompson, W. J. (1985). Activity and synapse elimination at the neuromuscular junction. *Cell Mol. Neurobiol., 5,* 167–182.

Trowe, T., Klostermann, S., Baier, H., Granato, M., Crawford, A. D., Grunewald, B., Hoffmann, H., Karlstrom, R. O., Meyer, S. U., Muller, B., Richter, S., Nusslein, V. C., and Bonhoeffer, F. (1996). Mutations disrupting the ordering and topographic mapping of axons in the retinotectal projection of the zebrafish, *Danio rerio. Development, 123,* 439–450.

Tuzi, N. L., and Gullick, W. J. (1994). eph, the largest known family of putative growth factor receptors. *Br. J. Cancer, 69,* 417–421.

VanEssen, D. C., Gordon, H., Soha, J. M., and Fraser, S. E. (1990). Synaptic dynamics at the neuromuscular junction: Mechanisms and models. *J. Neurobiol., 21,* 223–249.

Vielmetter, J., and Stuermer, C. A. (1989). Goldfish retinal axons respond to position-specific properties of tectal cell membranes *in vitro. Neuron, 2,* 1331–1339.

Vielmetter, J., Walter, J., and Stuermer, C. A. (1991). Regenerating retinal axons of goldfish respond to a repellent guiding component on caudal tectal membranes of adult fish and embryonic chick. *J. Comp. Neurol., 311,* 321–329.

Walter, J., Henke, F. S., and Bonhoeffer, F. (1987a). Avoidance of posterior tectal membranes by temporal retinal axons. *Development, 101,* 909–913.

Walter, J., Kern, V. B., Huf, J., Stolze, B., and Bonhoeffer, F. (1987b). Recognition of position-specific properties of tectal cell membranes by retinal axons *in vitro. Development, 101,* 685–696.

Wiesel, T. N., and Hubel, D. H. (1963). Single cell responses in striate cortex of kittens deprived of vision in one eye. *J. Neurophysiol., 26,* 1003–1017.

Williams, C. V., Davenport, R. W., Dou, P., and Kater, S. B. (1995). Developmental regulation of plasticity along neurite shafts. *J. Neurobiol., 27,* 127–140.

Wilson, M. A., and Tonegawa, S. (1997). Synaptic plasticity, place cells and spatial memory: Study with second generation knockouts. *Trends Neurosci., 20,* 102–106.

Winslow, J. W., Moran, P., Valverde, J., Shih, A., Yuan, J. Q., Wong, S. C., Tsai, S. P., Goddard, A., Henzel, W. J., Hefti, F., et al. (1995). Cloning of AL-1, a ligand for an Eph-related tyrosine kinase receptor involved in axon bundle formation. *Neuron, 14,* 973–981.

Wizenmann, A., Thies, E., Klostermann, S., Bonhoeffer, F., and Bahr, M. (1993). Appearance of target-specific guidance information for regenerating axons after CNS lesions. *Neuron, 11,* 975–83.

Zheng, J. Q., Poo, M. M., and Connor, J. A. (1996). Calcium and chemotropic turning of nerve growth cones. *Perspect. Dev. Neurobiol., 4,* 205–213.

Zheng, J. Q., Zheng, Z., and Poo, M. (1994). Long-range signaling in growing neurons after local elevation of cyclic AMP-dependent activity. *J. Cell. Biol., 127,* 1693–1701.

Zoubine, M. N., Ma, J. Y., Smirnda, I. V., Citron, B. A., and Festoff, B. W. (1996). A molecular mechanism for synapse elimination: Novel inhibition of locally generated thrombin delays synapse loss in neonatal mouse muscle. *Dev. Biol.* 179, 447–457.

2

Effects of Differential Experience on Brain and Cognition Throughout the Life Span

MARK R. ROSENZWEIG

The basic neural processes of learning and development are now considered by many to be intimately related to both normal development and developmental disorders. The last half century has seen remarkable advances in knowledge about these fields and their inter-relationships. This knowledge is also entering debates on public policy, as reflected by material in Hillary Rodham Clinton's book, *It Takes a Village* (1996, esp. pp. 57–61), in the President's 1997 State of the Union message, and in the White House Conference on Early Learning and the Brain, which took place April 17, 1997.

In the first part of this chapter I give some personal perspectives on the changes of knowledge and conceptualization during the last half century. Next, I take up research on the question of whether the neural mechanisms of learning and development are the same. This also includes the question of why some neurobiologists were reluctant to recognize the life-long plasticity of the nervous system. Then, I consider some applications of research on the plasticity of brain and cognition throughout the life span. Finally, I provide a coda on language learning, including some personal experiences.

The Outlook Around 1950

During my graduate studies at Harvard in the late 1940s and in my early postdoctoral years, I was aware of conflicting opinions about prospects for understanding the neural bases of learning and memory. Karl S. Lashley published a pessimistic review in 1950. When he surveyed the literature on possible synaptic changes as a result of training, he concluded that there was no solid evidence to support any of the "growth" theories. Specifically, Lashley offered these criticisms: *(1)* Neural cell growth appears to be too slow to account for the rapidity with which some learning can take place (we will return to this point later). *(2)* Because he was unable to localize the memory trace, Lashley held that there was no warrant to look for localized changes. A few years later, Hans-Lukas Teuber stated in an *Annual Review of Psychology* chapter on physiological psychology that

> . . . the absence of any convincing physiological correlate of learning is the greatest gap in physiological psychology. Apparently, the best we can do with learning is to prevent it from occurring, by intercurrent stimulation through implanted electrodes . . . , by cerebral ablation . . . , or by depriving otherwise intact organisms, early in life, of normal sensory influx . . . (Teuber 1955, p. 267).

Edwin G. Boring, the historian of psychology with whom I studied in the latter 1940s, also testified to the lack of progress in this area in the 1950 edition of his history of experimental psychology:

> Where or how does the brain store its memories? That is the great mystery. . . . The physiology of memory has been so baffling a problem that most psychologists in facing it have gone positivistic, being content with hypothesized intervening variables or with empty correlations (Boring, 1950, p. 670).

At the end of his chapter on the history of research on brain functions, Boring gave his view about what was needed for further progress:

> In general it seems safe to say that progress in this field is held back, not by lack of interest, ability or industry, but by the absence of some one of the other essentials for scientific progress. Knowledge of the nature of the nerve impulse waited upon the discovery of electric currents and galvanometers of several kinds. Knowledge in psychoacoustics seemed to get nowhere until electronics developed. The truth about how the brain functions may eventually yield to a technique that comes from some new field remote from either physiology or psychology. Genius waits on insight, but insight may wait on the discovery of new concrete factual knowledge (Boring, 1950, p. 688).

In fact, some major advances were beginning to occur in research on the neural mechanisms of learning and memory. Some of these resulted from application of recently developed techniques such as single cell electrophysiological recording, electron microscopy, and use of new neurochemical methods. Another major influence encouraging research on neural mechanisms of learning and memory was Donald O. Hebb's 1949 monograph *The Organization of Behavior.* I had the good fortune to be exposed to Hebb's optimistic perspective in a seminar he gave at Harvard in the summer of 1947, using a mimeographed version of his 1949 book as text.

Hebb (1949) was more positive about possible synaptic changes in learning than his mentor Lashley. Hebb noted some evidence for neural changes and did not let the absence of conclusive evidence deter him from reviving hypotheses about the conditions that could lead to formation of new synaptic junctions and underlie memory. In essence, Hebb's hypothesis of synaptic change underlying learning resembled William James' formulation of 1890: "When two elementary brain-processes have been active together or in immediate succession, one of them, on recurring, tends to propagate its excitement into the other" (James, 1890, p. 566). (So did the formulation of Hebb's contemporary, Ralph W. Gerard, in 1949.) Hebb's "dual trace hypothesis" also resembled the "consolidation-perseveration" hypothesis of Müller and Pilzecker (1900). Much current neuroscience research concerns properties of what are now known as *Hebb synapses*. Hebb was somewhat amused that his name was connected to this resurrected hypothesis rather than to concepts he considered original (Milner, 1993, p. 127).

Ten years after Hebb's 1949 book was published, his postulate of use-dependent neural plasticity had still not been demonstrated experimentally. It seemed to many that it would not be possible, with available techniques, to find changes in the brain induced by training or experience. Thus, even in the 1970s Agranoff et al. (1978, p. 628) spoke of a Catch 22 in research in this area: If a change is big enough to be detected, it is too big to be a specific correlate of memory. Or, more formally, any neurochemical change that could be detected in a whole-brain extract after training would probably be too large to be related specifically to learning and instead would probably reflect grosser and less specific concomitants of learning such as stress or attentiveness. At a symposium in 1957 my colleagues and I proposed that an approach to this problem would be to make neurochemical analyses of specific regions of trained and untrained brains. This might be able to integrate and permit measurement of small changes taking place over many thousands of neural units. If such changes were found within a region, then subsequent analyses might be able to focus more closely (Rosenzweig et al., 1958, p. 338).

The First Reports of Cerebral Effects of Training or Experience

In the early 1960s two experimental programs announced findings demonstrating that the brain can be altered measurably by training or differential experience. First were the demonstrations by our group at Berkeley that both formal training and informal experience in varied environments led to measurable changes in neurochemistry and neuroanatomy of the brains of laboratory rats (Krech et al., 1960; Rosenzweig et al., 1961, 1962). Soon after came the reports of Hubel and Wiesel that occluding one eye of a kitten led to reduction in the number of cortical cells responding to that eye, but only during an early critical period (Wiesel and Hubel, 1963, 1965; Hubel and Wiesel, 1965).

The original clues for the discovery of our Berkeley group came from data on rats given formal training in a variety of problems to examine possible relations between individual differences in brain chemistry and problem-solving ability. We did obtain significant correlations between levels of activity of the enzyme acetylcholinesterase (AChE) in the cerebral cortex and ability to solve spatial problems (e.g., Krech et al., 1956; Rosenzweig et al., 1958). When we tested the generality of this finding over six different behavioral tests, we found a surprise: As we reported at a 1959 symposium, total AChE activity was higher in the cerebral cortex of groups that had been trained and tested on more difficult problems than in those given easier problems, and all the tested groups measured higher in total cortical AChE activity than did groups given no training and testing (Rosenzweig et al., 1961, p. 102 and their Fig. 4). It appeared that formal training could alter the AChE activity of the cortex! To test this further, we conducted an experiment in which littermates were either trained on a difficult problem or left untrained; the trained rats developed significantly higher cortical AChE activity than did their untrained littermates (Rosenzweig et al., 1961, p. 103). Control experiments showed that the results could not be attributed to the fact that the trained rats were handled or were underfed to increase their motivation to perform the task.

Instead of continuing to train rats in problem-solving tests, a time-consuming and expensive procedure, we decided to house the animals in different environments that provided differential opportunities for informal learning. Measures made at the end of the experiment showed that informal enriched experience led to increased cortical AChE activity (Krech et al., 1960). The discovery that formal training or differential experience caused changes in cortical chemistry was soon followed by the even more surprising finding that enriched experience increased the *weights* of regions of the neocortex (Rosenzweig et al., 1962).

Work by students of Hebb (e.g., Forgays and Forgays, 1952) suggested the environments used in these experiments. Typically, we assigned littermates of the same sex by a random procedure among various laboratory environments, the three most common being these: *(1)* a large cage containing a group of 10–12 animals and a variety of stimulus objects, which were changed daily. This was called the enriched condition (EC) because it provided greater opportunities for informal learning than did the other conditions. *(2)* The standard colony or social condition (SC) had three animals in a standard laboratory cage. *(3)* SC-sized cages housing single animals was called the impoverished condition or isolated condition (IC). All three conditions provided food and water *ad libitum.*

Over the next several years, replications and extensions by us (e.g., Bennett et al., 1964a) and by others (e.g., Altman and Das, 1964; Geller et al., 1965; Greenough and Volkmar, 1973) added to the evidence that training or differential experience could produce measurable changes in the brain. Control experiments demonstrated that the cerebral differences could not be attributed to differential handling, locomotor activity, or diet. The brain weight differences caused by differential experience were extremely reliable, although they amounted to only about 4% in total cortex. Moreover, these differences were not uniformly distributed throughout the cerebral cortex: They were almost invariably largest in occipital cortex (6%) and smallest in the adjacent somesthetic cortex (about 2%). The rest of the brain outside the cerebral cortex tended to show very little effect (Bennett et al., 1964a,b; Rosenzweig et al., 1972a,b). Thus the experience caused changes in specific cortical regions and not undifferentiated growth of brain. Later work also showed effects of differential experience in other parts of the brain that have been implicated in learning and formation of memory—the cerebellar cortex (Pysh and Weiss, 1979) and the hippocampal dentate gyrus (Juraska et al., 1985, 1989).

Further early studies revealed experience-induced changes in other measures, especially in occipital cortex: These measures included cortical thickness (Diamond et al., 1964), sizes of neuronal cell bodies and nuclei (Diamond, 1967), size of synaptic contact areas (West and Greenough, 1972), an increase of 10% in numbers of dendritic spines per unit of length of basal dendrites (Globus et al., 1973), an increase in extent and branching of dendrites (Holloway, 1966) amounting to 25% or more (Greenough and Volkmar, 1973), and a parallel increase in numbers of synapses per neuron (Turner and Greenough, 1985). Mainly because of the increase in dendritic branching, the neuronal cell bodies are spaced farther apart in the cortex of EC than in IC rats. These effects indicate substantial increases in cortical volume and intracortical connections; they suggest greater processing capacity of the cortical region concerned. They contradict the speculation of Ramón y Cajal (1894) that, with training, neural cell bodies would shrink to allow neural arborizations to grow, thus allowing brain volume to remain constant. Instead, increased arborization requires *larger* cell bodies to maintain them, and the volume of the cortex increases as cell bodies and dendrites grow.

These experimental reports indicated growth of number and/or size of synaptic connections as results of training or enriched experience. Some workers declared for one or the other of these possibilities, as when neurophysiologist John C. Eccles (1965, p. 97) stated his belief that learning and memory storage involve "growth just of bigger and better synapses that are already there, not growth of new connections." But Rosenzweig et al. (1972c) reviewed findings and theoretical discussions suggesting that memory can be stored by negative as well as positive synaptic changes, including shedding neural connections and forming new connections. Depending on where one measures and the kind of training or differential experience employed, one may find an increase in number of synapses, an increase in their size, a decrease in number, or a decrease in size.

Skepticism or frank disbelief were the initial reactions to our reports that significant changes in the brain were caused by relatively simple and benign exposure of animals to differential experience. By the early 1970s some neurobiologists began to accept these results. Thus neurobiologist B. G. Cragg (1972, p. 42) wrote, "Initial incredulity that such differences in social and psychological conditions could give rise to significant differences in brain weight, cortical thickness, and glial numbers seems to have been overcome by the continued series of papers from Berkeley reporting consistent results. Some independent confirmation by workers elsewhere has also been obtained." Other neurobiologists continued into the 1980s to believe that neural connections in the adult brain remain fixed, discussed further in the section "Are the Neural Mechanisms of Learning and Development the Same?"

Soon after the early publications of neurochemical and anatomical plasticity came another kind of evidence of cortical plasticity—the announcement by Hubel and Wiesel that depriving one eye of light in a young animal, starting at the age at which the eyes open, reduced the number of cortical cells responding to stimulation of that eye (Wiescl and Hubel, 1963, 1965; Hubel and Wiesel, 1965). Depriving an eye of light is a rather severe and pathological condition. In contrast, giving animals different amounts of experience without depriving them of any sensory modality is a rather mild and natural treatment, yet it leads to measurable changes of neurochemistry and neuroanatomy, and it has significant effects on problem-solving ability. The report of Wiesel and Hubel (1965) that changes can be induced in the visual system only during a critical period early in the life of the kitten served to solidify the belief of many neurobiologists that neural connections in the adult brain are fixed and do not vary as a result of training.

Differential experience produces cerebral changes throughout the life span

Further experiments revealed that significant cerebral effects of enriched versus impoverished experience could be induced at any part of the life span and with relatively short periods of exposure. In contrast, Hubel and Wiesel reported that depriving an eye of light altered cortical responses only if the eye was occluded during a critical period early in life. Later, however, investigators found that modifying sensory experience in adult animals could alter both receptive fields of cortical cells and cortical maps, as reviewed by Kaas (1991) and Weinberger (1995).

Initially we supposed that cerebral plasticity might be restricted to the early part of the life span, so we assigned animals to differential environments at weaning (about 25 days of age) and kept them there for 80 days. Later, members of our group obtained similar effects in rats assigned to the differential environments for 30 days as juveniles at 50 days of age (Zolman and Morimoto, 1962) and as young adults at 105 days of age (Rosenzweig et al., 1963; Bennett et al., 1964a). Riege (1971) in our laboratory found that similar effects occurred in rats assigned to the differential environments at 285 days of age and kept there for periods of 30, 60, or 90 days. Two hours a day in the differential environments for a period of 30 or 54 days produced similar cerebral effects to 24-hour exposure for the same periods (Rosenzweig et al., 1968). Four days of differential housing produced clear effects on cortical weights (Bennett et al., 1970) and on dendritic branching (Kilman et al., 1988); Ferchmin and Eterovic (1986) reported that four 10-minute daily sessions in EC significantly altered cortical RNA concentrations.

The fact that differential experience can cause cerebral changes throughout the life span, and relatively rapidly, was consistent with our interpretation of these effects as due to learning. Recall also that our original observation of differences in cortical neurochemistry came from experiments on formal training. Later Chang and Greenough (1982) reported that formal visual training confined to one eye of rats caused increased dendritic branching in the visual cortex contralateral to the open eye. Recently single-trial peck-avoidance training in chicks has been found to result in changes in density of dendritic spines (Lowndes and Stewart, 1994).

Although the capacity for these plastic changes of the nervous system, and for learning, remain in older subjects, the cerebral effects of differential environmental experience develop somewhat more rapidly in younger than in older animals, and the magnitude of the effects is often larger in the younger animals. Also, continuing plasticity does not hold for all brain systems and types of experience. As noted earlier, changes in responses of cortical cells to an occluded eye are normally

restricted to early development, as Wiesel and Hubel (1963) found. But this restriction may itself be modifiable: Baer and Singer (1986) reported that plasticity
of the adult visual cortex could be restored by infusing acetylcholine and noradrenaline. Further work showed that the plastic response of the young kitten brain
to occlusion of one eye also depends on glutamate transmission, because treating
the striate cortex with an inhibitor of the glutamate NMDA receptor prevented the
changes (Kleinschmidt et al., 1987). Thus, the extent to which the brain shows
plastic changes in response to a particular kind of experience depends on the age
of the subject, the brain region, the kind of experience, and special circumstances
or treatments that enhance or impair plasticity. A recent review shows the diversity of temporal constraints on plasticity (Rosenzweig et al., 1999, pp. 557–561).

Enriched experience improves ability to learn and solve problems

Hebb (1949) reported briefly that when he allowed laboratory rats to explore his
home for some weeks as pets of his children and then returned the rats to the laboratory, they showed better problem-solving ability than rats that had remained in
the laboratory throughout. Furthermore, they maintained their superiority or even
increased it during a series of tests. Hebb (1949, pp. 298–299) concluded that "*the
richer experience of the pet group during development made them better able to
profit by new experience at maturity*—one of the characteristics of the 'intelligent'
human being" (italics in the original). Moreover, the results seemed to show a *permanent* effect of early experience on problem-solving at maturity.

We and others have found that experience in an enriched laboratory environment improves learning and problem-solving ability on a wide variety of tests, although such differences have not been found invariably. One general finding is that
the more complex the task, the more likely it is that animals with EC experience
will perform better than animals from SC or IC groups (see a review and different
explanations offered for this effect in Renner and Rosenzweig, 1987, pp. 46–48).

We were unable, however, to replicate an important aspect of Hebb's report—
that over a series of tests, EC rats maintain or increase their superiority over IC
rats. On the contrary, we found that IC rats tend to catch up with EC rats over a series of trials; this occurred with each of three different tests, including the Hebb-
Williams mazes (Rosenzweig, 1971, p. 321). Thus we did not find that early deprivation of experience caused a permanent deficit, at least for rats tested on spatial
problems. Also, decreases in cortical weights induced by 300 days in the IC (versus the EC) environment could be overcome by a few weeks of training and testing in the Hebb-Williams mazes (Cummins et al., 1973). Later we will see a similar effect in birds.

Similar neuroanatomical effects of training and experience
occur in all species tested to date

Experiments with several strains of rats showed similar effects of EC versus IC experience on both brain values and problem-solving behavior, as reviewed by Renner and Rosenzweig (1987, pp. 53–54). Similar effects on brain measures have

been found in several species of mammals—mice, gerbils, ground squirrels, cats, and monkeys (reviewed by Renner and Rosenzweig, 1987, pp. 54–59), and effects of training on brain values of birds have also been found. Thus the cerebral effects of experience that were surprising when first found in rats have now been generalized to several mammalian and avian species. Anatomical effects of training or differential experience have been measured in specific brain regions of *Drosophila* (Davis, 1993; Heisenberg et al., 1995). Synaptic changes with training have also been found in the nervous systems of the molluscs *Aplysia* and *Hermissenda,* as reviewed by Krasne and Glanzman (1995). In *Aplysia,* long-term habituation led to decreased numbers of synaptic sites, whereas long-term sensitization led to an increase (Bailey and Chen, 1983); this is a case where either a decrease or an increase in synaptic numbers stores memory. Thus, as noted by Greenough et al. (1990, p. 164), "experience-dependent synaptic plasticity is more widely reported, in terms of species, than any other putative memory mechanisms."

In the human brain, noninvasive imaging is beginning to detect changes in the brain map caused by learning. Thus, in a recent study I discuss further in the Coda below, learning a second language by adolescents was found to establish a second motor speech area in the left hemisphere, adjacent to the speech area for the primary language (Kim et al., 1997).

Similar neurochemical cascades occur in different kinds of learning and in different species

By what mechanisms do enriched experience or formal training lead to plastic changes in the nervous system? We found early that enriched experience causes increased rates of protein synthesis and increased amounts of protein in the cortex (Bennett et al., 1964a). Later, imprinting was reported to increase the rates of incorporation of precursors into RNA and protein in the forebrain of the chick (Haywood et al., 1970). We viewed these and related findings in the light of the hypothesis, perhaps first enunciated by Katz and Halstead (1950), that protein synthesis is required for memory storage.

Tests of the protein-synthesis hypothesis of memory formation were initiated by Flexner and associates in the early 1960s (e.g., Flexner et al., 1962, 1965). I have reviewed elsewhere (e.g., Rosenzweig, 1996) difficulties in confirming this hypothesis and how our group in Berkeley contributed decisive evidence for it.

Having demonstrated that protein synthesis soon after training is necessary for formation of long-term memory (LTM), we then designed further experiments to find the neurochemical processes that underlie the formation of short-term memory (STM) and intermediate-term memory (ITM), since neither of these earlier stages requires protein synthesis. The basic distinction between STM and LTM was apparent to psychologists as early as William James. Lashley, however, failed to take this distinction into account when, as we noted earlier, he argued that cell growth could not account for memory because growth is too slow to account for some learning.

Much of our early work on stages of memory formation used rodent subjects (e.g., Mizumori et al., 1987), but STM and ITM are short-lived and difficult to dissociate from each other in rodents. Cherkin (1969) and Gibbs and Ng (1977) had found that the early stages of memory last on the order of tens of minutes in chicks. Moreover, in experiments with chicks, STM and ITM can be affected separately by several amnestic agents, and young chicks have many advantages as subjects in this type of experiment. After replicating and extending some of the reports with chicks (Rosenzweig, 1990), we then concentrated on this preparation.

Using the chick system, several investigators have traced parts of a cascade of neurochemical events from initial stimulation to synthesis of protein and structural changes (e.g., Gibbs and Ng, 1977; Ng and Gibbs, 1991; Rose, 1992a,b; Rosenzweig et al., 1992). At some if not all stages, parallel processes occur. In brief, here are some of the stages: The cascade is initiated when sensory stimulation activates receptor organs, which stimulate afferent neurons by using various synaptic transmitter agents such as acetylcholine (ACh) and glutamate. Inhibitors of ACh synaptic activity, such as scopolamine and pirenzepine, can prevent STM. So can inhibitors of glutamate receptors, including both the NMDA and AMPA receptors. Alteration of regulation of ion channels in the neuronal membrane can inhibit STM formation, as seen in effects of lanthanum chloride on calcium channels and of ouabain on sodium and potassium channels. Inhibition of second messengers is also amnestic, for example, inhibition of adenylate cyclase by forskolin or of diacylglycerol by bradykinin. These second messengers can activate protein kinases—enzymes that catalyze addition of phosphate molecules to proteins. We found that two kinds of protein kinases are important in formation, respectively, of ITM or LTM. Agents that inhibit calcium–calmodulin protein kinases (Cam kinases) prevent formation of ITM, whereas agents that do *not* inhibit Cam kinases but *do* inhibit protein kinase A (PKA) or protein kinase C (PKC) prevent formation of LTM (Rosenzweig et al., 1992; Serrano et al., 1994). From this research, Serrano et al. (1995) were able to predict for a newly available inhibitor of PKC its effective amnestic dose and how long after training it would cause memory to decline. One-trial training leads to increase of immediate early gene messenger RNA in the chick forebrain (Anokhin and Rose, 1991) and to increase in the density of dendritic spines (Lowndes and Stewart, 1994). Many of these effects occur only in the left hemisphere of the chick or are more prominent in the left than in the right hemisphere. (Observations of hemispheric differences in learning have recently been extended to humans: Hemispheric differences in both encoding and retrieval have been found in human subjects using noninvasive imaging [e.g., Nyberg et al., 1996; Tulving 1998].) Thus, learning in the chick system permits study of many steps that lead from sensory stimulation to formation of neuronal structures involved in memory.

The neurochemical cascade involved in formation of memory in the chick is similar to the cascade involved in long-term potentiation in the mammalian brain (e.g., Colley and Routtenberg, 1993) and in the nervous systems of invertebrates (e.g., Krasne and Glanzman, 1995). In a recent review, DeZazzo and Tully (1995) discuss STM, ITM, and LTM and compare the characteristics of the three stages in fruitflies, chicks, and rats.

Experience may be necessary for full growth of brain
and of behavioral potential

Sufficiently rich experience may be necessary for full growth of species-specific brain characteristics and behavioral potential. This is seen in recent research on differential experience conducted with different species of the crow family. Species that cache food in a variety of locations for future use are found to have significantly larger hippocampal formations than related species that do not cache food (Krebs et al., 1989; Sherry et al., 1989). But the difference in hippocampal size is not found in young birds who are still in the nest; it appears only after food storing has started, a few weeks after the birds have left the nest (Healy and Krebs, 1993). Even more interesting is the finding that this species-typical difference in hippocampal size depends on experience; it does not appear in birds that have not had the opportunity to cache food (Clayton and Krebs, 1994). Different groups of hand-raised birds were given experience in storing food at three different ages: either 35–59 days, 60–83 days, or 115–138 days posthatch. Experience at each of these periods led to increased hippocampal size, much as we had found for measures of occipital cortex in the rat. Thus, both birds and rats appear to retain considerable potential for experience-induced brain growth if it does not occur at the usual early age.

Are the Neural Mechanisms of Learning and Development the Same?

Some historical background

The hypothesis that the mechanisms of learning and development are the same was proposed separately by neurologist Eugenio Tanzi (1893) and by neuroanatomist Santiago Ramón y Cajal (1894). This hypothesis was also advanced from time to time during the present century, and it is undergoing a current wave of popularity as more is being learned about the mechanisms of both learning and development. Some of the current investigators recognize that this is an old hypothesis. Thus, Marcus et al. (1994, p. 179) start their article in this way: "At the turn of the century, Ramón y Cajal (1911) articulated the hypothesis that growth processes involved in the development of the nervous system persist into the adult where they subserve learning and memory." Others treat this hypothesis as being much more recent. Thus, Kandel and O'Dell (1992, p. 243) start the second paragraph of their article ("Are adult learning mechanisms also used for development?") with the following statement:

> Perhaps the most interesting clues to shared mechanisms [of learning and development] are evidenced in the current revisions in our thinking about how connections in the vertebrate brain are formed in development. Until 10 or 15 years ago, most neurobiologists believed, as Roger Sperry proposed for cold-blooded vertebrates, that connections in the brain are formed independently of activity or experi-

ence and are programmed by a set of recognition molecules on each pre- and post-synaptic neuron of the synapse (Sperry, 1963).

This statement requires comments in two respects. First, how is it that "most neurobiologists" took until the later 1970s or early 1980s to recognize that activity and experience affect connections in the brain? Accounts of the effects of experience on brain measures appeared in many neurobiological as well as psychological journals in the 1960s and early 1970s. This research was also reported in a cover article in the February 1972 *Scientific American* that discussed effects of experience on dendritic spine numbers and synaptic sizes, as well as other neural measures (Rosenzweig et al., 1972b). Some neurobiologists, such as Cragg (1972), cited above, overcame their initial skepticism and accepted these reports by the early 1970s.

Second, although mentioning Sperry's conclusion about predetermined connections, Kandel and O'Dell (1992) ignored the fact that Sperry limited this inflexibility to the basic neural projection systems and believed that learning could alter connections in higher brain regions. In a presentation and discussion of his results and those of others, Sperry (1951, p. 237) tried to partial out the extent to which neural connections are "(1) preformed directly by processes of growth and cell differentiation and (2) patterned by functional regulation through experience and training." After concluding that the basic patterns of connections "are organized for the most part by intrinsic forces of development without the aid of learning," Sperry asked where effects of learning could be found. "By process of elimination the interneuronal relations patterned by learning would seem to be relegated to those circuits farthest removed from the conduction pathways which, in the mammal, would be confined mainly to the cerebral cortex." It is true that Sperry's evidence that the connections in the lower parts of the nervous systems of amphibians are preformed attracted more attention than his complementary conclusion of plasticity in the higher parts of the nervous system, but to ignore the latter conclusion misrepresents his views.

Accepting evidence that the adult brain can change neural connections throughout the life span was a paradigm shift, and such shifts are usually resisted strongly. It was more comfortable to accept Sperry's evidence of fixity of connections in the lower parts of the nervous system than to consider his conclusion that plasticity underlying learning must occur in upper regions of the brain. Hubel and Wiesel's evidence for plasticity in the cortex could be accepted, since it was restricted to an early critical period of life, but life-long plasticity is another matter. We are still exploring the ramifications and implications of the idea that the brain is plastic throughout the life span.

Tests of the hypothesis that the neural mechanisms of learning and development are the same

The main method used so far to investigate the hypothesized identity between neural mechanisms of development and of learning has been to compile lists of mechanisms that are involved in both. But, as Marcus et al. (1994, p. 179) point out, "to date no single experimental system has been extensively studied from both a developmental and a learning perspective. For this reason, comparisons between the mechanisms of learning and development often resort to analogies and inferences drawn across diverse systems." They therefore focus attention on research with *Aplysia,* using the growing "understanding of the cellular and molecular mechanism of learning in *Aplysia* as a basis for comparison with the three principle [sic] stages of neuronal development: differentiation, neurite outgrowth and synapse formation (p. 180)." From their review, Marcus et al. (1994, p. 181) cite five specific neurochemical points of similarity between learning and development in *Aplysia:*

> (i) the role of serotonergic axosomatic contacts; (ii) the activation of transcription factors including immediate early genes and perhaps differentiation-inducing genes; (iii) the necessity of an appropriate post-synaptic target; (iv) the role of cAMP as a second messenger in the signal transcription cascade; and (v) the common role of cell adhesion molecules and other growth related proteins. During development, activation of these pathways leads to differentiation and neurite outgrowth; in adult learning, reactivation of these same pathways results in a growth-mediated increase in synaptic strength.

Beyond identifying similar processes involved in development and learning, Marcus et al. (1994, p. 186) point out that "the real test of the relationship between development and learning will ultimately come from studies that ask whether the same process is *required* for both neuronal development and synaptic plasticity." They see hope for such tests in studies that can now be made with genetic manipulation in both vertebrates and invertebrates. For example, investigators are using homologous recombination technology in mice where knocking out the gene for a specific kinase produces both developmental abnormalities in the nervous system and a deficiency in long-term synaptic plasticity in the adult. In this regard Marcus et al. (1994) cite both Grant et al. (1992) and Silva et al. (1992). Kandel and O'Dell (1992) cite the same authors. Although knocking out a gene can impair some kinds of learning, it does not completely prevent the learning, raising questions about the necessity of the mechanism and the possibility that alternative mechanisms can accomplish learning. Two problems in interpreting knockout studies are these: *(1)* The genes that have mutated or been knocked out usually affect cells throughout the nervous system and perhaps in other organs as well, so the effects cannot be pinpointed to specific regions or processes in the nervous system; and *(2)* the alterations are present throughout the development of the animals, so they may involve developmental abnormalities or special compensations for the missing gene products.

Recently investigators in the laboratory of Susumu Tonegawa at MIT (Tsien et al., 1996a) have overcome some of the problems in this area by eliminating a mouse gene with highly specific effects: Knocking it out inactivates a subunit of the NMDA R1 receptor, but only in pyramidal neurons in the CA1 region of the hippocampus. Furthermore, the gene begins to be expressed only a few days after birth, so eliminating it does not affect prenatal or early postnatal development of the brain. Both the anatomy of the brain and the general behavior of the mice were normal; however, the knockout mice were impaired on a spatial problem but not on a nonspatial one, showing that the genetic "lesion" had highly specific effects. The knockout mice also failed to show long-term potentiation in the CA1 region (Tsien et al., 1996b).

As the mapping of genes progresses and techniques advance, we can expect to see more instances of manipulation of genes with highly specific behavioral effects. For example, work is underway to knock out genes in adult animals by injecting a specific antibiotic that triggers disruption of the gene; this will produce specific "time-and-place" knockouts that should greatly aid in studying the contributions of particular genes. Nevertheless, as is true of all ablation techniques, the knockout technique studies the effects of the *absence* of the gene, not the direct effects of the gene itself.

Some Applications of Research on Plasticity of Brain and Cognition Throughout the Life Span

Early in our research on plasticity of brain and cognition, we began to point out possible applications, and many others have contributed in this direction. Space permits mentioning only a few examples here. Animal research on effects of experience on brain plasticity and learning is being applied to several areas of human behavior, and in other cases it is being used as converging or supporting evidence. Thus, it is being used to promote child development, successful aging, and recovery from brain damage; it is also being applied to benefit animals in laboratories, zoos, and farms. Let us consider a few of these kinds of application or influence briefly below. Over more than 30 years, our group has tried to make knowledge of our work available to stimulate applications by publishing in a variety of locations and by taking part in interdisciplinary conferences and symposia, including meetings and/or publications on fostering mental development (Rosenzweig, 1966), mental retardation (Rosenzweig, 1964), psychopathology of mental development (Rosenzweig, 1976; Rosenzweig et al., 1967), brain damage (Rosenzweig et al., 1984), recovery from brain damage (Rosenzweig, 1980), applications of neuroscience advances to education (Rosenzweig, 1981; Rosenzweig and Bennett, 1976; Rosenzweig et al., 1968), aging (Bennett and Rosenzweig, 1979), nutrition and development (Bennett and Rosenzweig, 1971), behavioral medicine (Rosenzweig and Bennett, 1980), and Alzheimer's disease (Rosenzweig and Bennett, 1996; Rosenzweig et al., 1993).

Applications to child development

The findings of effects of differential experience in animals have influenced some research on child development and have been offered as supporting evidence for the necessity of giving adequate experience to ensure normal development. The importance of this approach is shown in a major report, *Starting Points: Meeting the Needs of our Youngest Children* (Carnegie Task Force on Meeting the Needs of Young Children, 1994). The tenor of the findings is indicated by this quotation:

> Beginning in the 1960s, scientists began to demonstrate that the quality and variety of the environment have direct impact on brain development. Today, researchers around the world are amassing evidence that the role of the environment is even more important than earlier studies had suggested. For example, histological and brain scan studies of animals show changes in brain structure and function as a result of variations in early experience.
>
> These findings are consistent with research in child development that has shown the first eighteen months of life to be an important period of development. Studies of children raised in poor environments—both in this country and elsewhere—show that they have cognitive deficits of substantial magnitude by eighteen months of age and that full reversal of these deficits may not be possible. These studies are based on observational and cognitive assessments; researchers say that neurobiologists using brain scan technologies are on the verge of confirming these findings.
>
> In the meantime, more conventional studies of child development—using cognitive and observational measures—continue to show short- and long-term benefits of an enriched early environment (Carnegie Task Force on Meeting the Needs of Young Children, 1994, p. 8).

This is one of the latest contributions to a back-and-forth debate between those who hold that child development proceeds mainly from innate factors with only a small influence of the environment and those who hold that environment can make a major contribution. Gall and Spurzheim differed on this question early in the 19th century, as I have discussed elsewhere (Rosenzweig, 1996).

It is rather disheartening to see, on the one hand, how often during the past 30 years investigators have shown that lack of adequate intellectual stimulation can cause mental retardation and that appropriate stimulation can foster normal development, and, on the other, how little sustained attempt has been made to apply these findings. Hunt (1979), for example, presented evidence for the importance of early experience on children's intellectual development. He reviewed several studies showing substantial effects of specific kinds of environmental interventions on particular aspects of child development. One was his own study (Hunt et al., 1976) demonstrating the importance of specific caretaking to ensure language development of infants in a Teheran orphanage. Hunt also reviewed animal research on effects of differential experience on problem-solving, neuroanatomy, and neurochemistry—research whose inspiration he attributed to Hebb's 1949 book and that included some of the experiments of the 1960s and 1970s described above.

Several factors have complicated attempts to apply research on environmental enrichment to improve the cognitive status of children raised in poor environments. One is that some proponents have overestimated the potential effects of relatively short periods of enrichment and then have been disappointed that the effects were not larger. This has been one of the problems confronting the Head Start program that began in 1963 in the United States (Zigler and Muenchow,

1992). Although this and related programs have proved to be beneficial and cost effective, they were unable to bring participating children up to the scholastic levels of children living in better environments. Another problem is that the human programs involve a variety of aspects, so it is difficult to determine whether the positive effects are attributable to enriched experience and training or to other causes such as improved nutrition and health care. On this point, however, a recent review of effects of nutrition on child development states that "Adequacy of the social and educational environment is as significant as nutrition for mental development (or possibly more significant)" (Sigman, 1995, p. 54).

The authors of a recent series of studies conducted in Atlanta (Drews et al., 1995; Murphy et al., 1995; Yeargin-Allsopp et al., 1995) conclude that the principal causes of mild retardation (IQ scores between 50 and 70) appear to be poverty and lack of education of mothers, that is, fewer than 12 years of education. Thus they claim that many cases of mild retardation are preventable and/or treatable by appropriate early training and experience. Dr. David Satcher, then the Director of the Centers for Disease Control and Prevention, which supported these studies, and now the U.S. Surgeon General, announced that the Centers would start a demonstration program in 1996 "aimed at promoting the cognitive, communicative, and behavioral development, as well as the health, of children born to women with fewer than 12 years of education" (Satcher, 1995, p. 305). In this connection, Satcher cited the report of the Carnegie Corporation, mentioned above: "[It] goes beyond questions of intellectual function and underscores the importance of early (birth to 3 years) experiential and social factors in brain development. The report emphasizes long-lasting effects of early environmental experience on both brain structure and cognitive function" (Satcher, 1995, p. 305).

The problems of finding exactly what factors are most important in enhancing cognitive development should not overshadow the clear beneficial effects of programs to provide environmental enrichment to children in need of it. I believe that current programs need to be expanded to include more children and to retain them for longer periods of years. In the 1997 State of the Union address, an announcement that won applause was a plan that "expands Head Start to one million children by 2002." What President Clinton failed to mention was that those one million amount to only half of the children who are eligible for the program (Bennet, 1997), and, in the present political climate, even that increase is not sure to be adopted.

Enriched experience aids "successful aging"

Enriched experience, beginning early in life, also helps to ensure maintenance of ability into old age. Thus, infantile handling or later enriched experience help prevent hippocampal damage caused by stress in rats. Meaney et al. (1988, 1991) handled some neonatal rat pups each of their first 21 days and left other rats unhandled. They examined the cognitive function of the rats at different ages from 3 months to 24 months and also measured basal and stress levels of glucocorticoids, numbers of hippocampal neurons, and numbers of glucocorticoid receptors.

Chronic excess of glucocorticoids is toxic to neurons, particularly those of the hippocampus, and aged rats are particularly vulnerable (Sapolsky, 1992). Handling improved spatial memory, increased the numbers of hippocampal corticoid receptors, and led to a more rapid return of corticosterone to basal levels after response to a stressful situation. In old age, the handled animals, as compared to the unhandled, had lower basal levels of corticosterone and lost fewer hippocampal neurons.

Young adult rats given 30 days of EC or IC experience beginning at 50 days of age, like rats given infantile handling, showed higher expression of the gene encoding glucocorticoid receptors in the hippocampus, and they also showed induction of genes for nerve growth factors in the hippocampus (Mohammed et al., 1993; Olsson et al., 1994). The investigators suggest that enriched experience in adulthood, like infantile handling, may protect the aging hippocampus from glucocorticoid neurotoxicity.

Although some kinds of learning and performance decline with age after middle adulthood, this is not true of other kinds of learning and memory. People who continue to learn actively can maintain high levels of performance. For example, professors in their 60s perform as well as professors in their 30s on many tests of learning and memory (Shimamura et al., 1995).

Beyond the age of retirement, stimulation and activity continue to contribute to health and mental status. This is borne out in a longitudinal study that has assessed mental abilities of more than 5,000 adults and has followed some for as long as 35 years (Schaie, 1994). Among the eight variables found to reduce the risk of cognitive decline in old age, three are particularly relevant here:

> Living in favorable environmental circumstances as would be the case for persons characterized by high socio-economic status. These circumstances include above-average education, histories of occupational pursuits that involve high complexity and low routine, above-average income, and the maintenance of intact families.
>
> Substantial involvement in activities typically available in complex and intellectually stimulating environments. Such activities include extensive reading habits, travel, attendance at cultural events, pursuit of continuing education activities, and participation in clubs and professional associations.
>
> Being married to a spouse with high cognitive status. Our studies of cognitive similarity in married couples suggest that the lower functioning spouse at the beginning of marriage tends to maintain or increase his or her level vis à vis the higher functioning spouse (Schaie, 1994, p. 312).

Enriched experience may also cushion the brain and intellectual function against the effects of Alzheimer's disease. Terry et al. (1991) report that loss of synapses correlates more strongly than other brain measures with the severity of symptoms in Alzheimer's disease. Enriched experience produces richer neural networks in the brains of all species that have been studied in this regard, as reported earlier in this chapter. If similar effects occur in humans, as seems likely, then this may set up reserves of connections that protect intellectual function from the signs of Alzheimer's disease.

From this review, what should we conclude with regard to Swaab's query (1991) whether, in adulthood and old age, use of the nervous system is better characterized by the phrase "wear and tear" or by the phrase "use it or lose it"? It seems to me that the research reviewed here, and in some of the articles that commented on Swaab's paper, mainly support the conclusion "use it or lose it." But we should add that use and experience are especially effective early in life and set the basis for later use and maintenance of the brain and of ability. This supports a formulation that includes both early experience and later sustained use. At a 1994 symposium in Freiburg on Alzheimer's disease, we put it in the form of a limerick (Rosenzweig and Bennett, 1996, p. 63):

It's a fortunate person whose brain
Is trained early, again and again,
And who continues to use it
To be sure not to lose it,
So the brain, in old age, may not wane.

Applications to recovery from brain damage or compensation for brain damage

In all parts of the life span, training and enriched experience promote recovery from or compensation for effects of brain damage. We showed this in experiments with rats in the 1970s (Will et al., 1977), and research along this line continues. One of the major questions is the extent to which experience actually aids in recovery or only in compensation for the effects of brain injury. At a minimum, behavioral techniques aid the quality of life of people with injuries of the brain or of the spinal cord. Beyond this, there may be interaction between physiological and behavioral interventions.

In attempts to promote recovery from brain damage, some neuroscientists are transplanting fetal brain cells into the region of a brain lesion. Many psychologists along with other neuroscientists are taking part in this research. Sometimes the neural transplants or implants are successful and help to restore function. But often the neural implants do not work, for reasons that are not yet fully understood.

A few years ago, investigators started to combine the two methods by studying the separate and the combined effects of enriched environment and neural transplants (Kelche et al., 1988). Under some conditions, neither the enriched experience nor the transplant alone had a beneficial effect, but the combination of the two treatments yielded significant improvement in learning. Further work indicates that formal training of rats may be more effective than enriched environment in promoting the effects of brain cell grafts on recovery of learning ability (Kelche et al., 1995). These results of animal research may find application in attempts to aid human patients. At present one sees quite varied reports of attempts to aid patients with Parkinson's disease by implanting brain cells. Perhaps some of the differences among clinics in success of cell grafts reflect the kinds and amounts of training and stimulation given the patients; this may interact with the skill of the neurosurgeon. The combination of brain implants with training and stimulation may become an increasingly important area of interaction between research and application in the field of plasticity of brain and behavior.

Research on enriched environments is benefitting animals
in laboratories, zoos, and farms

Animals not only contribute to research on mechanisms of memory and effects of environmental enrichment, but they also benefit from such research, as I have described in somewhat more detail elsewhere (Rosenzweig, 1984). Newer standards for housing animals in laboratories reflect findings that animals benefit in development of brain and behavior from adequate space and facilities for exercise and for species-specific activities of running, investigating, and so forth. Zoos are also providing more natural settings and apparatus that permits animals to engage in species-specific activities. Two of my former students who studied rats in enriched laboratory environments have since worked to improve settings for zoo animals. Research on some farms has found that animals thrive better in more natural settings, so some farms are providing them.

Coda on Language Learning

Personal experiences with language learning have expanded my understanding of life-long learning. My wife (whose native language is French) and I decided to raise our three children bilingually in French and English. Living in the United States, where we all spoke English most of the day, our main method to teach French was to make it the language of the evening meal. My own French was weak when we married, particularly the faulty pronunciation I acquired in high school. That improved significantly, and I learned as an adult to speak French fluently and without offending critical French ears. I still make errors, but I have given lecture courses at the University of Paris. Our children were never misled by my errors, recognizing my wife's French as the gold standard. The fact that we were conversing in French encouraged the children to acquire French at the same time they learned English. And I enriched my adult knowledge of French by learning children's songs, sayings, and games. Later the children's learning of Spanish was facilitated by their knowledge of French. One child also went on to learn German, and another, Chinese. Recently my wife and I had the visit of an almost four-year-old grandson who lives in Switzerland and is learning English and French from the start. He speaks both languages well and replies in whichever language he is spoken to. These personal observations have impressed me with the capacity of young children to learn languages rapidly and skillfully and even to acquire more than one language system from the start.

An adult or even an adolescent learner cannot expect to achieve the flawless performance of one who starts a language early, although it is certainly possible for an adult to gain a useful, expressive command of another language. Psychologists Jacqueline Johnson and Elisa Newport (1989) pinpointed the ages at which native mastery of a second language can occur. They tested the English proficiency of native Chinese or Korean speakers who had arrived in the United States between the ages of 3 and 39. Those who arrived in the age range 3–7 had scores equal to a native American control group. Those who arrived at ages 8–10 had slightly but significantly lower scores, and successively lower scores were obtained by the 11–16 and 17–39 year groups. A scatterplot showed an approximately linear decline in performance as age of arrival increased from 7 to 16 years; thereafter there was no clear effect of age of arrival on test scores within the age range studied.

A recent study using functional magnetic resonance imaging found that those who acquire a second language beginning about age 11 form a separate Broca's area (motor speech area) for their second language, whereas those who acquire two languages together in infancy use essentially the same Broca's area for both (Kim et al., 1997). The fact that learning a language as an adolescent changes the human brain map in a measurable way is further striking evidence that the brain is malleable well past infancy and that training can produce significant changes in the brain.

Perhaps the exercise of using two or more languages will even be found to slow the processes of cerebral aging! It certainly adds to the quality of life and may increase intelligence. Recent support for the latter claim comes from David Dalby, director of the Observatoire Linguistique, based in Wales. Dalby states that the benefit of bilingual training for intelligence is shown by comparisons of bilingually trained and monolingual children in Wales. He maintains that "Monolingualism is a disadvantage like illiteracy, and this is a serious danger for anglophones. Bilingualism should be regarded as an educational norm" (see Carvel, 1997, p. 1). This is a far cry from early studies that claimed that bilingualism impaired cognition, but those studies suffered from methodological faults—they compared children of socially disadvantaged immigrants with native-born children. Although subsequent better designed studies have produced mixed results, many have reported superior performance in cognitive tasks by bilingual groups versus properly selected monolingual control groups (e.g., Hamers and Blanc, 1989; Bialystok, 1992).

Concluding Comment

The last half century has been a fascinating period in which to observe and take part in research on plasticity of brain and behavior. The invention of new concepts and the emergence of new experimental techniques has allowed important progress and rejection of inadequate hypotheses. Exciting new techniques promise new insights. Attempts to apply the insights from basic research of the 1960s and 1970s are both testing our current understanding and offering hope to those who suffer from developmental disorders and diseases and injuries of the nervous system. The next half century promises many more surprises and advances in this complex and engrossing field.

References

I am happy to thank Dr. Edward L. Bennett for his knowledgeable, insightful, and friendly collaboration during more than 40 years. It is also a pleasure to thank the colleagues, students, and postdoctoral fellows who collaborated with us.

The research of our laboratories received indispensable grant support from the National Science Foundation, the Department of Energy, the National Institute of Mental Health, the Easter Seal Foundation, and the National Institute on Drug Abuse.

Agranoff, B. W., Burrell, H. R., Dokas, L. A., and Springer, A. D. (1978). Progress in biochemical approaches to learning and memory. In M. A. Lipton, A. DiMascio, and K. F. Killam (eds.): *Psychopharmacology: A Generation of Progress.* New York: Raven, pp. 623–635.

Altman, J., and Das, G. D. (1964). Autoradiographic examination of the effects of enriched environment on the rate of glial multiplication in the adult rat brain. *Nature, 204,* 1161–1163.

Anokhin, K. V., and Rose, S. P. R. (1991). Learning-induced increase of early immediate gene messenger RNA in the chick forebrain. *Eur. J. Neurosci., 3,* 162–167.

Baer, M. F., and Singer, W. (1986). Modulation of visual cortical plasticity by acetylcholine and noradrenaline. *Nature, 320,* 172–176.

Bailey, C. H., and Chen, M. (1983). Morphological basis of long-term habituation and sensitization in *Aplysia. Science, 220,* 91–93.

Bennet, J. (1997). In evolution of Clinton, a few echoes survive. *New York Times,* February 6, p. A13.

Bennett, E. L., Diamond, M. C., Krech, D., and Rosenzweig, M. R. (1964a). Chemical and anatomical plasticity of brain. *Science, 164,* 610–619.

Bennett, E. L., Krech, D., and Rosenzweig, M. R. (1964b). Reliability and regional specificity of cerebral effects of environmental complexity and training. *J. Comp. Physiol. Psychol., 57,* 440–441.

Bennett, E. L., and Rosenzweig, M. R. (1971). Potentials of an intellectually enriched environment. In S. Margen (ed.): *Progress in Human Nutrition.* Westport, CT: Avi Publishing Company, pp. 210–224.

Bennett, E. L., and Rosenzweig, M. R. (1979). Brain plasticity, memory, and aging. In A. Cherkin et al. (eds.): *Physiology and Cell Biology of Aging, vol. 8, Aging.* New York: Raven, pp. 141–150.

Bennett, E. L., Rosenzweig, M. R., and Diamond, M. C. (1970). Time courses of effects of differential experience on brain measures and behavior of rats. In W. L. Byrne (ed.): *Molecular Approaches to Learning and Memory.* New York: Academic Press, pp. 69–85.

Bialystok, E. (1992). Selective attention in cognitive processing: The bilingual edge. In R. J. Harris (ed.): *Cognitive Processing in Bilinguals.* Amsterdam: North-Holland, pp. 501–513.

Boring, E. G. (1950). *A History of Experimental Psychology.* New York: Appleton-Century-Crofts.

Cajal, S. (1894). La fine structure des centres nerveux. *Proc. R. Soc. Lond., 55,* 444–468.

Cajal, S. (1911). *Histologie du système nerveux de l'homme et des vertébrés.* Paris: A. Maloine.

Carnegie Task Force on Meeting the Needs of Young Children. (1994). *Starting Points: Meeting the Needs of Our Youngest Children.* New York: Carnegie Corporation of New York.

Carvel, J. (1997). Global study finds world speaking in 10,000 tongues. *The Manchester Guardian Weekly,* July 27, 1997, p. 1.

Chang, F.-L. F., and Greenough, W. T. (1982). Lateralized effects of monocular training on dendritic branching in adult split-brain rats. *Brain Res., 232,* 283–292.

Cherkin, A. (1969). Kinetics of memory consolidation: Role of amnesic treatment parameters. *Proc. Natl. Acad. Sci., U.S.A., 63*, 1094–1101.

Clayton, N. S., and Krebs, J. R. (1994). Hippocampal growth and attrition in birds affected by experience. *Proc. Natl. Acad. Sci. U.S.A., 91*, 7410–7414.

Clinton, H. R. (1996). *It Takes a Village*. New York: Simon and Schuster.

Colley, P. A., and Routtenberg, A. (1993). Long-term potentiation as synaptic dialogue. *Brain Res. Rev., 18*, 115–122.

Cragg, B. G. (1972). Plasticity of synapses. In G. H. Bourne (ed.): *The Structure and Function of Nervous Tissue*, vol. 4. New York: Academic Press, pp. 2–60.

Cummins, R. A., Walsh, R. N., Budtz-Olsen, O. E., Konstantinos, T., and Horsfall, C. R. (1973). Environmentally-induced changes in the brains of elderly rats. *Nature, 243*, 516–518.

Davis, R. (1993). Mushroom bodies and *Drosophila* learning. *Neuron, 11*, 1–14.

Diamond, M. C. (1967). Extensive cortical depth measurements and neuron size increases in the cortex of environmentally enriched rats. *J. Comp. Neurol. 131*, 357–364.

Diamond, M. C., Krech, D., and Rosenzweig, M. R. (1964). The effects of an enriched environment on the histology of the rat cerebral cortex. *J. Comp. Neurol., 123*, 111–119.

DeZazzo, J., and Tully, T. (1995). Dissection of memory formation: From behavioral pharmacology to molecular genetics. *TINS, 18*, 212–218.

Drews, C. D., Yeargin-Allsopp, M., Decouflé, P., and Murphy, C. C. (1995). Variation in the influence of selected sociodemographic risk factors for mental retardation. *Am. J. Public Health, 85*, 329–334.

Eccles, J. C. (1965). Comment. In D. P. Kimble (ed.): *The Anatomy of Memory*. Palo Alto, CA: Science and Behavior Books, p. 97.

Ferchmin, P., and Eterovic, V. (1986). Forty minutes of experience increase the weight and RNA content of cerebral cortex in periadolescent rats. *Dev. Psychobiol., 19*, 511–519.

Flexner, J. B., Flexner, L. B., de la Haba, G., and Roberts, R. B. (1962). Inhibition of protein synthesis in brain and learning and memory following puromycin. *J. Neurochem., 9*, 595–605.

Flexner, J. B., Flexner, L. B., de la Haba, G., and Roberts, R. B. (1965). Loss of memory as related to inhibition of cerebral protein synthesis. *J. Neurochem., 12*, 535–541.

Forgays, D. G., and Forgays, J. W. (1952). The nature of the effect of free-environmental experience on the rat. *J. Comp. Physiol. Psychol., 45*, 747–750.

Geller, E., Yuwiler, A., and Zolman, J. F. (1965). Effects of environmental complexity on constituents of brain and liver. *J. Neurochem., 12*, 949–955.

Gerard, R. W. (1949). Physiology and psychiatry. *Am. J. Psychiatry, 105*, 161–173.

Gibbs, M. E., and Ng, K. T. (1977). Psychobiology of memory: Towards a model of memory formation. *Biobehav. Rev., 1*, 113–136.

Globus, A., Rosenzweig, M. R., Bennett, E. L., and Diamond, M. C. (1973). Effects of differential experience on dendritic spine counts in rat cerebral cortex. *J. Comp. Physiol. Psychol., 82*, 175–181.

Grant, S. G., O'Dell, T. J., Karl, K. A., Stein, P. L., Soriano, P., and Kandel, E. R. (1992). Impaired long-term potentiation, spatial learning, and hippocampal development in *fyn* mutant mice. *Science, 258*, 1903–1910.

Greenough, W. T. and Volkmar, F. R. (1973). Pattern of dendritic branching in occipital cortex of rats reared in complex environments. *Exp. Neurol., 40*, 491–504.

Greenough, W. T., Withers, G. S., and Wallace, C. S. (1990). Morphological changes in the nervous system arising from behavioral experience: What is the evidence they are involved in learning and memory? In L. R. Squire and E. Lindenlaub (eds.): *The Biology of Memory.* Stuttgart: F. K. Schattauer Verlag, pp. 159–185.

Hamers, J. F., and Blanc, M. H. (1989). *Bilinguality and Bilingualism.* Cambridge: Cambridge University Press.

Haywood, J., Rose, S. P. R., and Bateson, P. P. G. (1970). Effects of an imprinting procedure on RNA polymerase activity in the chick brain. *Nature, 288,* 373–374.

Healy, S. D., and Krebs, J. R. (1993). Development of hippocampal specialisation in a food-storing bird. *Behav. Brain Res., 53,* 127–130.

Hebb, D. O. (1949). *The Organization of Behavior: A Neuropsychological Theory.* New York: John Wiley & Sons.

Heisenberg, M., Heusipp, M., and Wanke, C. (1995). Structural plasticity in the *Drosophila* brain. *J. Neurosci., 15,* 1951–1960.

Holloway, R. L. (1966). Dendritic branching: Some preliminary results of training and complexity in rat visual cortex. *Brain Res., 2,* 393–396.

Hubel, D. H., and Wiesel, T. N. (1965). Binocular interaction in striate cortex of kittens reared with artificial squint. *J. Neurophysiol., 28,* 1041–1059.

Hunt, J. M. (1979). Psychological development: Early experience. *Annu. Rev. Psychol., 30,* 103–143.

Hunt, J. M., Mohandessi, K., Ghodssi, M., and Akiyama, M. (1976). The psychological development of orphanage-reared infants: Interventions with outcomes (Tehran). *Genet. Psychol. Monogr., 94,* 177–226.

James W. (1890). *Principles of Psychology,* vol. 1. New York: Henry Holt.

Johnson, J. S., and Newport, E. L. (1989). Critical period effects in second language learning: The influence of maturational state on the acquisition of English as a second language. *Cognitive Psychol., 21,* 60–99.

Juraska, J. M., Fitch, J. M., Henderson, C., and Rivers, N. (1985). Sex differences in dendritic branching of dentate granule cells following differential experience. *Brain Res., 333,* 73–80.

Juraska, J. M., Fitch, J. M., and Washburne, D. L. (1989). The dendritic morphology of neurons in the rat hippocampus CA3 area. II. Effects of gender and the environment. *Brain Res., 479,* 115–119.

Kaas, J. (1991). Plasticity of sensory and motor maps in adult mammals. *Annu. Rev. Neurosci., 14,* 137–167.

Kandel, E. R., and O'Dell, T. J. (1992). Are adult learning mechanisms also used for development? *Science, 258,* 243–245.

Katz, J. J., and Halstead, W. G. (1950). Protein organization and mental function. *Comp. Psychol. Monogr., 20,* 1–38.

Kelche, C., Dalrymple-Alford, J. C., and Will, B. (1988). Housing conditions modulate the effects of intracerebral grafts in rats with brain lesions. *Behav. Brain Res., 53,* 287–296.

Kelche, C., Roeser, C., Jeltsch, H., Cassel, J. C., and Will, B. (1995). The effects of intrahippocampal grafts, training, and postoperative housing on behavioral recovery after septohippocampal damage in the rat. *Neurobiol. Learning Memory, 63,* 155–166.

Kilman, V. L., Wallace, C. S., Withers, G. S., and Greenough, W. T. (1988). 4 days of differential housing alters dendritic morphology of weanling rats. *Soc. Neurosci. Abstr., 14,* 1135.

Kim, K. H. S., Relkin, N., Lee, K.-M., and Hirsh, J. (1997). Distinct cortical areas associated with native and second languages. *Nature, 388,* 171–174.

Kleinschmidt, A., Baer, M. F., and Singer, W. (1987). Blockade of NMDA receptors disrupts experience-dependent plasticity of kitten striate cortex. *Science, 238,* 355–358.

Krasne, F. B., and Glanzman, D. L. (1995). What we can learn from invertebrate learning. *Annu. Rev. Psychol., 46,* 585–624.

Krebs, J. R., Sherry, D. F., Healy, S. D., Perry, V. H., and Vaccarino, A. L. (1989). Hippocampal specialisation of food-storing birds. *Proc. Natl. Acad. Sci. U.S.A., 86,* 1388–1392.

Krech, D., Rosenzweig, M. R., and Bennett, E. L. (1956). Dimensions of discrimination and level of cholinesterase activity in the cerebral cortex of the rat. *J. Comp. Physiol. Psychol., 82,* 261–268.

Krech, D., Rosenzweig, M. R., and Bennett, E. L. (1960). Effects of environmental complexity and training on brain chemistry. *J. Comp. Physiol. Psychol., 53,* 509–519.

Lashley, K. S. (1950). In search of the engram. *Symp. Soc. Exp. Biol., 4,* 454–482.

Lowndes, M., and Stewart, M. G. (1994). Dendritic spine density in the lobus parolfactorius of the domestic chick is increased 24 h after one-trial passive avoidance training. *Brain Res., 654,* 129–136.

Marcus, E. A., Emptage, N. J., Marois, R., and Carew, T. J. (1994). A comparison of the mechanistic relationships between development and learning in *Aplysia. Prog. Brain Res., 100,* 179–188.

Meaney, M. J., Aitkin, D. H., Bhatnagar, S., Van Berkel, C., and Sapolsky, R. M. (1988). Postnatal handling attenuates neuroendocrine, anatomical, and cognitive impairments related to the aged hippocampus. *Science, 238,* 766–768.

Meaney, M. J., Mitchell, J. B., Aitkin, D. H, Bhatnagar, S., Bodnoff, S. R., Iny, L. J., and Sarrieu, A. (1991). The effects of neonatal handling on the development of the adrenocortical response to stress: Implications for neuropathology and cognitive deficits in later life. *Psychoneuroendocrinology, 16,* 85–103.

Milner, P. M. (1993). The mind and Donald O. Hebb. *Sci. Am., 268*(1), 124–129.

Mizumori, S. J. Y., Sakai, D. H., Rosenzweig, M. R,, Bennett, E. L., and Wittreich, P. (1987). Investigations into the neuropharmacological basis of temporal stages of memory formation in mice trained in an active avoidance task. *Behav. Brain Res., 23,* 239–250.

Mohammed, A. H., Henriksson, B. G., Soderstrom, S., Ebendal, T., Olsson, T., and Seckl, J. R. (1993). Environmental influences on the central nervous system and their implications for the aging rat. *Behav. Brain Res., 23,* 182–191.

Müller, G. E., and Pilzecker, A. (1900). Experimentelle Beiträge zur Lehre vom Gedächtnis [Experimental research on memory]. *Zeitschrift für Psychologie, Suppl.,* 1–288.

Murphy, C. C., Yeargin-Allsopp, M., Decouflé, P., and Drews, C. D. (1995). The administrative prevalence of mental retardation in 10-year-old children in metropolitan Atlanta, 1985 through 1987. *Am. J. Public Health, 85,* 319–323.

Ng, K. T., and Gibbs, M. E. (1991). Stages in memory formation: A review. In R. J. Andrew (ed.): *Neural and Behavioural Plasticity: The Use of the Domestic Chick as a Model.* Oxford, England: Oxford University Press, pp. 351–369.

Nyberg, L., Cabeza, R., and Tulving, E. (1996). PET studies of encoding and retrieval: The HERA model. *Psychonomic Bull. Rev., 3*(2), 135–148.

Olsson, T., Mohammed, A. H., Donaldson, L. F., Henriksson, B. G., and Seckl, J. R. (1994). Glucocorticoid receptor and NGFI-A gene expression are induced in the hippocampus after environmental enrichment in adult rats. *Mol. Brain Res., 23,* 349–353.

Pysh, J. J., and Weiss, M. (1979). Exercise during development induces an increase in Purkinje cell dendritic tree size. *Science, 206,* 230–232.

Renner, M. J., and Rosenzweig, M. R. (1987). *Enriched and Impoverished Environments: Effects on Brain and Behavior.* New York: Springer-Verlag

Riege, W. H. (1971). Environmental influences on brain and behavior of old rats. *Dev. Psychobiol., 4,* 157–167.

Rose, S. [P. R.]. (1992a). *The Making of Memory.* New York: Doubleday.

Rose, S. P. R. (1992b). On chicks and Rosetta stones. In L. R. Squire and N. Butters (eds.): *Neuropsychology of Memory,* 2nd ed. New York: Guilford, pp. 547–556.

Rosenzweig, M. R. (1964). Effects of heredity and environment on brain chemistry, brain anatomy and learning ability in the rat. In A. J. Edwards and J. F. Cawley (eds.): *Symposium on Physiological Determinates of Behavior: Implications for Mental Retardation. Kansas Stud. Educ., 14,* 3–34.

Rosenzweig, M. R. (1966). Environmental complexity, cerebral change, and behavior. *Am. Psychologist, 21,* 321–332.

Rosenzweig, M. R. (1971). Effects of environment on development of brain and of behavior. In E. Tobach, E. L. Aronson, and E. Shaw (eds.): *The Biopsychology of Development.* New York: Academic Press, pp. 303–342.

Rosenzweig, M. R. (1976). Effects of environment on brain and behavior in animals. In E. Schopler and R. J. Reichler (eds.): *Psychopathology and Child Development.* New York: Plenum Press, pp. 33–49.

Rosenzweig, M. R. (1980). Animal models for effects of brain lesions and for rehabilitation. In P. Bach-y-Rita (ed.): *Recovery of Function Following Brain Injury: Theoretical Considerations.* Bern, Switzerland: Hans Huber, pp. 127–172.

Rosenzweig, M. R. (1981). Neural bases of intelligence and training. *J. Spec. Educ., 15,* 106–123.

Rosenzweig, M. R. (1984). Experience, memory, and the brain. *Am. Psychologist, 39,* 365–376.

Rosenzweig, M. R. (1990). The chick as a model system for studying neural processes in learning and memory. In L. Erinoff (ed.): *Behavior as an Indicator of Neuropharmacological Events: Learning and Memory.* Washington, DC: NIDA Research Monographs, pp. 1–20.

Rosenzweig, M. R. (1996). Aspects of the search for neural mechanisms of memory. *Annu. Rev. Psychol., 47,* 1–32.

Rosenzweig, M. R., and Bennett, E. L. (eds.). (1976). *Neural Mechanisms of Learning and Memory.* Cambridge, MA: MIT Press.

Rosenzweig, M. R., and Bennett, E. L. (1980). How plastic is the nervous system? In B. Taylor and J. Ferguson (eds.): *A Comprehensive Handbook of Behavioral Medicine,* vol. 1. Jamaica, NY: Spectrum Publications, pp. 149–185.

Rosenzweig, M. R., and Bennett, E. L. (1996). Psychobiology of plasticity: Effects of training and experience on brain and behavior. *Behav. Brain Res., 78,* 57–65.

Rosenzweig, M. R., Bennett, E. L., and Alberti, M. (1984). Multiple effects of lesions on brain structure in young rats. In C. R. Almli and S. Finger (eds.): *The Behavioral Biology of Early Brain Damage, vol. 2. Neurobiology and Behavior.* New York: Academic Press, pp. 49–70.

Rosenzweig, M. R., Bennett, E. L., Colombo, P. J., Lee, D. W., and Serrano, P. A. (1993). Short-term, intermediate-term, and long-term memories. Special Issue: Alzheimer's disease: Animal models and clinical perspectives. *Behav. Brain Res., 57,* 193–198.

Rosenzweig, M. R., Bennett, E. L., and Diamond, M. C. (1967). Effects of differential environments on brain anatomy and brain chemistry. In J. Zubin and G. Jervis (eds.): *Psychopathology of Mental Development.* New York: Grune and Stratton, pp. 45–56.

Rosenzweig, M. R., Bennett, E. L., and Diamond, M. C. (1968). Modifying brain chemistry and anatomy by enrichment or impoverishment of experience. In G. Newton and S. Levine (eds.): *Early Experience and Behavior.* Springfield, IL: C. C. Thomas, pp. 258–298.

Rosenzweig, M. R., Bennett, E. L., and Diamond, M. C. (1972a). Chemical and anatomical plasticity of brain: Replications and extensions, 1970. In J. Gaito (ed.): *Macromolecules and Behavior,* 2nd ed. New York: Appleton-Century-Crofts, pp. 205–277.

Rosenzweig, M. R., Bennett, E. L., and Diamond, M. C. (1972b). Brain changes in response to experience. *Sci. Am., 226,* 22–29.

Rosenzweig, M. R., Bennett, E. L., Martinez, J. L., Colombo, P. J., Lee, D. W., and Serrano, P. A. (1992). Studying stages of memory formation with chicks. In L. R. Squire and N. Butters (eds.): *Neuropsychology of Memory,* 2nd ed. New York: Guilford, pp. 533–546.

Rosenzweig, M. R., Diamond, M. C., Bennett, E. L., and Mollgaard, K. (1972c). Negative as well as positive synaptic changes may store memory. *Psychol. Rev., 79,* 93–96.

Rosenzweig, M. R., Krech, D., and Bennett, E. L. (1958). Brain enzymes and adaptive behaviour. In *Ciba Foundation Symposium on Neurological Basis of Behaviour.* London: J., and A. Churchill, pp. 337–355.

Rosenzweig, M. R., Krech, D., and Bennett, E. L. (1961). Heredity, environment, brain biochemistry, and learning. In *Current Trends in Psychological Theory.* Pittsburgh: University of Pittsburgh Press, pp. 87–110.

Rosenzweig, M. R., Krech, D., and Bennett, E. L. (1963). Effects of differential experience on brain AChE and ChE and brain anatomy in the rat, as a function of stain and age. *Am. Psychologist, 18,* 430.

Rosenzweig, M. R., Krech, D., Bennett, E. L., and Diamond, M. C. (1962). Effects of environmental complexity and training on brain chemistry and anatomy: A replication and extension. *J. Comp. Physiol. Psychol., 55,* 429–437.

Rosenzweig, M. R., Leiman, A. L., and Breedlove, S. M. (1999). *Biological Psychology: An Introduction to Behavioral, Cognitive, and Clinical Neuroscience* (2nd ed.) Sunderland, MA: Sinauaer Associates.

Sapolsky, R. M. (1992). *Stress, the Aging Brain and Mechanisms of Neuronal Death.* Cambridge, MA: MIT Press.

Satcher, D. (1995). Annotation: The sociodemographic correlates of mental retardation. *Am. J. Public Health, 85,* 304–306.

Schaie, K. W. (1994). The course of adult intellectual development. *Am. Psychologist, 49,* 304–313.

Serrano, P. A., Beniston, D. S., Oxonian, M. G., Rodriguez, W. A., Rosenzweig, M. R., and Bennett, E. L. (1994). Differential effects of protein kinase inhibitors and activators on memory formation in the 2-day-old chick. *Behav. Neural Biol., 61,* 60–72.

Serrano, P. A., Rodriguez, W. A., Pope, B., Bennett, E. L., and Rosenzweig, M. R. (1995). Protein kinase C inhibitor chelerythrine disrupts memory formation in chicks. *Behav. Neurosci., 109,* 1–7.

Sherry, D. F., Vaccarino, A. L., Buckenham, K., and Herz, R. S. (1989). The hippocampal complex of food-storing birds. *Brain Behav. Evol., 34,* 308–317.

Shimamura, A., Berry, J. M., Mangels, J. A., Rusting, C. L., and Jurica, P. J. (1995). Memory and cognitive abilities in university professors: Evidence for successful aging. *Psychol. Sci., 6,* 271–277.

Sigman, M. (1995). Nutrition and child development. *Curr. Dir. Psychol. Sci., 4,* 52–55.

Silva, A. J., Stevens, C. F., Tonegawa, S., and Wang, Y. (1992). Deficient hippocampal long-term potentiation in alpha-calcium–calmodulin kinase II mutant mice. *Science, 257,* 201–206.

Sperry, R. W. (1951). Mechanisms of neural maturation. In S. S. Stevens (ed.): *Handbook of Experimental Psychology.* New York: Wiley, pp. 236–280.

Sperry, R. W. (1963). Chemoaffinity in the orderly growth of nerve fiber patterns and connections. *Proc. Natl. Acad. Sci. U.S.A., 50,* 703–710.

Swaab, D. F. (1991). Brain aging and Alzheimer's disease, "wear and tear" versus "use it or lose it." *Neurobiol. Aging, 12,* 317–324.

Tanzi, E. (1893). I fatti e le induzioni nell'odierna isologia del sistema nervoso. *Rev. Sper. Freniatria Med. Legale, 19,* 419–472.

Terry, R. D., Masliah, E., Salmon, D. P., Butters, N., DeTeresa, R., Hill, R., Hansen, L. A., and Katzman, R. (1991). Physical basis of cognitive alterations in Alzheimer's disease: Synapse loss is the major correlate of cognitive impairment. *Ann. Neurol., 30,* 572–580.

Teuber, H.-L. (1955). Physiological psychology. *Annu. Rev. Psychol., 6,* 267–296.

Tsien, J. Z., Chen, D. F., Gerber, D., Tom, C., Mercer, E. H., Anderson, D. J., Mayford, M., Kandel, E. R., and Tonegawa, S. (1996a). Subregion- and cell type-restricted gene knockout in mouse brain. *Cell, 87,* 1317–1326.

Tsien, J. Z., Huerta, P. T., and Tonegawa, S. (1996b). The essential role of hippocampal CA1 NMDA receptor-dependent synaptic plasticity in spatial memory. *Cell, 87,* 1327–1338.

Tulving, E. (1998). Brain/mind correlates of human memory. In M. Sabourin, F. Craik, and M. Robert (eds.): *Advances in Psychological Research, vol. 2, Biological and Cognitive Aspects.* Proceedings of the XXVI International Congress of Psychology. Hove, East Sussex: Psychology Press, pp. 441–480.

Turner, A. M., and Greenough, W. T. (1985). Differential rearing effects on rat visual cortex synapses. I. Synaptic and neuronal density and synapses per neuron. *Brain Res., 329,* 195–203.

Weinberger, N. M. (1995). Dynamic regulation of receptive fields and maps in the adult sensory cortex. *Annu. Rev. Neurosci., 18,* 1291–1358.

West, R. W., and Greenough, W. T. (1972). Effects of environmental complexity on cortical synapses of rats: Preliminary results. *Behav. Biol., 7,* 279–284.

Wiesel, T. N., and Hubel, D. H. (1963). Single-cell responses in striate cortex of kittens deprived of vision in one eye. *J. Neurophysiol., 26,* 1003–1017.

Wiesel, T. N., and Hubel, D. H. (1965). Comparison of the effects of unilateral and bilateral eye closure on cortical unit responses in kittens. *J. Neurophysiol., 28,* 1029–1040.

Will, B. E., Rosenzweig, M. R., Bennett, E. L., Hebert, M., and Morimoto, H. (1977). Relatively brief environmental enrichment aids recovery of learning capacity and alters brain measures after postweaning brain lesions in rats. *J. Comp. Physiol. Psychol., 91,* 33–50.

Yeargin-Allsopp, M., Drews, C. D., Decouflé, P., and Murphy, C. C. (1995). Mild mental retardation in black and white children in metropolitan Atlanta: A case–control study. *Am. J. Public Health, 85,* 324–328.

Zigler, E., and Muenchow, S. (1992). *Head Start: The Inside Story of America's Most Successful Educational Experiment.* New York: Basic Books.

Zolman, J. F., and Morimoto, H. (1962). Effects of age of training on cholinesterase activity in the brains of maze-bright rats. *J. Comp. Physiol. Psychol., 55,* 794–800.

3

Experience and Plasticity in Brain Structure: Possible Implications of Basic Research Findings for Developmental Disorders

WILLIAM T. GREENOUGH, JAMES E. BLACK,
ANNA KLINTSOVA, KATHY E. BATES,
AND IVAN JEANNE WEILER

This chapter reviews research on the effects of postnatal experience on the structure of the developing and adult brain. Because rare developmental disorders often occur with either genetic defects or prenatal neuropathology, we briefly discuss how early development establishes the foundation for neural plasticity systems and also influences the quality of experience utilized. The chapter then focuses on neural plasticity systems that appear predictably to incorporate aspects of experience into brain development or other systems that appear more individualized and not closely tied to development. Then we propose an integrative perspective of neural plasticity that moves beyond synapses to consideration of local tissue elements, cooperative neural circuits, and endocrine modulatory effects. We next describe a molecular process that may be involved in synaptic development and plasticity that appears to require the fragile X mental retardation protein (FMRP), the absence of which is associated with the fragile X mental retardation syndrome, a relatively rare (1:2,000) developmental disorder (Brown, 1996). Finally, we present an example of an experiential therapy for an acquired brain disorder, the effect of fetal alcohol exposure on the developing brain.

51

Structural and Functional Plasticity

Early brain development and neural plasticity systems

Although this volume focuses on neural plasticity, it is nonetheless important to acknowledge briefly the importance of developmental processes that are relatively *insensitive* to experience. As discussed below, such processes are probably central to interactions of neurodevelopmental disorders with neural plasticity during development. Genetically determined processes set up the structural framework in which neural plasticity systems operate, and at the molecular level many developmental processes appear similar to neural plasticity in later development. Our knowledge of these processes has expanded rapidly over the last decade, and we now know much of the molecular biology of neuron migration, cell differentiation, and neural regulation and signaling. In some circumstances, these genetically driven processes are capable of building enormously complex neural structures without any input from the external environment. Indeed, the basic organization of most nervous systems is impervious to experience to protect brain development from minor perturbations of pH or temperature, for example. Correspondingly, many species find it also adaptive for aspects of brain development to be insensitive to variations in postnatal nutrition or experience. Waddington (1971) termed such entrenchment (or resistance to environmental influences) during embryonic development *canalization*.

In contrast to canalization, some species have found considerable advantage in adapting their brains to their environment or incorporating information from it. Indeed, many mammalian species have evolved specialized brain structures that constrain and organize experiential information and sometimes can incorporate truly massive amounts of information (e.g., human language or graduate training in neuroscience). Because they have a long evolutionary history, the specialized plasticity systems vary across species and occur in multiple brain regions such that there is not a single "place" or "process" for neural plasticity. Although such plasticity systems may have many molecular components in common, their long phylogenetic history may have produced substantial diversity in their adaptive function, timing, and control.

From this perspective, human brain development results from complex interactions of gene-driven processes providing much of the basic structure of the brain, neural plasticity systems that are intrinsic components of the brain's developmental schedule, and other systems that have evolved to serve the individual's needs by incorporating information unique to its environment. Although for didactic purposes writers often resort to metaphors of "schedules" and "scaffolding," a more contemporary model of brain development is derived from the study of dynamic, nonlinear systems (Thelen and Smith, 1995; Boldrini et al., 1998). From the dynamic systems perspective, the interaction of genetic constraints and environmental information can self-organize highly complex systems (especially brains). Each organism follows a potentially unique and partly self-determined developmental path of brain assembly to the extent that they have unique experiences. Genetically determined restrictions (e.g., the initial cortical architecture) serve as constraints to the system, allowing environmental information interacting with existing neural structures to organize and refine neural connections.

Both canalization and neural plasticity processes can contribute directly to the behavioral and neural pathology of rare developmental disorders (Black et al., 1998). Genetic disorders or neuropathology can affect the starting point of canalized processes, resulting in brain development being dragged down a maladaptive path while remaining relatively impervious to any corrective experience or therapeutic interventions. In callosal agenesis, for example, early deviation results in the loss of nearly all interhemispheric connections with no realistic hope of their structural or functional restoration using these pathways (Lassonde et al., 1995). At another level, pathology in the structural foundation for neural plasticity systems can have a profound impact on how experience shapes the brain, as well as how later experience is incorporated. At yet another level, early stress or psychological trauma can have lasting effects on both brain and behavior (e.g., van der Kolk et al., 1996). Much of our therapeutic efforts to help restore brain development to a more adaptive path necessarily utilize the neural plasticity mechanisms we emphasize in this chapter.

Categories of neural plasticity

There is an extensive body of data relating to neuronal and synaptic plasticity during development and throughout the life span. There appear to be two basic mechanisms whereby the brain becomes organized by experience, which are described here using terms coined by Black and Greenough (1986). *Experience-expectant* brain information storage refers to a process in which the brain appears to ready itself to store relatively specific information at a specific time by overproducing synapses relative to the number that ultimately survive and "stabilizing" those that have been validated in some manner by function. For example, the developing visual system appears to extend geniculocortical axons from the two eyes to layer IV in an initially intermingled pattern and then subsequently to retract axons to yield the segregated projections of the eyes into the monocular "columns" of the adult (LeVay et al., 1980). The idea of synapse overproduction and selection, which has been evident in a number of studies of developing sensory systems (e.g., Cragg, 1975; Boothe et al., 1979; Huttenlocher and de Courten, 1987), will become important later in this chapter when we discuss the fragile X mental retardation syndrome. Studies that merely show a developmental increase and subsequent decrease in synapse *density* may or may not reflect equivalent processes because density changes in other tissue components, such as glial hypertrophy or hyperplasia, could generate the synapse density decreases that have been reported later in development (Huttenlocher and Dabholkar, 1997; Zecevic et al., 1989). *Experience-dependent* brain information storage describes a lifelong mechanism for incorporating effects of experience that appears to involve *de novo* formation of synapses and is discussed in more detail below.

Black and Greenough (1986) hypothesized that the *experience-expectant* mechanism was utilized largely for information that is reliably available in the environments of all normally reared members of a species such that the intrinsic developmental process can be enhanced by using externally originating information. If the externally originating information is abnormal, as in the absence of focused pattern vision in one or both eyes, the system incorporates this information, and development is abnormal (e.g., Mitchell et al., 1973). It seems likely that the overproduction and loss mechanism is even more pervasive in early development than has been previously believed. Our studies of mouse somatosensory cortex, for example, reveal that the overproduction and regression of dendrites during development is significantly masked in quantitative measures of the net amount of dendrite per neuron because growth and regression occur simultaneously on different parts of the same cell (Greenough and Chang, 1988; Greenough et al., 1998). Similarly, spine loss occurs in different temporal patterns on different parts of the dendritic field of the same neurons (Juraska, 1982). While evidence in humans can be interpreted to indicate that the ages over which these overproduction and loss processes are operative may vary widely across brain regions, with primary sensory regions completing the cycle largely within the first year or two and frontal association regions exhibiting protracted overproduction and regression across several years, these interpretations are based on synaptic density, as opposed to synapse number per neuron, and hence must be regarded with caution (Huttenlocher, 1990; Huttenlocher and Dabholkar, 1997). Interestingly, an area thought to be centrally involved in language production (but see Bates, Chapter 10) exhibits relatively protracted overproduction and loss. It may be that, even though the particular language is unique to the individual, the brain utilizes a generalized information capture mechanism to acquire aspects of it, as appears to be the case for phonemic perception and production (Kuhl, 1994; Werker and Tees, 1992). The prolonged development of human cortical development may reflect an adaptive characteristic that evolved to allow the (slow) incorporation of vast amounts of information (Bjorklund, 1997). Recently we have found evidence that the synthesis of FMRP at synapses may play a role in the synapse stabilization–elimination process; this is elaborated later in this chapter.

Experience-dependent plasticity

Experience-dependent plasticity is hypothesized to be involved in storing information unique to the individual member of the species. Unlike experience-expectant mechanisms, the time course of which appear to be heavily governed by intrinsic forces, experience-dependent information storage exhibits minimal age constraints beyond sequential dependencies (e.g., the need to learn letters before learning words). The model for the experience-dependent information storage process that has received the greatest attention in our laboratory is the complex or "enriched" environment paradigm also discussed by Rosenzweig (Chapter 2). Rats are reared from weaning to late adolescence or young adulthood in groups in large cages with a changing array of objects for play and exploration (EC rats). In various brain regions such as visual cortex, EC rats have larger neuronal dendritic fields (e.g., Volkmar and Greenough, 1972; Greenough and Volkmar, 1973; Juraska et al., 1980; Juraska, 1984) compared with rats reared individually (IC) or socially (SC) in standard laboratory cages without play objects. This result is paralleled by a greater number of synapses per neuron in EC rats than in SC and IC rats (e.g., Turner and Greenough, 1983, 1985).

Until recently, the only direct indication that these morphological differences arising from differential experience had any *functional* manifestations arose from behavioral measurements. There have been numerous indications, following the original report of pet-reared rats by Hebb (1949), that animals reared under relatively more enriched circumstances perform better than those housed in standard laboratory cages on a variety of complex, appetitively motivated tasks (e.g., Forgays and Read, 1962; Brown, 1968; Greenough, 1976; Greenough et al., 1973). These effects appear particularly pronounced in tasks involving spatial navigation and utilizing distal cues (Juraska et al., 1984; Brown, 1968), although other cognitive dimensions such as object perception appear to be affected as well (Thinus-Blanc, 1981). While this work clearly indicates the overall impact of the rearing environment on behavior, none of these studies really addresses the issue of the functional interpretation of particular brain measurements, such as the morphological alterations in the visual cortex, in a manner that allows possible attribution of the structural changes to processes such as information acquisition or learning.

We have begun to examine functional effects of complex environment rearing on visual cortex organization in rats using electrophysiological measures. The initial question is a simple but very important one: Does the physiological organization of the visual cortex of the EC rat reflect the structural differences it exhibits in comparison to the IC rat? A positive answer to this question would indicate that the differential experience did not merely bring into existence a set of nonfunctional or "silent" synapses but instead created "working" synapses of the sort that could represent added functional information. In one experiment, Wang (Greenough and Wang, 1993) recorded responses from layer II–III of visual cortex evoked by stimulation of lateral subcortical white matter that contained visual cortex afferents including the optic radiations from the lateral geniculate nucleus. The responses to these stimuli revealed two components, an apparent synaptic response (population EPSP) evoked exclusively at low stimulating currents and an apparent population spike (PS), the timing of which corresponded to individual cell firing, superimposed as a reverse inflection on the EPSP at higher stimulus intensities. When the responses for EC and IC rats were compared, the EC rats showed a greater population spike, indicating that more neurons were brought to threshold by the stimulus, as would be expected with a higher synapse number per neuron. This result, and comparable ones in other paradigms, indicates that the synapses that arise as a result of experience affect the functional organization of the brain region in which they occur.

An important issue is whether *learning* might trigger the formation of new synapses while a more general reflection of *neural activity* might regulate components potentially more relevant to activity level, such as the vasculature. To examine this, Black et al. (1990) exposed middle-aged rats to one of four conditions: an acrobatic condition (AC), in which animals were trained to perform complex visuomotor tasks, such as with rope ladders and balance beams, with relatively little physical exercise; a forced exercise (FX) condition in which rats had to exercise on a treadmill but had little to learn; a voluntary exercise (VX) condition in which rats could run freely in wheels and with little learning or stress; and an inactive condition (IC), living in standard laboratory caging with no opportunities for either learning or exercise. Morphological measures of the paramedian lobule of the cerebellum (an area associated with visuomotor activity) showed that the AC animals had substantially more synapses per Purkinje neuron than the other three groups. This indicates that learning of new visuomotor tasks caused synaptogenesis, in contrast to robust physiological activation of the same areas by exercise. Although repetitive, dull exercise had no apparent effect on synaptic connections, the substantial running done by the VX group increased the amount of capillaries, presumably to support increased neural activity. The AC animals also apparently added capillaries to compensate for the expanded cortical volume and dilution of existing vessels. Using the same animals, Anderson et al. (1994) compared the volume of astrocyte per Purkinje cell with the number of synapses per Purkinje cell and found a striking correlation across treatment groups with synapse numbers, suggesting that the increase in astrocytic processes was driven by synapse formation or synaptic activity.

Subsequently, Kleim et al. (1997) examined the persistence of both synaptic and astrocytic responses to 10 days of intense motor skill training in animals sacrificed immediately, animals that languished without training for a subsequent 4 weeks, and animals that continued training for the same 4-week period, in each case comparing AC rats to a yoked motor control (MC) condition in which rats walked in a closed alleyway and received a "prod" from the experimenter (usually a gentle squeeze of the hindquarters) each time it was necessary to do this to encourage the AC rat with which the MC was paired. (This was usually necessary only for the first few days of training.) The result for the number of synapses per Purkinje cell was clear-cut: Whether or not animals had continued training from day 11 to day 38 or not, the AC groups retained synapses to a degree statistically indistinguishable from the numbers seen in the 10-day, immediate sacrifice group (Fig. 3-1). That is, there was no statistical or apparent loss of cerebellar cortical synapses in the absence of continued training over a 4-week period. This result was paralleled by behavioral data: The latency to complete the obstacle course for the group that continued training over 4 weeks and those that were not trained over this period was statistically indistinguishable. Thus both the memory for the motor skill and the synapses that appear to subserve it persisted in the absence of continued training. In contrast, the glial response was significantly diminished after the 28-day hiatus from training (Kleim et al., 1999), while the animals that continued to train did not differ from those sacrificed after 10 days, suggesting that maintained activity of neurons and their synapses is necessary to maintain the full astrocytic response to training.

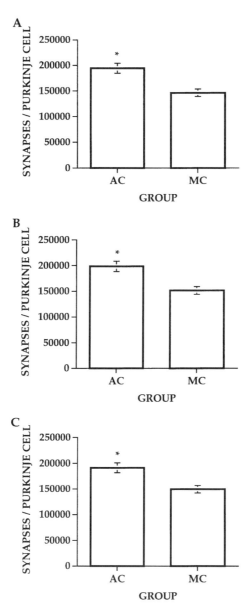

Figure 3-1. There is no decrement in the number of synapses per neuron compared with motor controls (MC) in the absence of additional motor skill training for 4 weeks following an initial training period of 10 days (AC, *B*) compared with a group examined immediately after 10 days' training (AC, *A*) or after 4 weeks' additional training (AC, *C*). Number of synapses per Purkinje cell (±SEM) within the paramedian lobule. Multiple comparisons (*Student-Newman-Keuls, *p* < 0.05) showed that the AC animals had significantly more synapses per Purkinje cell than the MC animals in the EARLY (*A*), DELAY (*B*), and CONTINUOUS (*C*) conditions.

An integrative perspective on neural plasticity

While much of our emphasis has been on changes in synaptic connectivity, it is important to emphasize that these changes occur in the context of other supporting and modulating tissue elements, as well as at more global levels of cooperative systems. This has particular pertinence with regard to neurodevelopmental disorders, as disruptions in these other elements (e.g., genetic lesions leading to mitochondrial encephalopathies; DiMauro and Schon, 1998) could substantially affect both brain structure and function, including neural plasticity systems. Our work has focused on experience-driven changes in two types of non-neural components that are associated with neural plasticity: vasculature and glia. If neural plasticity results in long-term increases in neural activity and metabolism, one would expect that the vasculature must be correspondingly altered to support it. Similarly, glia play important supportive and regulatory roles in neuron function (e.g., Anderson et al., 1994; Wenzel et al., 1991), so long-term structural changes in neuronal architecture should elicit associated structural changes in glia. Collectively, these components form an interdependent and interactive system, which might be called a "memory organ" to distinguish it from simple synaptic modifications, such that changes in one component are likely to affect the others in a homeostatic fashion.

When rats are provided with complex experience, the synaptic changes described above are associated with vascular changes. Early studies of vascular development in the brain had used animals raised in standard laboratory housing, and without exposure to complex experience it appeared that angiogenesis was completed before weaning age. An early study of EC rats reported that the increase in cortical thickness and the spreading apart of neuron cell bodies caused capillaries to be spread further apart (Diamond et al., 1964), but this study had substantial methodological problems (see Sirevaag et al., 1988, for further discussion). With better techniques (Black et al., 1987; Sirevaag et al., 1988), it became clear that young EC rats actually have closer spacing of capillaries in spite of the expanded cortical volume, clearly indicating that enough new capillaries had formed to actually improve the vascular support in this region. Parallel work suggested that the capacity for angiogenesis in response to cortical expansion was diminished in older EC animals (Black et al., 1989a), and such impairment could conceivably limit the brain's ability to build or maintain new synaptic connections. Correspondingly, syndromes that impair vascular development (and thus interfere with neural plasticity) could potentially disrupt a child's ability to benefit from experience.

The role of glia in neural plasticity has been relatively neglected until recently. Early reports of glial changes in EC rats had methodological problems (e.g., Altman and Das, 1964; Diamond et al., 1964, 1966; Szeligo and Leblond, 1977), but improved stereological methods demonstrated increased glia volume-to-neuron ratios in visual cortex (Sirevaag and Greenough, 1987), suggesting the production of new glial cells in association with new synapses. In addition, the nuclei of both the myelinating oligodendrocytes and astrocytes increased their proportion of cortical volume, suggesting an increase in functional activity. Stereological methods also allowed reliable determination that astrocytes first increased their average surface area in response to complex experience, then increased their numerical density (Sirevaag and Greenough, 1991). Suggestive of their direct role in neural plasticity, astrocytes wrap and cover substantially more of the surface of individual synapses after complex experience (Jones and Greenough, 1996). This relationship appears to be complex, however, as suggested by the finding of a close relationship between glial hypertrophy and synaptogenesis after EC in visual cortex layer II–III with a looser coupling in layer IV (Jones et al., 1996). Because the glial population is strikingly diverse in structure and function, it is likely that a wide variety of glial disorders could have both direct and indirect effects on neural plasticity.

Another aspect of our motor skill training paradigm is also of interest. A parallel study of *motor* cerebral cortex by Kleim et al. (1996) indicated a pattern of response to training, in terms of the number of synapses per neuron, comparable with that seen in cerebellar paramedian lobule by Black et al. (1990) and Kleim et al. (1997). This suggests a distributed representation of the motor skill across brain regions, possibly with the cerebral cortex playing roles in fine motor movements and the cerebellar cortex orchestrating general body movement patterns in accordance (Brodal, 1975; Hrycyshyn et al., 1982; Kunzle, 1975; Santori et al., 1986; Sharp and Ryan, 1984). Thus, at a global level, multiple neural plasticity systems appear to work cooperatively to store information. Although laboratory paradigms can sometimes isolate one memory system, real-world learning and memory are likely to involve multiple systems working together, as suggested by the finding of brain changes after complex experience in multiple cerebral cortical regions, hippocampus, basal ganglia, and cerebellum (see Black and Greenough, 1998, for review).

An integrative perspective is also suggested by numerous findings that the animal's hormonal milieu can strongly influence brain development and neural plasticity processes (McEwen, 1997). Growth and thyroid hormones have complex interactions and a strong influence on brain development (Bernal and Nunez, 1995; Noguchi, 1996). Sex differences in neural responses to complex experience are presumably modulated by sex hormones (Juraska, 1984). Surprisingly, young rats placed in EC have *retarded* somatic development in a number of organ systems (Black et al., 1989b). Collectively these data reflect the capacity of endocrine factors, most of which do not directly act on the synapse, to affect neural plasticity.

A concept that helps to integrate this broad pattern of multiple brain responses to experience is that of *brain adaptation*. Simplistically put, the role of the brain is to adapt itself so as to maximize the organism's fitness in its environment, a process that will likely involve multiple systems working at multiple levels. Although there is still an enormous amount of research to do at the synaptic level, the adaptations of other tissue components and more global systems that allow neurons to function efficiently may be equally important. Collectively, all of these findings support an integrated perspective on neural plasticity, moving beyond synaptic connections to consideration of local tissue support, cooperative regional networks, and diffuse modulation by endocrine factors.

Links to Fragile X Mental Retardation

In the course of studying structural responses to complex environment exposure, Greenough et al. (1985) found increased numbers of polyribosomal aggregates, the entities that synthesize protein, in spines of EC compared with IC and SC rats. This supported the hypothesis that protein synthesis at synapses might be involved in synaptogenesis in development and in plastic synaptic change (Steward and Levy, 1982; Steward and Falk, 1986), and it prompted a series of experiments directed at understanding synaptic protein synthesis. These experiments have shown that synthesis of protein in an *in vitro* synaptoneurosome preparation is regulated by activation of metabotropic receptors for the neurotransmitter glutamate and that a cascade involving receptor-coupled phospholipase C and subsequent activation of protein kinase C leads to local protein synthesis at the synapse (Weiler and Greenough, 1991, 1993; Weiler et al., 1996). Of particular interest is that one of the proteins whose synthesis appears to be stimulated via this pathway is the FMRP (Weiler et al., 1997) (see Fig. 3-2).

The specific function(s) of FMRP are unknown. Individuals who cannot produce the protein, due to an elongated triplet repeat that leads to hypermethylation of a 5′ CpG island and thus impedes gene transcription (Fu et al., 1991; Oberle et al., 1991), exhibit moderate to severe mental retardation (Hagerman and Cronister, 1996), as does a unique patient with a structural mutation in the RNA-binding domain of the protein (DeBoulle et al., 1993). The protein has three domains that bind to mRNA and to ribosomes and is associated with polyribosomal aggregates (Corbin et al., 1997), suggesting that it may influence the translation of other pro-

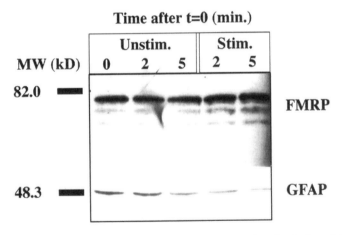

Figure 3-2. Western blot of protein from synaptoneurosomes lysed at indicated intervals (minutes) after $t = 0$, either untreated (control) or stimulated by 10^{-4} M DHPG. (*Upper*) Staining by anti-FMRP showing increases in bands of fragile X mental retardation protein (FMRP) in the stimulated groups over time (rightmost 2 lanes). (*Lower*) Same blot restained with anti-GFAP as a control protein that should not change across time.

teins, or even its own, as it binds its own mRNA (Ashley et al., 1993). It has also been speculated that FMRP may regulate transport of mRNA from nuclear to cytoplasmic locations, as it contains both nuclear localization (NLS) and nuclear export signal amino acid sequences (Eberhart et al., 1996). In our own work using electron microscopic immunocytochemistry, the appearance of immunoreactivity in neuronal nuclei is relatively rare, while it is present at some synapses in the postsynaptic spine (but rarely in axonal terminals), in dendrites, and in neuronal somata (Weiler et al., 1997).

Indications of the possible functions of FMRP have also come from autopsy studies of fragile X patient brain tissue and from our work on a new FMR-1 knockout mouse recently produced by Oostra, Willems, and their colleagues (see Consortium, 1994). Hinton et al. (1991) and, earlier, Rudelli et al. (1985) reported a higher than normal number of thin, tortuously shaped, long postsynaptic spines on cortical neurons of patients. In electron microscopy, these spines exhibited immature-appearing synapses. In the knockout mice, we (Comery et al., 1997) initially observed longer, thinner spines compared with wild type, but subsequently learned that the FVB strain containing the knockout carried a retinal degeneration mutation (Farber, 1995) that could also have affected the spines we studied, which were in the visual cortex. A replication of that work using mice with wild-type retinae has now repeated these findings. In both replications, however, we have noted that the density of spines on pyramidal cell apical dendrites was *higher* in the knockout mice. This, combined with the apparent immaturity of synapses, led us to propose that FMRP may be necessary for the normal developmental processes of synapse maturation and elimination discussed above. That is, the overproduction and loss of connections often associated with what was called *experience-expectant plasticity* above may be impaired in the fragile X mental retardation syndrome because there is an impairment of the ability for some synapses to become mature and stable while others disappear in the course of experience-guided development. If so, the fragile X child might have a "noisy" brain that has not acquired the fine patterning normally available through daily experience. Sensory, motor, emotional, social, and cognitive systems might all be affected if this failure to acquire fine structural organization were a general property of brain systems. The sensitivity to intense or multiple stimuli and the occasionally seen susceptibility to seizures might similarly reflect an excess of excitatory synapses in various brain regions. Developmental deficits might be evident at early ages in abilities that appear to be shaped by experience early in development, such as phonemic perception (e.g., Kuhl, 1994) and cortical visual ability (e.g., Banks et al., 1975).

Experiential Therapy for a Developmental Disorder

Fetal alcohol syndrome (FAS), the more severe consequence of prenatal alcohol exposure, manifests with characteristic facial abnormalities, growth deficiency, and CNS impairment (Jones and Smith, 1975; Abel, 1996; Harris et al., 1993; Buljan et al., 1996). Alcohol-related neurodevelopmental disorder (ARND, or "fetal alcohol effect") constitutes a milder disorder without evident facial malformation, with less evident developmental delays (sometimes detected only in follow-up studies), and less severe mental retardation and neurobehavioral impairment (Stratton et al., 1996). The ARND diagnosis can be made only if maternal drinking during pregnancy is confirmed. Both in the human disorder (Mattson and Riley, 1996; Mattson et al., 1996; Sowell et al., 1996) and in animal models (e.g., Bauer-Moffett and Altman, 1977; Davies and Smith, 1981; Barnes and Walker, 1981; West et al., 1984; Hannigan, 1996) there is a gross brain tissue loss, along with neuronal and synaptic loss, the location varying with the period of exposure to alcohol. Third trimester human exposure to binge drinking, which may result in childhood motor deficits and deficient fine motor control (Hanson et al., 1978; Streissguth et al., 1978, 1991; Conry, 1990; Autti-Ramo and Granstrom, 1991; Jacobson et al., 1993) is modeled by neonatal exposure (PD 4–9) of rats to high peak blood alcohol concentrations, which is associated with motor deficits and cerebellar cortical cell loss (Meyer et al., 1990; Goodlett et al., 1991; Goodlett and Lundhal, 1996).

Both animal and human studies have suggested that human infants exposed *in utero* to alcohol may be resistant to some kinds of behaviorally based therapeutic interventions. Some literature on humans (e.g., Streissguth et al., 1991; Streissguth and Kanter, 1997) has emphasized the importance of structuring the environment of the FAS/ARND child to maximize the influence of extrinsic protective factors (living in a stable and nurturant home, in nonalcoholic families) and to minimize the effects of risk factors (such as abuse or neglect). These interventions are expected to diminish the lifelong problems that can be significantly more severe in FAS/ARND patients than would be expected solely on the basis of their mental retardation or delayed development (Streissguth et al., 1996). At the present time the concept of a demanding, challenging intervention appears not to have been applied successfully at the human level with FAS/ARND children. In animal models, exposure to interventions such as a complex environment or early handling has been shown to have ameliorative effects at the level of behavioral assessment (Osborne et al., 1980; Hannigan et al., 1993; Wainwright et al., 1993). Behavioral recovery may be more sensitive to intervention after low doses of alcohol and become more resistant when the alcohol level to which the prenatal or neonatal animal is exposed is increased (Osbourne et al., 1980). The failure to find brain effects of a complex environment in alcohol-exposed rats compared with controls has led to the suggestion that fetal alcohol-exposed animals may be relatively more resistant to interventive approaches (Berman et al., 1996; Wainwright et al., 1993) or that the response to intervention in ethanol-exposed animals is significantly decreased and delayed in comparison with controls (West et al., 1990; Berman et al., 1996). If so, this may occur because the alcohol-induced damage impedes full interaction with the intervention. Issues pertaining to intervention studies in humans are discussed by Landry (Chapter 14).

We used the acrobatic motor skill learning procedure described above as an adult therapeutic intervention focusing on the symptoms of impaired motor skills in neonatally alcohol-exposed rats (Klintsova et al., 1997, 1998). We reasoned that the weak brain effect in the complex environment animal studies could result from the fact that these environments can allow alcohol-exposed subjects to minimize or avoid challenging interactions with the environment. Motor skill learning, by contrast, *forced involvement* of our animal subjects in the program of therapy and *focused on one critically affected domain* of alcohol impairment—motor performance.

In this study, alcohol was delivered in two consecutive feedings 2 hours apart, a model of binge-like maternal drinking through implanted intragastric cannulae to alcohol-exposed rats. Both alcohol-exposed rats and gastrostomy controls fed isocaloric carbohydrate were artificially reared in individual warmed styrofoam cups from days 4 to 9 postnatal. The other 10 feedings per day were milk formulae. A separate suckling control was also used to assess effects of the artificial rearing procedure. Peak blood alcohol concentrations of approximately 260 mg/dl were achieved, which has been previously associated with substantial cerebellar cortical Purkinje cell loss (Goodlett and West, 1992; West et al., 1989). In an initial study, the effects of 10 days of intense acrobatic motor skill learning rehabilitation compared with inactive individual cage housing on cerebellar cortical morphology were assessed in alcohol-exposed, gastrostomy controls, and suckling control rats at 6 months of age. Significant increases in the numbers of synapses per Purkinje cell were evident in the alcohol-exposed and suckling control groups, while the gastrostomy control group did not exhibit a significant synaptic response to this therapy (Klintsova et al., 1997). In a subsequent behavioral study, we increased the duration of the motor skill training to 20 days and added a motor control group that merely walked a continuous course in a closed alleyway in response to experimenter encouragement to control for the effects of handling. On three tests of motor performance, ability to walk on parallel bars, ability to climb a rope to a platform, and ability to traverse a rotating drum, female alcohol-exposed rats were improved by rehabilitative intervention to levels of performance nearly comparable to suckling and gastrostomy rats given equivalent rehabilitative intervention training (see Fig. 3-1), and male alcohol-exposed rats demonstrated significant improvement after rehabilitation on the parallel bar test, whereas performances on the rotating rod test and on rope climbing were negatively influenced by the excessive body weight of the 7-month-old male rats. In general, there was a clear behavioral effect of this forced intervention. Current studies are underway to evaluate the effects of this 20-day period of intervention on the brain.

The results of this series of studies suggest that a program of intervention that challenges the alcohol-exposed subjects by forcing them to become involved in the procedure may have therapeutic efficacy, at least in this highly controlled animal model. It should be noted that this program focused on the specific domain of motor performance and may not reflect the kind of gains that can be obtained through conceptually similar interventions in other performance domains (e.g., language or emotional regulation). Nonetheless, we feel that the implications of these findings should be given serious consideration in the design of experimental interventions in the human syndrome.

Summary and Conclusions

We have illustrated here some of the ways in which a program of basic research can have meaningful impact at the clinical or preclinical levels with regard to developmental disorders. It is of interest that, in addition to the apparent synaptic role of the FMRP described here, other previously poorly understood developmental syndromes involving delay or retardation have been recently tied to mutations affecting specific signaling and other pathways within nerve cells (e.g., Petrij et al., 1995). This sort of finding seems likely to recur with increasing frequency as we better understand the molecular and cellular bases of brain information storage.

We have also drawn attention to the concept of "brain adaptation," which stresses the multifaceted nature of brain plasticity, involving not just neurons and their interconnections but also the networks of vasculature and of glia supporting neuronal function. The roles of these components deserve increasing attention in understanding of and rehabilitative efforts with regard to rare developmental disorders.

Finally, we have presented an example of active, challenging experiential therapy in the treatment of an animal model for alcohol-induced brain damage during the third trimester of pregnancy. Together these provide a range of examples of how basic research can address problems from the level of causation to the level of rehabilitation of rare developmental disorders.

References

Preparation of this chapter and recent work described herein was supported by grants MH35321, AG10154, and AA09838, the Retirement Research Foundation; the FRAXA Research Foundation; the Iowa/Illinois Kiwanis Spastic Paralysis and Allied Diseases of the Central Nervous System Research Foundation; and the National Association for Research in Schizophrenia and Affective Disorders.

Abel, E. A. (ed.) (1996). *Fetal Alcohol Syndrome: From Mechanism to Prevention.* Boca Raton, FL: CRC Press, Inc.

Altman, J., and Das, G. D. (1964). Autoradiographic examination of the effects of enriched environment on the rate of glial multiplication in the adult rat brain. *Nature, 204,* 1161–1163.

Anderson, B. J., Li, X., Alcantara, A. A., Isaacs, K. R., Black, J. E., and Greenough, W. T. (1994). Glial hypertrophy is associated with synaptogenesis following motor-skill learning, but not with angiogenesis following exercise. *GLIA, 11,* 73–80.

Ashley, C. T., Wilkinson, K. D., Reines, D., et al. (1993). FMR1 protein: Conserved RNP family domains and selective RNA binding. *Science, 262,* 563–566.

Autti-Ramo, I., and Granstrom, M. L. (1991). The effect of intrauterine alcohol exposition in various durations on early cognitive development. *Neuropediatrics, 22,* 203–210.

Banks, M. S., Aslin, R. N., and Letson, R. D. (1975). Sensitive period for the development of human binocular vision. *Science, 190,* 675–677.

Barnes, D. E., and Walker, D. W. (1981). Prenatal ethanol exposure permanently reduces the number of pyramidal neurons in the hippocampus. *Dev. Brain Res., 1,* 333–340.

Bauer-Moffet, C., and Altman, J. (1977). The effect of ethanol chronically administered to preweanling rats on cerebellar development: A morphological study. *Brain Res., 119,* 249–268.

Berman, R. F., Hannigan, J. H., Sperry, M. A., and Zajac, C. S. (1996). Prenatal alcohol exposure and the effects of environmental enrichment on hippocampal dendritic spine density. *Alcohol Int. Biomed. J., 13,* 209–216.

Bernal, J., and Nunez, F. (1995). Thyroid hormones and brain development. *Eur. J. Endocrinol., 133,* 390–398.

Bjorklund, D. F. (1997). The role of immaturity in human development. *Psychol. Bull., 122,* 153–169.

Black, J. E., and Greenough, W. T. (1986). Induction of pattern in neural structure by experience: Implications for cognitive development. In Lamb, M. E., Brown, A. L., and Rogoff, B. (eds.): *Advances in Developmental Psychology,* vol. 4. Hillsdale, NJ: Lawrence Earlbaum Assoc., pp. 1–50.

Black, J. E., and Greenough, W. T. (1998). Developmental approaches to the memory process. In J. L. Martinez and R. P. Kesner (eds.): *Learning and Memory: A Biological View,* 3rd ed. New York: Academic Press, pp. 55–88.

Black, J. E., Isaacs, K. R., Anderson, B. J., Alcantara, A. A., and Greenough, W. T. (1990). Learning causes synaptogenesis, whereas motor activity causes angiogenesis, in cerebellar cortex of adult rats. *Proc. Natl. Acad. Sci. U.S.A., 87,* 5568–5572.

Black, J. E., Jones, T. A., Nelson, C. A., and Greenough, W. T. (1998). Neural plasticity. In N. Alessi (ed.): *The Handbook of Child and Adolescent Psychiatry, vol. IV, Varieties of Development* (Section I, Developmental Neuroscience). New York: John Wiley and Sons, pp. 31–53.

Black, J. E., Polinsky, M., and Greenough, W. T. (1989a). Progressive failure of cerebral angiogenesis supporting neural plasticity in aging rats. *Neurobiol. Aging, 10,* 353–358.

Black, J. E., Sirevaag, A. M., and Greenough, W. T. (1987). Complex experience promotes capillary formation in young rat visual cortex. *Neurosci. Lett., 83,* 351–355.

Black, J. E., Sirevaag, A. M., Wallace, C. S., Savin, M., and Greenough, W. T. (1989b). Effects of complex experience on somatic growth and organ development in rats. *Dev. Psychobiol., 22,* 727–752.

Boldrini, M., Placidi, G. P. A., and Marazziti, D. (1998). Applications of chaos theories to psychiatry: A review and future perspectives. *CNS Spectrum, 3,* 22–29.

Boothe, R. G., Greenough, W. T., Lund, J. S., et al. (1979). A quantitative investigation of spine and dendrite development of neurons in the visual cortex (area 17) of *Macaca nemestrina* monkeys. *J. Comp. Neurol., 186,* 473–490.

Brodal, P. (1975). Demonstration of somatotopically organized projection onto the paramedial lobule and the anterior lobe from the lateral reticular nucleus: An experimental study with the horseradish peroxidase method. *Br. Res., 95,* 221–239.

Brown, R. T. (1968). Early experience and problem solving ability. *J. Comp. Physiol. Psychol., 65,* 433–440.

Brown, W. T. (1996). The FRAXE syndrome: Is it time for routine screening? *Am. J. Hum. Genet., 58,* 903–905.

Buljan, D., Thaller, V., and Breitenfeld, D. (1996). Fetal alcohol syndrome: Influence of alcohol on the fetuses of alcoholic mothers. *Alcoholism J Alcoholism Rel Addictions, 32,* 69–78.

Comery, T. A., Harris, J. B., Willems, P. J., Oostra, B. A., Irwin, S. A., Weiler, I. J., and Greenough, W. T. (1997). Abnormal dendritic spines in fragile-X knockout mice: Maturation and pruning deficits. *Proc. Natl. Acad. Sci. U.S.A., 94,* 5401–5404.

Conry, J. (1990). Neuropsychological deficits in fetal alcohol syndrome and fetal alcohol effects. *Alcoholism Clin. Exp. Res. 14*, 650–655.

Consortium, D.-B. F. X. (1994). FMR1 knockout mice: A model to study fragile X mental retardation. *Cell, 7,* 23–33.

Corbin, F., Bouillon, M., Fortin, A., Morin, S., Rousseau, F., and Khandjian, E. W. (1997). The fragile X mental retardation protein is associated with poly(A)+ mRNA in actively translating polyribosomes. *Hum. Mol. Genet., 6,* 1465–1472.

Cragg, B. G. (1975). The development of synapses in the visual system of the cat. *J. Comp. Neurol., 160,* 147–166.

Davies, D. L., and Smith, D. E. (1981). A Golgi study of mouse hippocampal CA1 pyramidal neurons following perinatal ethanol exposure. *Neurosci. Lett., 26,* 49–54.

De Boulle, K., Verker, A. J. M. H., Reyniers, E., et al. (1993). A point mutation in the FMR-1 gene associated with fragile X mental retardation. *Nature Genet., 3,* 31–35.

Diamond, M. C., Krech, D., and Rosenzweig, M. R. (1964). The effects of enriched environment on the histology of the rat cerebral cortex. *J. Comp. Neurol., 123,* 111–120.

Diamond, M. C., Law, F., Rhodes, H., Lindner, B., Rosenzweig, M. R., Krech, D., and Bennett, E. L. (1966). Increases in cortical depth and glial numbers in rats subjected to enriched environment. *J. Comp. Neurol., 128,* 117–126.

DiMauro, S., and Schon, E. A. (1998). Mitochondrial DNA and disease of the nervous system: The spectrum. *Neuroscientist, 4,* 53–63.

Eberhart, D. E., Malter, H. E., Feng, Y., and Warren, S. T. (1996). The fragile X mental retardation protein is a ribonucleoprotein containing both nuclear localization and nuclear export signals. *Hum. Mol. Genet., 5,* 1083–1092.

Farber, D. B. (1995). From mice to men: The cyclic GMP phosphodiesterase gene in vision and disease. *Invest. Ophthalmol. Vis. Sci., 36,* 263–275.

Forgays, D. G., and Read, J. M. (1962). Crucial periods for free-environmental experience in the rat. *J. Comp. Physiol. Psychol., 55,* 816–818.

Fu, Y. H., Kuhl, D. P. A., Pizzuti, A., et al. (1991). Variation of the CGG repeat at the fragile X site results in genetic instability: Resolution of the Sherman paradox. *Cell, 67,* 1047–1058.

Goodlett, C. R., and Lundahl, K. R. (1996). Temporal determinants of neonatal alcohol-induced cerebellar damage and motor performance deficits. *Pharmacol. Biochem. Behav., 55,* 531–540.

Goodlett, C. R., Thomas, J. D., and West, J. R. (1991). Long-term deficits in cerebellar growth and rotarod performance of rats following "binge-like" alcohol exposure during the neonatal brain growth spurt. *Neurotoxicol. Teratol., 13,* 69–74.

Goodlett, C. R., and West, J. R. (1992). Fetal alcohol effects: Rat model of alcohol exposure during the brain growth spurt. In I. S. Zagon and T. Slotkin (eds.): *Maternal Substantial Abuse and the Developing Nervous System.* New York: Academic Press, pp. 45–75.

Greenough, W. T., and Chang, F.-L. F. (1988). Plasticity of synapse structure and pattern in the cerebral cortex. In E. G. Jones and A. Peters (eds.): *Cerebral Cortex,* vol. 7. New York: Plenum, pp. 391–440.

Greenough, W. T., Comery, T. A., Irwin, S. I., Black, J. E., and Weiler, I. J. (1999). Discussion: Synapse stabilization and fragile X protein synthesis in the rodent brain. In D. M. Hann et al. (eds): *Advancing Research on Developmental Plasticity: Integrating the Behavioral Science and Neuroscience of Mental Health.* (DHHS Publication No. NIH 98-xxxx). Washington DC: U.S. Government Printing Office, in press.

Greenough, W. T., Hwang, H.-M., and Gorman, C. (1985). Evidence for active synapse formation, or altered postsynaptic metabolism, in visual cortex of rats reared in complex environments. *Proc. Natl. Acad. Sci., 82,* 4549–4552.

Greenough, W. T., and Volkmar, F. R. (1973). Pattern of dendritic branching in rat occipital cortex after rearing in complex environments. *Exp. Neurol., 40,* 491–504.

Greenough, W. T., and Wang, X. (1993). Altered post-synaptic response in the visual cortex in vivo of rats reared in complex environments. *Society for Neuroscience Abstracts, 69,* 11, 19, 164.

Greenough, W. T., Yuwiler, A., and Dollinger, M. (1973). Effects of post-trial eserine administration on learning in "enriched" and "impoverished" reared rats. *Behav. Biol., 8,* 261–272.

Hagerman, R. J., and Cronister, A. (eds). (1996). *Fragile X Syndrome: Diagnosis, Treatment, and Research.* Baltimore: Johns Hopkins University Press.

Hannigan, J. H. (1996). What research with animals is telling us about alcohol-related neurodevelopmental disorder. *Pharmacol. Biochem. Behav., 55,* 489–499.

Hannigan, J. H., Berman, R. F., and Zajac, C. S. (1993). Environmental enrichment and the behavioral effects of prenatal exposure to alcohol in rats. *Neurotoxicol. Teratol., 15,* 261–266.

Hanson, J. W., Streissguth, A. P., and Smith, D. W. (1978). The effects of moderate alcohol consumption during pregnancy on fetal growth and morphogenesis. *J. Pediatr., 92,* 457–460.

Harris, S. I. R., Osborn, J. A., Weinberg, J., Loock, C., and Junaid, K. (1993). Effects of prenatal alcohol exposure on neuromotor and cognitive development during early childhood: A series of case reports. *Phys. Ther., 73,* 608–617.

Hebb, D. O. (1949). *The Organization of Behavior.* New York: Wiley.

Hinton, V. J., Brown, W. T., Wisniewski, K., and Rudelli, R. D. (1991). Analysis of neocortex in three males with the fragile X syndrome. *Am. J. Med. Genet., 41,* 289–294.

Hrycyshyn, A. W., Flumerfelt, B. A., and Anderson, W. A. (1982). A horseradish peroxidase study of the projections from the lateral reticular nucleus to the cerebellum in the rat. *Anat. Embryol., 165,* 1–18.

Huttenlocher, P. R. (1990). Morphometric study of human cerebral cortex development. *Neuropsychologia, 28,* 517–527.

Huttenlocher, P. R., and Dabholkar, A. S. (1997). Regional differences in synaptogenesis in human cerebral cortex. *J. Comp. Neurol., 387,* 167–178.

Huttenlocher, P. R., and de Courten, C. (1987). The development of synapses in striate cortex of man. *Hum. Neurobiol., 6,* 1–9.

Jacobson, S. W., Jacobson, J. L., Sokol, R. J., Martier, S. S., and Ager, J. W. (1993). Prenatal alcohol exposure and infant information processing ability. *Child Dev., 64,* 1706–1721.

Jones, T. A., and Greenough, W. T. (1996). Ultrastructural evidence for increased contact between astrocytes and synapses in rats reared in a complex environment. *Neurobiol. Learn. Mem., 65,* 48–56.

Jones, T. A., Hawrylak, N., and Greenough, W. T. (1996). Rapid laminar-dependent changes in GFAP immunoreactive astrocytes in the visual cortex of rats reared in a complex environment. *Psychoneuroendocrinology, 21,* 189–201.

Jones, K. L., and Smith, D. W. (1975). The fetal alcohol syndrome. *Teratology, 12,* 1.

Juraska, J. (1982). The development of pyramidal neurons after eye opening in the visual cortex of hooded rats: A quantitative study. *J. Comp. Neurol., 212,* 208–213.

Juraska, J. (1984). Sex differences in dendritic response to differential experience in the rat visual cortex. *Brain Res., 295,* 27–34.

Juraska, J. M., Greenough, W. T., Elliott, C., Mack, K. J., and Berkowitz, R. (1980). Plasticity in adult rat visual cortex: An examination of several cell populations after differential rearing. *Behav. Neurol. Biol., 29,* 157–167.

Juraska, J. M., Henderson, C., and Muller, J. (1984). Differential rearing experience, gender, and radial maze performance. *Dev. Psychobiol., 17,* 209–215.

Kleim, J. A., Lussnig, E., Schwarz, E. R., Comery, T. A., and Greenough, W. T. (1996). Synaptogenesis and Fos expression in the motor cortex of the adult rat following motor skill learning. *J. Neurosci., 16,* 4529–4535.

Kleim, J. A., Vij, K., Ballard, D. H., and Greenough, W. T. (1997). Learning dependent synaptic modifications in the cerebellar cortex of the adult rat persist for at least four weeks. *J. Neurosci., 17,* 717–721.

Kleim, J. A., Vij, K., Kelly, J. L., Ballard, D. H., and Greenough, W. T. (1999). The persistence of training-induced astrocytic hypertrophy within the cerebellar cortex. In revision.

Klintsova, A. Y., Cowell, R. M., Swain, R. A, Napper, R. M. A., Goodlett, C. R., and Greenough, W. T. (1998). Therapeutic effect of complex motor skill learning on neonatal alcohol-induced motor performance deficits: I. Behavioral results. *Brain Research, 800,* 48–61.

Klintsova, A. Y., Matthews, J. T., Goodlett, C. R., Napper, R. M. A., and Greenough, W. T. (1997). Therapeutic motor training increases parallel fiber synapse number per Purkinje neuron in cerebellar cortex of rats given postnatal binge alcohol exposure: Preliminary report. *Alcoholism Clin. Exp. Res., 21,* 1257–1263.

Kuhl, P. K. (1994). Learning and representation in speech and language. *Curr. Opin. Neurobiol., 4,* 812–822.

Kunzle, H. (1975). Autoradiographic tracing of the cerebellar projections from the lateral reticular nucleus in the cat. *Exp. Br. Res., 38,* 125–135.

Lassonde, M., Lepore, F., and Sauerwein, H. C. (1995). Extent and limits of callosal plasticity: Presence of disconnection syndromes in callosal agenesis. *Neuropsychology, 33,* 989–1007.

LeVay, S, Wiesel, T. N., and Hubel, D. H. (1980). The development of ocular dominanace columns in normal and visually deprived monkeys. *J. Comp. Neurol., 191,* 1–51.

Mattson, S. N., and Riley, E. P. (1996). Brain anomalies in fetal alcohol syndrome. In E. L. Abel (ed.), *Fetal Alcohol Syndrome: From Mechanism to Prevention.* Boca Raton, FL: CRC Press, pp. 51–68.

Mattson, S. N., Riley, E. P., Sowell, E. R., Jernigan, T. L., Sobel, D. F., and Jones, K. L. (1996). A decrease in the size of the basal ganglia of children with fetal alcohol syndrome. *Alcoholism Clin. Clin. Res., 20,* 1088–1093.

McEwen, B. S. (1997). Hormones as regulators of brain development: Lifelong effects related to health and disease. *Acta Pediatr. Suppl., 422,* 41–44.

Meyer, L. S., Kotch, L. E., and Riley, E. P. (1990). Alterations in gait following ethanol exposure during the brain growth spurt in rats. *Alcoholism Clin. Exp. Res., 14,* 23–27.

Mitchell, D. E., Freeman, R. D., Millodot, M., and Haegerstrom, G. (1973). Meridional amblyopia: Evidence for modification of the human visual system by early visual experience. *Vision Res., 13,* 535–558.

Noguchi, T. (1996). Effects of growth hormone on cerebral development: Morphological studies. *Hormone Res., 45,* 5–17.

Oberle, I., Rousseau, F., Heitz, D., et al. (1991). Instability of a 550-base pair DNA segment and abnormal methylation in fragile X syndrome. *Science, 252,* 1097–1102.

Osborne, G. L., Caul, W. F., and Fernandez, K. (1980). Behavioural effects of prenatal ethanol exposure and differential early experience in rats. *Pharmacol. Biochem. Behav.,* *12,* 393–401.

Petrij, F., Giles, R. H., Dauwerse, H. G., Saris, J. J., Hennekam, R. C. M., Masuno, M., Tommerup, N., et al. (1995). Rubenstein-Taybi syndrome caused by mutations in the transcriptional co-activator CBP. *Nature, 376,* 348–351.

Rudelli, R. D., Brown, W. T., Wisniewski, K., et al. (1985). Adult fragile X syndrome. Cliniconeuropathologic findings. *Acta Neuropathol. (Berl.), 67,* 289–295.

Santori, E. M., Der, T., and Collins, R. C. (1986). Functional metabolic mapping during forelimb movement in rat. II. Stimulation of forelimb muscles. *J. Neurosci., 6,* 463–474.

Sharp, F. R., and Ryan, A. F. (1984). Regional (14C) 2-deoxyglucose uptake during forelimb movements evoked by rat motor cortex stimulation: Pons, cerebellum, medulla, spinal cord, muscle. *J. Comp. Neurol., 224,* 286–306.

Sirevaag, A. M., Black, J. E., Shafron, D., and Greenough, W. T. (1988). Direct evidence that complex experience increases capillary branching and surface area in visual cortex of young rats. *Dev. Brain Res., 43,* 299–304.

Sirevaag, A. M., and Greenough, W. T. (1987). Differential rearing effects on rat visual cortex synapses. III. Neuronal and glial nuclei, boutons, dendrites, and capillaries. *Brain Res., 424,* 320–332.

Sirevaag, A. M., and Greenough, W. T. (1991). Plasticity of GFAP-immunoreactive astrocyte size and number in visual cortex of rats reared in complex environments. *Brain Res., 540,* 273–278.

Sowell, E. R., Jernigan, T. L., Mattson, S. N., Riley, E. P., Sobel, D. F., and Jones, K. L. (1996). Abnormal development of the cerebellar vermis in children prenatally exposed to alcohol: Size reduction in lobules I–V. *Alcoholism Clin. Exp. Res., 20,* 31–34.

Steward, O., and Falk, P. (1986). Protein-synaptic machinery at postsynaptic sites during synaptogenesis: A quantitative study of the association between polyribosomes and developing synapses. *J. Neurosci., 6,* 412–423.

Steward, O., and Levy, W. (1982). Preferential localization of polyribosomes under the base of dendritic spines in granule cells of the dentate gyrus. *J. Neurosci., 2,* 284–291.

Stratton, K., Howe, C., and Battaglia, F. (eds.). (1996). *Fetal Alcohol Syndrome: Diagnosis, Epidemiology, Prevention, and Treatment.* Washington, D. C.: National Academy Press.

Streissguth, A. P., Aasi, J. M., Clarren, S. K., Randels, S. P., LaDue, R. A., and Smith, D. F. (1991). Fetal alcohol syndrome in adolescents and adults. *JAMA, 265,* 1961–1967.

Streissguth, A. P., Bookstein, F. L., and Barr, H. M. (1996). Dose–response study of enduring effects of prenatal alcohol exposure: Birth to 14 years. In H. L. Spohr and H. C. Steinhausen (eds.): *Alcohol, Pregnancy and the Developing Child.* Cambridge: England, pp. 141–168.

Streissguth, A. P., Herman, C. S., and Smith, D. W. (1978). Intelligence, behavior and dysmorphogenesis in the fetal alcohol syndrome: A report on 20 patients. *J. Pediatr., 92,* 363–367.

Streissguth, A. P., and Kanter, J. W. (eds.). (1997). *Selected Papers From: Overcoming and Preventing Secondary Disabilities in FAS and FAE.* Seattle: University of Washington Press.

Szeligo, F., and Leblond, C. P. (1977). Response of the three main types of glial cells of cortex and corpus callosum in rats handled during suckling or exposed to enriched, control and impoverished environments following weaning. *J. Comp. Neurol., 172,* 247–263.

Thelen, E., and Smith, A. (1995). *A Dynamic Systems Approach to the Development of Cognition and Action.* Cambridge, MA: MIT Press.

Thinus-Blanc, C. (1981). Volume discrimination learning in golden hamsters: Effects of the structure of complex rearing cages. *Dev. Psychobiol., 14,* 397–403.

Turner, A. M., and Greenough, W. T. (1983). Synapses per neuron and synaptic dimensions in occipital cortex of rats reared in complex, social, or isolation housing. *Acta Stereol., 2(suppl. 1),* 239–244.

Turner, A. M., and Greenough, W. T. (1985). Differential rearing effects on rat visual cortex synapses. I. Synaptic and neuronal density and synapses per neuron. *Brain Res., 329,* 195–203.

van der Kolk, B. A., McFarlane, A. C., and Weisaeth (eds.). (1996). *Traumatic Stress: The Effects of Overwhelming Experience on Mind, Body, and Society.* New York: Guilford Press.

Volkmar, F. R., and Greenough, W. T. (1972). Rearing complexity affects branching of dendrites in the visual cortex of the rat. *Science, 176,* 1445–1447.

Wainwright, P. E., Levesque, S., Krempulec, L., Bulman-Fleming, B., and McCutcheon, D. (1993). Effects of environmental enrichment on cortical depth and Morris-Maze performance in B6D2F2 mice exposed prenatally to ethanol. *Neurotoxicol. Teratol., 15,* 11–20.

Weiler, I. J., Childers, W. S., and Greenough, W. T. (1996). Calcium ion impedes translation initiation at the synapses. *J. Neurochem., 66,* 197–202.

Weiler, I. J., and Greenough, W. T. (1991). Potassium ion stimulation triggers protein translation in synaptoneurosomal polyribosomes. *Mol. Cell. Neurosci., 2,* 305–314.

Weiler, I. J., and Greenough, W. T. (1993). Metabotropic glutamate receptors trigger postsynaptic protein synthesis. *Proc. Natl. Acad. Sci. U.S.A., 90,* 7168–7171.

Weiler, I. J., Irwin, S. A., Klintsova, A. Y., Spencer, C. M., Brazelton, A. D., Miyashiro, K., Comery, T. A., Patel, B., Eberwine, J., and Greenough, W. T. (1997). Fragile-X mental retardation protein is translated near synapses in response to neurotransmitter activation. *Proc. Natl. Acad. Sci. U.S.A., 94,* 5395–5400.

Wenzel, J., Lammert, G., Meyer, U., and Krug, M. (1991). The influence of long-term potentiation on the spatial relationship between astrocytic processes and potentiated synapses in the dentate gyrus neuropil of the rat brain. *Brain Res., 560,* 122–131.

Werker, J. F., and Tees, R. C. (1992). The organization and reorganization of human speech perception. *Annu. Rev. Neurosci., 15,* 377–402.

West, J. R., Goodlett, C. R., Bonthius, G. D. J., and Pierce, D. R. (1989). Manipulating peak blood alcohol concentrations in neonatal rats: Review of an animal model for alcohol-related developmental effects. *Neurotoxicology, 10,* 347–366.

West, J. R., Goodlett, C. R., and Brandt, J. P. (1990). New approaches to research on the long-term consequences of prenatal exposure to alcohol. *Alcohol Clin. Exp. Res., 14,* 684–689.

West, J. R., Hamre, K., and Pierce, D. R. (1984). Delay in brain growth induced by alcohol in artificially reared rat pups. *Alcohol, 1,* 213–222.

Zecevic, N., Rakic, P., and Bourgeois, J. P. (1989). Changes in synaptic density in motor cortex of rhesus monkey during fetal and postnatal life. *Dev. Brain Res., 50,* 11–32.

II

MECHANISMS OF
REORGANIZATION

4

Structural Changes Underlying Long-Term Memory

CRAIG H. BAILEY

Recent studies of the biological basis of learning and memory, in both higher invertebrates and vertebrates, have demonstrated that aspects of long-term memory storage are associated with altered gene expression, new protein synthesis, and the growth of synaptic connections (for review, see Bailey et al., 1996). Such changes also appear to accompany the *de novo* synapse formation that occurs during development and in the adult brain could reflect the recruitment, by environmental stimuli, of developmental processes that are latent or inhibited in the fully differentiated neuron. The ability to study learning and memory at the cellular and molecular levels now makes it possible to examine the degree to which the central nervous system may utilize a similar set of cell biological mechanisms to achieve learning-related plasticity in the mature animal as it does for the reorganization of synaptic connections during the later stages of development.

In this brief review I consider possible relationships between the mechanisms that may underlie the structural changes expressed during both memory storage and neuronal development by focusing on studies of the synaptic growth that is associated with long-term sensitization in the marine mollusk *Aplysia californica*.

Structural Organization of the Synapse in *Aplysia*

A synaptic contact in *Aplysia* consists of a single presynaptic component, which is usually an irregularly shaped varicose expansion occurring along or at the end of a fine neurite, and a single postsynaptic element, which is typically a small diameter spine (Bailey et al., 1979). The functional architecture of these sites is similar to the synaptic morphology described in other higher invertebrates as well as in the vertebrate central nervous system.

As is the case in other species, only a restricted portion of the contact in *Aplysia* appears to be specialized for synaptic transmission (Fig. 4-1). These focal and

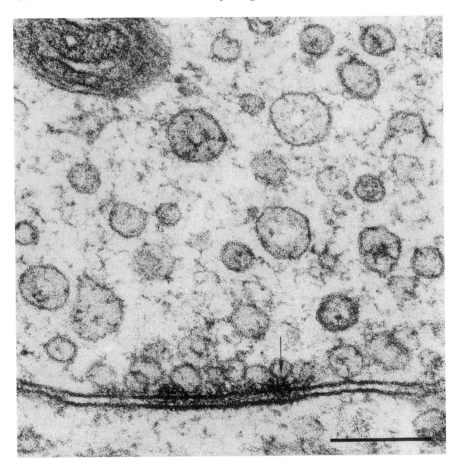

Figure 4-1. Structure of the central nervous system synapse in *Aplysia*: organization of the presynaptic active zone. The active zone at *Aplysia* synapses is characterized by rigidly parallel pre- and postsynaptic membranes bounding a widened synaptic cleft containing electron-dense material. Within the presynaptic terminal small lucent vesicles preferentially cluster at these specialized sites and are often found in close association with condensed filamentous material (dense projections, arrow) that appears to arise from the cytoplasmic leaflet of the presynaptic membrane. Bar = 0.25 μm. (From Bailey et al., 1981.)

modified regions appear analogous to the active zones described at other central synapses and consist of a presynaptic secretory component, which is thought to participate in the translocation of vesicles prior to their fusion and subsequent exocytotic release, and a postsynaptic recognition component, which is modified for the reception and transduction of this chemical information (Couteaux and Pecot-Dechavassine, 1970; Heuser et al., 1979).

    The organization of the axoplasm contiguous to the presynaptic active zone is replete with fine-diameter filaments and small electron-lucent synaptic vesicles. In fact, the number of vesicles at these specialized sites is roughly 12 times greater than at unspecialized regions of the synaptolemma. Clumps of electron-dense fib-rillar material can be found adherent to the cytoplasmic leaflets of both the pre- and postsynaptic membrane. These paramembranous components of the active zone can be isolated and studied in detail by the application of a variety of selec-tive cytochemical stains (Bailey et al., 1981; Bloom and Aghajanian, 1968). When such approaches are utilized, the presynaptic specialization at *Aplysia* synapses can be seen to consist of a series of small, truncated, dense projections that prob-ably represent a condensed form of the filamentous material that is present near the active zone membrane in conventionally fixed material. Rapid freezing and shallow freeze-etch studies of central synapses in the mammalian brain suggest that this filamentous mesh work in the vicinity of the presynaptic active zone may serve to concentrate vesicles and perhaps modulate their availability for exocytot-ic release (Landis et al., 1988). In contrast, the postsynaptic specialization at *Aplysia* synapses is typically more modest and consists of a thin, fairly continuous sheet-like density.

Based on these cytochemical and ultrastructural studies, synaptic connections in *Aplysia* appear to have clearly differentiated, discrete active zones similar to those described in other species. Our next goal was to determine what effect, if any, learning and memory might have on the structure of these specialized trans-mitter release sites.

Long-Term Sensitization in *Aplysia*: A Simple Behavioral Model for Studying Molecular and Structural Mechanisms Underlying Memory Storage

One of the major surprises in the modern study of behavior has been the realization that learning and memory are probably universal features of the nervous system (Thorpe, 1956). In recent years, this realization has encouraged the use of several higher invertebrate preparations where the advantages of a tractable central nervous system and identified neurons have facilitated the study of learning and memory at the cellular and molecular levels (Kandel, 1976; Kandel and Schwartz, 1982; Alkon, 1984; Carew and Sahley, 1986; Byrne, 1987; Bailey and Kandel, 1993).

One such model system has been the gill- and siphon-withdrawal reflex of *Aplysia*. This reflex is analogous to vertebrate defensive escape and withdrawal reflexes and like them can be modified by a variety of nonassociative and asso-ciative forms of learning. One elementary form of nonassociative learning exhib-ited by this reflex is sensitization.* Sensitization is a process by which an animal

*Behavioral sensitization of the gill- and siphon-withdrawal reflex in *Aplysia* is quantitatively assessed by comparing the duration of gill or siphon withdrawal elicited by brief jets of seawater delivered to the siphon both before and 24 hours after sensitization training. Sensitization training trials consist of electric stimuli delivered to another site such as the neck or tail. Following sensitization training, the responsiveness of the reflex to previously neutral stimuli is enhanced. This strengthening of the reflex is characterized by significantly longer siphon withdrawal times compared with each animal's own pre-training score as well as to control animals that received no shocks (for a more detailed explanation of experimental protocol, see Pinsker et al., 1970, 1973; Frost et al., 1985).

learns about the properties of a novel, usually noxious stimulus. Through it an animal learns to strengthen its defensive reflexes and to respond vigorously to what was previously a neutral or indifferent stimulus. In both invertebrates and vertebrates, sensitization can exist in both a short-term form and a long-term form. The duration of the memory is dependent on the number of training trials; that is, the memory is graded. In *Aplysia,* for example, a single training trial produces short-term sensitization that lasts from minutes to hours (Pinsker et al., 1970). Repeated training trials can produce a long-term memory that persists for at least several weeks (Pinsker et al., 1973; Frost et al., 1985).

Among the great advantages of the invertebrate brain for the cellular analysis of behavior and its modification is a greatly reduced cell number and the presence of large, invariant, identified nerve cells. In *Aplysia,* certain elementary behaviors that can be modified by learning may use fewer than 100 cells. This neural parsimony makes it possible to delineate in detail the wiring diagram of the behavior and thus pinpoint the contribution of individual nerve cells to the behavior in which they participate.

Exploiting this reductionist approach, Eric Kandel and his colleagues have analyzed the neuronal circuits responsible for sensitization of the gill- and siphon-withdrawal reflex (Kandel, 1976). Short- and long-term sensitization lead to enhanced synaptic transmission at the monosynaptic connection between identified mechanoreceptor sensory neurons and their follower cells. Although this component accounts for only part of the behavioral modification measured in the intact animal, its simplicity has facilitated the cellular and molecular analysis of both the short- and long-term forms of sensitization. For example, this monosynaptic pathway can be reconstituted in dissociated cell culture (Rayport and Schacher, 1986; Montarolo et al., 1986) by serotonin (5-HT), a modulatory neurotransmitter normally released by sensitizing stimuli in the intact animal. In parallel to behavioral sensitization, a single application of 5-HT produces short-term changes in synaptic effectiveness, whereas four or five applications of 5-HT over a period of 1.5 hours (or continuous application of 5-HT for 1.5–2 hours) produces long-term changes lasting one or more days (Montarolo et al., 1986). These findings of an elementary cellular representation of the short- and long-term memory for sensitization has allowed the mechanisms underlying each form to be addressed directly. Biophysical and biochemical studies of this monosynaptic connection suggest that both the similarities and differences in memory reflect, at least in part, intrinsic cellular mechanisms of the nerve cells participating in memory storage. Thus, studies of the connections between sensory and motor neurons in both the intact animal and in cells in culture indicate that the short- and long-term changes share aspects of a common mechanism. Both processes are initiated by 5-HT, and a component of the increase in synaptic strength observed during both short- and long-term facilitation (Frost et al., 1985; Montarolo et al., 1986) is due to an enhancement in transmitter release by the sensory neuron. This presynaptic increase in excitability is attributable to the spike broadening that results from the modulation by 5-HT of potassium currents (Dale et al., 1987; Klein and Kandel, 1980; Hochner et al., 1986; Scholz and Byrne, 1987).

Despite these similarities, the short-term cellular changes differ from the long-term modifications in two important ways. First, the short-term change involves only covalent modification of preexisting proteins and an alteration of preexisting connections. Both short-term behavioral sensitization in the animal and short-term facilitation in dissociated cell culture do not require ongoing macromolecular synthesis and are not blocked by inhibitors of transcription or translation (Montarolo et al., 1981; Schwartz et al., 1971). In contrast, these inhibitors selectively block the induction of the long-term changes both in the semi-intact animal (Castellucci et al., 1989) and in primary cell culture (Montarolo et al., 1986).

Second, as detailed below, the long-term but not the short-term process involves a structural change. Bailey and Chen (1983, 1988a,b, 1989) have demonstrated that long-term sensitization is associated with the growth of new synaptic connections by the sensory neurons onto their follower cells. Similar changes can be reconstituted in sensorimotor co-cultures by repeated presentations of the modulatory neurotransmitter 5-HT (Glanzman et al., 1990; Bailey et al., 1992b).

The finding that long-term memory involves structural remodeling and requires new macromolecular synthesis raises the following questions: How closely do the cellular and molecular changes recruited for learning-related structural plasticity in the mature animal resemble the activity-dependent fine tuning of synaptic connections that characterize the initial construction of the nervous system? Are a common set of molecules and mechanisms shared between memory storage and development?

In this chapter, I address these issues by examining the nature, extent, and time course of structural changes at sensory neuron synapses that accompany long-term sensitization in *Aplysia*. I then consider the subcellular and molecular mechanisms that might give rise to this learning-related synaptic growth. Since structural changes appear to be one of the key signatures of the long-term process throughout the animal kingdom, principles derived from this reductionist approach may be applicable to more complex systems and ultimately to human memory.

Morphological Basis of Long-Term Sensitization in *Aplysia*

An increasing body of anatomical data, emanating originally from studies on mammalian development, and more recently embodying results from studies on nonmammalian vertebrates and higher invertebrates, suggests that long-term memory resembles a process of neuronal growth and differentiation (for reviews, see Greenough, 1984; Greenough and Bailey, 1988; Bailey and Kandel, 1993).

In *Aplysia,* Bailey and Chen first demonstrated that long-term behavioral sensitization is associated with significant structural plasticity. By combining selective intracellular labeling techniques with complete serial reconstructions, they have shown that the memory for long-term sensitization is accompanied by a family of alterations at identified sensory neuron synapses. These changes reflect structurally detectable modifications at two different levels of synaptic organization: *(1)* alterations in focal regions of membrane specialization of the synapse (the

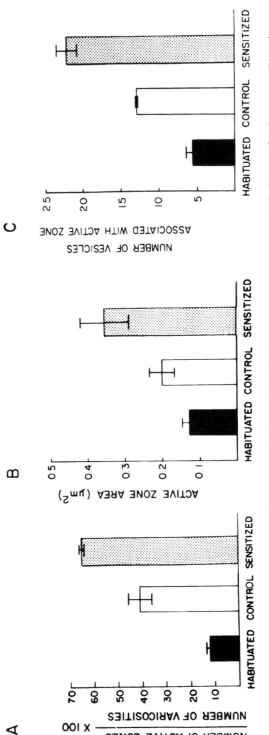

Figure 4-2. Effects of long-term memory on active zone morphology at identified sensory neuron synapses. (A) Incidence of active zones. (B) Active zone area. (C) Vesicle complement. Each bar represents the mean score of two animals ±SEM in each behavioral group (data from Bailey and Chen, 1983). (From Bailey and Kandel, 1985.)

number, size, and vesicle complement of sensory neuron active zones are larger in sensitized animals than in control animals) (Fig. 4-2) (Bailey and Chen, 1983, 1988b) and *(2)* a parallel but more pronounced and widespread effect involving modulation of the total number of presynaptic varicosities per sensory neuron (Bailey and Chen, 1988a). Sensory neurons from long-term sensitized animals exhibited a twofold increase in the total number of synaptic varicosities as well as an enlargement in the size of each neuron's axonal arbor within the neuropil (Fig. 4-3).

The increase in the number of sensory neuron varicosities and the enlarged neuropil arbor observed after behavioral training for long-term sensitization can also be induced in the intact ganglion by intracellular injection of adenosine $3'5'$-cyclic phosphate (cAMP) (Nazif et al., 1991) and can be reconstituted in dissociated sensorimotor neuron co-cultures by the repeated presentation of 5-HT that evokes long-term facilitation (Glanzman et al., 1990; Bailey et al., 1992b). In culture, this increase can be correlated with long-term (24-hour) enhancement of the amplitude of the sensory-to-motor neuron synaptic potential and depends on the presence of an appropriate target cell, similar to the synapse formation that occurs during development (Glanzman et al., 1989).

Transient and Enduring Components of the Structural Change

As a first step in examining the mechanisms that might give rise to the growth of new synaptic connections during long-term sensitization, Bailey and Chen (1989) compared the time courses of each class of structural changes with the behavioral duration of the memory. Such a temporal analysis is important because it can not only serve as a framework for bringing the structural changes into register with the behavioral and physiological components of long-term sensitization but may also provide useful insights into the underlying cellular and molecular events responsible for learning-related synaptic remodeling at different stages of the long-term process. For example, this approach allows one to distinguish between transient and more permanent effects and thereby determine which class of structural changes at the synapse might underlie long-term memory rather than being a stage in its development or a by-product of its formation. By examining the morphology of sensory neuron synapses at 1–2 days, 1 week, and 3 weeks after the completion of behavioral training, these researchers found that not all the structural changes persisted as long as the memory. The increased size and vesicle complement of sensory neuron active zones present 24 hours after the completion of training were found to have returned to control levels when tested 1 week later. These data indicate that, insofar as modulation of active zone size and associated vesicles is one of the mechanisms underlying long-term sensitization, it may represent only a transient structural component of the increased synaptic responsiveness underlying the long-term process. In contrast, the duration of changes in varicosity and active zone number, which persisted unchanged for at least 1 week and were only partially reversed at the end of 3 weeks, endured in parallel with

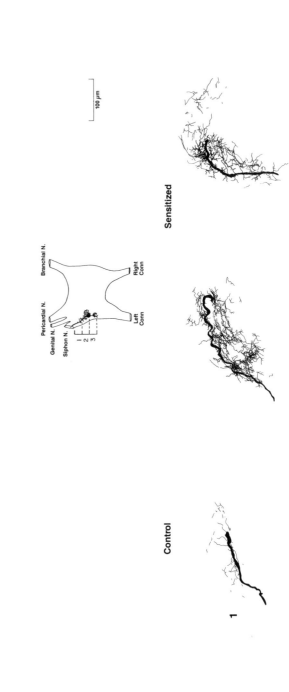

100 μm

Pericardial N.   Branchial N.

Genital N.

Siphon N.

1
2
3

Left
Conn

Right
Conn

Control

Sensitized

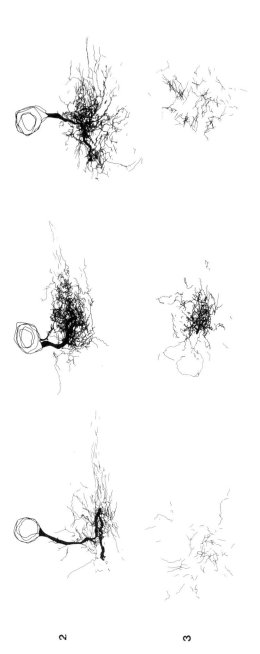

2

3

Figure 4-3. Effects of long-term sensitization on the neuritic arbor of sensory neurons. Represented are complete serial reconstructions of identified sensory neurons taken from long-term sensitized and untrained, control animals. In each case the rostral (*row 3*) to caudal (*row 1*) extent of the arbor is divided roughly into thirds. Each panel was produced by the superimposition of camera lucida tracings of all horseradish peroxidase (HRP)–labeled processes present in 17 consecutive slab-thick sections and represents a linear segment through the ganglion of roughly 340 μm. For each composite, ventral is up, dorsal is down, lateral is to the left, and medial is to the right. By examining images across each row (*rows 1, 2, and 3*), the viewer is comparing similar regions of each sensory neuron. In all cases, the arbor of long-term sensitized cells is markedly increased compared with control. Siphon N., Genital N., and so forth, are various peripheral nerves of the abdominal ganglion; Left and Right Conn are left and right connectives, fiber tracts connecting the abdominal ganglion with other ganglia. (From Bailey and Chen, 1988a.)

the behavioral time course of memory, suggesting that only the increases in the number of sensory neuron synapses contribute to the maintenance of long-term sensitization.

In addition to characterizing the structural changes that contribute to the onset and maintenance of long-term sensitization, the work of Bailey and Chen indicates that the decay of these changes during the process of forgetting, the period during which reflex strength returns to baseline levels, is paralleled by a reduction of similar magnitude in the number of sensory neuron synapses. These findings support the idea that the stability of long-term memory storage may be achieved, in part, because of the relative stability of synaptic structure, and suggest that the structural change may represent the final, perhaps most persistent phase of the long-term process.

The finding that some components of the changes in synaptic architecture are transient while others endure suggests that not all of these modifications are regulated synchronously. At the structural level, the sensory neuron appears to have multiple mechanisms and parameters of plasticity available to it. Thus, during the later phases of long-term memory storage for sensitization, although there are now more synapses, each individual synapse may recruit all of the mechanisms of plasticity that were present before training. The neurons have passed from an initial pretrained state, through a transient growth state induced by training, to a new baseline state in which long-term sensitization has been established and maintained. At this new baseline the neuron again has multiple mechanisms of plasticity, and new parameters of plasticity have been established.

Subcellular and Molecular Mechanisms Underlying the Learning-Related Growth of New Synaptic Connections in *Aplysia*

To explore further the specific molecules and mechanisms that may contribute to the growth process that accompanies long-term facilitation in *Aplysia*, Barzilai et al. (1989) examined changes in the expression of specific gene products induced by 5-HT. By focusing on the 1–1.5 hour period of training and studying the incorporation of labeled amino acids into proteins in the sensory neurons, they found that 5-HT produces three temporally discrete sets of changes in specific proteins that could be resolved on two-dimensional gels. First, 5-HT induces a rapid and transient increase at 30 minutes in the rate of synthesis of 10 proteins and a transient decrease in 5 proteins that subside within 1 hour and are in all cases dependent on transcription. These early changes are followed by at least two further rounds of changes in the expression of specific proteins, some of which are transient and some of which persist for at least 24 hours. The 15 early proteins induced by repeated exposure to 5-HT can also be induced by cAMP. These features—rapid induction, transcriptional dependence, and cAMP mediation—suggest the possibility that this control might involve a gene cascade, whereby early regulatory proteins activate later effector genes. The early proteins induced by 5-HT and cAMP during the acquisition phase of long-term facilitation in *Aplysia* may, therefore, resemble the immediate-early gene products induced in vertebrate cells by growth factors.

A comprehensive series of studies by Kandel and his colleagues has demonstrated that long-term facilitation is mediated by the activation of cAMP-responsive genes. Repeated presentations of 5-HT to sensorimotor co-cultures produce a long-term enhancement in transmitter release that lasts for 1 or more days and requires for its induction both translation and transcription (Montarolo et al., 1986). Injection of cAMP into sensory neurons can induce long-term facilitation (Scholz and Byrne, 1987; Schacher et al., 1988), and inhibitors of protein kinase A (PKA) block long-term facilitation (Ghirardi et al., 1992), suggesting that the long-term enhancement of the transmitter release requires cAMP-mediated gene activation. Consistent with this idea, Dash et al. (1990) demonstrated that injection of an oligonucleotide containing the cAMP-responsive element (CRE) into sensory neurons selectively blocked long-term facilitation, suggesting that the long-term process requires the recruitment of one or more cAMP-inducible genes via the CRE and CRE-like binding proteins (CREBS). Kaang et al. (1993) have further shown that the 5-HT–activated transcription is achieved through the PKA-mediated phosphorylation of CREB on Ser[119], suggesting that the phosphorylation of CREB-like proteins and the consequent activation of transcription represents a key component of the molecular switch for extending the short-term process, which is independent of protein synthesis, into the long-term process, which requires gene expression.

What genes are important for the induction of long-term facilitation? To address this question, Alberini et al. (1994) cloned and studied the *Aplysia* homologue of the mammalian family of CCAAT enhancer-binding protein (C/EBP) transcription factors. They have found that the *Aplysia* C/EBP (ApC/EBP) has a CRE in its upstream region and has the properties of an immediate-early gene. Moreover, blocking the expression of the gene selectively blocks long-term facilitation without affecting short-term facilitation. These experiments demonstrate a role for immediate-early genes in learning-related synaptic plasticity and suggest that the activation of C/EBP, and perhaps other immediate-early genes, may account for the critical time window of long-term facilitation, as well as for the induction of its maintenance phase. According to this scheme, Kandel and colleagues have suggested that long-term facilitation requires constitutively expressed transcription factors—perhaps including CRE-binding proteins that activate immediate early genes, one of which has been shown to be ApC/EBP that then acts on effector genes. Once the early phase is induced, the expression of late target genes may then contribute to the structural changes that appear to be required for the stabilization phase of long-term facilitation.

Modulation of Cell Adhesion Molecules and Induction of the Structural Change

What is the role of gene activation in the growth of new sensory neuron synapses that is a signature of long-term facilitation in *Aplysia*? How are these new synaptic connections formed? A series of studies has begun to explore the roles of early proteins in the induction of the structural change by attempting to characterize and identify each of the 15 proteins that Barzilai et al. (1989) observed to be specifically altered in expression during the acquisition of long-term facilitation. Six have now been identified. Surprisingly, the two proteins that increase (clathrin and tubulin) and the four proteins that decrease their level of expression (NCAM-related cell adhesion molecules) all seem to relate to structural changes.

Mayford et al. (1992) focused on the four proteins (D1–D4) that decrease their expression following the application of 5-HT or cAMP. Cloning and sequencing their cDNAs indicate they encode different isoforms of an immunoglobulin-related cell adhesion molecule, designated *Aplysia* cell adhesion molecule (apCAM), which shows greatest homology to neuronal cell adhesion molecules (NCAMs) in vertebrates and fasciclin II in *Drosophila*. Imaging of fluorescently labeled monoclonal antibodies bound to apCAM shows that a percentage of these cell adhesion molecules is lost from the surface membrane of the sensory neurons within 1 hour after the addition of 5-HT. This transient down-regulation of cell adhesion molecules induced by 5-HT may represent an early molecular step of learning-related synaptic growth. For example, blocking the surface expression of apCAM with monoclonal antibodies causes defasciculation, a process that may precede the formation of synapses during development in *Aplysia* (Glanzman et al., 1989; Keller and Schacher, 1990).

Findings in other invertebrate systems and in the mammalian brain have strengthened the idea that cell adhesion molecules may play a role in various forms of synaptic modification (reviewed by Doherty et al., 1995; Fields and Itoh, 1996; Martin and Kandel, 1996). For example, in *Drosophila,* down-regulation of the cell adhesion molecule fasciclin II is both necessary and sufficient for activity-dependent presynaptic outgrowth at the postembryonic nerve–muscle synapse (Davis et al., 1996; Schuster et al., 1996a, b). These studies in *Aplysia* and *Drosophila* suggest that down-regulation may be a general mechanism underlying the modulation of cell adhesion molecules during physiological forms of synaptic plasticity and growth and raise two important and interrelated questions: *(1)* What are the subcellular and molecular mechanisms that lead to the down-regulation of adhesion molecules, and *(2)* how does this down-regulation signal synaptic growth?

To examine the mechanisms by which 5-HT modulates apCAM, and the significance this modulation might have for the structural changes that are induced by 5-HT, Bailey et al. (1992a) combined thin-section electron microscopy with immunolabeling using a gold-conjugated monoclonal antibody specific to apCAM. They found that a 1-hour application of 5-HT led to a 50% decrease in the density of gold-labeled apCAM complexes at the surface membrane of the sensory neuron. There is no comparable change in the postsynaptic cell. This presynaptic down-regulation of preexisting cell adhesion molecules is particularly prominent at adherent processes of the sensory neurons and is achieved by a rapid and transient activation of the endosomal pathway leading to a protein synthesis-dependent internalization of apCAM and its rerouting from a pathway of apparent recycling to a pathway that seems distinct for degradation (Fig. 4-4). Concomitant

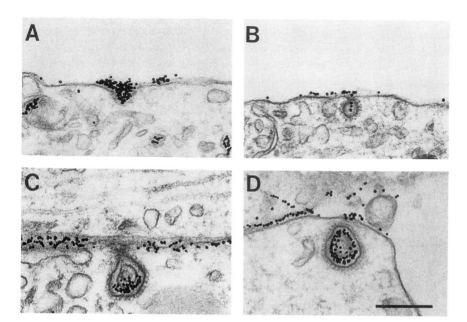

Figure 4-4. Serotonin-mediated endocytosis of apCAM: an early step of learning-related synaptic growth in *Aplysia*. A 1-hour exposure to the modulatory neurotransmitter 5-HT leads to a 50% decrease in the density of gold-labeled complexes bound to apCAM at the surface membrane of sensory neuron axons. This down-regulation is achieved by the transient activation of a coordinated program of clathrin-mediated endocytosis leading to the internalization of these cell adhesion molecules. *(A)* Even during the earliest steps of coated pit formation induced by 5-HT, there is already a prominent accumulation of gold particles, suggesting that, as with other forms of receptor-mediated endocytosis, these specialized depressions function as molecular sieves that can concentrate certain surface proteins and exclude others. The mechanisms for internalization of apCAM utilized at regions of contact between axonal fascicles of the sensory neurons seem to differ in several ways from those utilized at naked, unapposed segments of the axon. *(B)* At unapposed sites, the morphology of coated pits is simple and consists only of the conventional cup-like invagination of the surface membrane. *(C)* In contrast, at apposed sites the coated pits were consistently larger and more complex. In particular, they display a striking internal morphology often containing one or more smooth, membrane-bound vesicular profiles within the principle invagination. Occasionally, the membranes of these small, internal vesicles appear continuous with the surface membrane of the apposed neurite. These observations are consistent with the pinching off and internalization of small segments of the plasma membrane of the apposing neurite. *(D)* Indeed, after the formation of coated pits, at sites of membrane appositions, these complex invaginations separate from the surface membrane to form large, coated vesicles, which still contain internal membranous profiles and a heavy concentration of gold particles consistent with the internalization of two apposed membrane surfaces. Bar = 0.25 (μm. (From Bailey et al., 1992a.)

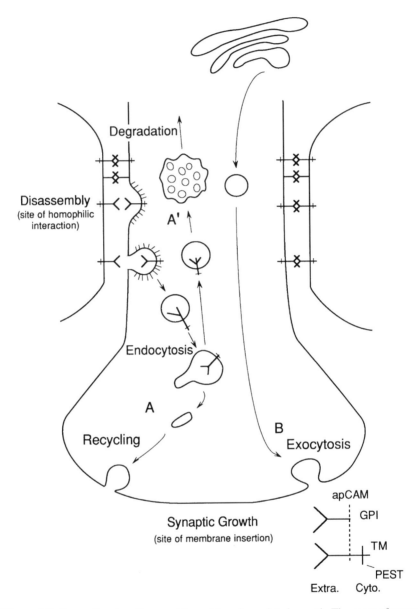

Figure 4-5. Internalization, disassembly, and learning-related growth. The onset of synaptic growth is triggered by the facilitating neurotransmitter 5-HT. Serotonin leads to a down-regulation of NCAM-related cell adhesion molecules (apCAMs). Part of this down-regulation occurs at the presynaptic membrane, where disassembly is achieved by a transient internalization involving the endosomal pathway. Internalization seems to be particularly active at sites of apposition (depicted here as stable, nongrowing regions where one neurite abuts and adheres to another) and is characterized there by intense endocytic activity. These focal endocytic bursts begin at coated pits and proceed through a series of endosomal pre-

with the down-regulation of apCAM, 5-HT and cAMP also induce in the sensory neurons an increase in the expression of the light chain of clathrin (apClathrin), one of the proteins whose expression is increased following long-term training, as well as an increase in the number of coated pits and coated vesicles (Hu et al., 1993). Since the apClathrin light chain contains the important functional domains of both LCa and LCb of mammalian clathrin thought to be essential for coated pit assembly and disassembly (Brodsky et al., 1991), the increase in clathrin may be an important component in the activation of the endocytic cycle required for the internalization of apCAM.

The ability of 5-HT to modify the structure of the surface and internal membrane systems of sensory neurons in *Aplysia,* by initiating a rapid, protein synthesis-dependent sequence of steps, bears a striking similarity to the ruffling of the cell surface and membrane remodeling induced in non-neuronal systems by epidermal growth factor and other well-characterized growth factors (Bretscher, 1989; Dadabay et al., 1991) or by nerve growth factor in PC12 cells (Connolly et al., 1984). These similarities suggest that modulatory transmitters important for learning, such as serotonin, may serve a double function. In addition to producing transient regulation of the excitability of neurons, repeated or prolonged exposure of a modulatory transmitter can also produce an action comparable with that of a growth factor, resulting in more persistent regulation of the architecture of the neuron.

Based on these findings, Bailey et al. (1992a) have suggested that the 5-HT–induced internalization of apCAM and consequent membrane remodeling may represent the first morphological steps in the structural program underlying long-term facilitation (Fig. 4-5). According to this view, learning-related synapse formation is preceded by and perhaps requires endocytic activation, which can then serve a double function. First, endocytic activation could remove cell adhesion molecules from the neuronal surface at sites of apposition, thereby destabilizing adhesive contacts between axonal processes of the sensory neuron normally inhibiting growth and perhaps facilitating defasciculation, a process that may be im-

---

cursors, including uncoupling (CURL) vesicles. Here, the internalized plasma membrane can follow one of two pathways. In pathway *A,* internalized endocytic membrane components are retrieved from sites of apparent adhesion in the tubular extension of the CURL and reinserted at the surface at sites of new synapse formation. In pathway *A',* the apCAM molecules are targeted for degradation and become segregated within the swollen, vesicular portion of the CURL, which ultimately fuses with or matures into late endosomal compartments such as multivesicular bodies. Additional membrane inserted into the terminal for growth may also come by means of recruitment of new transport vesicles from the trans-Golgi network and the insertion of membrane by exocytosis (pathway *B*). The cytoplasmic domain of apCAM contains a prominent PEST sequence, which may be proteolytically cleaved and lead to enhanced turnover of newly synthesized protein, as well as contribute to the rapid internalization that accounts for the altered expression of apCAM at the surface membrane. The internalization of the transmembrane (TM) but not the GPI-linked isoforms of apCAM suggest that the process of outgrowth is initiated by a selective down-regulation of cell adhesion isoforms at extrasynaptic sites of membrane apposition. (Modified from Bailey et al., 1992a.)

portant in disassembly. Second, the massive endocytic activation might lead to a redistribution of membrane components that favors synapse formation. The assembly of membrane components required for initial synaptic growth may involve insertion, by means of targeted exocytosis, of endocytic membrane retrieved from sites of adhesion and recycled to sites of new synapse formation. Synapse formation may require, in addition, the recruitment of new transport vesicles from the trans-Golgi network. Thus, the growth of synaptic connections that accompanies long-term facilitation in *Aplysia* may be dependent on a coordinated program of clathrin-mediated endocytosis leading to the internalization of NCAM-related cell adhesion molecules.

How is the 5-HT–induced internalization of apCAM achieved? The partial down-regulation of apCAM (only approximately 50% is removed from the surface membrane of the sensory neuron following a 1-hour exposure to 5-HT) may be explained by some heterogeneity in internalization exhibited by the different isoforms of apCAM. One of the isoforms is transmembrane in disposition, while the others are attached to the membrane by a glycosylphosphoinositol (GPI) linkage. To examine the specificity of the 5-HT–induced down-regulation of these different isoforms and to further characterize the molecular steps that may underlie their internalization, Bailey et al. (1997) utilized a highly efficient neuronal expression vector (Kaang et al., 1992) to selectively overexpressed hemagglutinin epitope-tagged (HA-tagged) constructs of either the transmembrane or the GPI-linked isoforms of apCAM in cultured sensory neurons. By combining thin-section electron microscopy with immunolabeling of gold-conjugated antibodies, they found that only the transmembrane form is internalized following exposure to 5-HT. Whereas both isoforms of apCAM have identical extracellular domains, the cytoplasmic tail of the transmembrane form provides a substrate for intracellular signal transduction and cytoskeletal interactions. Overexpression of epitope-tagged transmembrane constructs with specific deletions of or mutations in the cytoplasmic domain has demonstrated further that the 5-HT–induced down-regulation and concomitant internalization can be blocked by removing either the entire cytoplasmic tail or just the spanning region of the intracellular domain containing a sequence enriched in proline, glutamic acid, serine, and threonine residues (PEST) and thought to target degradation or by simply substituting alanine for threonine in the two mitogen-activated protein kinase (MAPK) consensus sites. Moreover, injection of a specific inhibitor of MAPK into sensory neurons, which blocks long-term facilitation (Martin et al., 1997), also blocks down-regulation and internalization of the endogenous form of apCAM. These data suggest that activation of the MAPK pathway is important for the internalization of apCAM and thus may represent one of the initial regulatory steps underlying learning-related synaptic growth in *Aplysia*.

An Overall View

How information is stored in the brain is a question central to both neurobiology and psychology. Since the insightful proposals of Ramon y Cajal and others at the turn of the century, it has seemed almost axiomatic that learning and memory must be expressed as a change in synaptic function and form. However, prior to the last few decades there was little direct evidence either to support this hypothesis or to indicate precisely what aspects of synaptic change might be important for information storage.

Recently studies on several higher invertebrates have enhanced our knowledge about the specific synaptic loci and mechanisms that are involved in the acquisition and retention of various elementary forms of learning and memory. One such model system, the gill- and siphon-withdrawal reflex in *Aplysia,* has proven particularly advantageous for examining the cellular and molecular events that underlie both short- and long-term memory. We have exploited the cellular specificity of this reflex and have begun to examine the functional relationship between synaptic architecture and the prolonged changes in synaptic effectiveness that accompany long-term behavioral modifications.

Toward that end we have developed a variety of cell marking and quantitative techniques for studying the morphological basis of synaptic transmission, with the idea of relating synaptic structure to behavior. Because aspects of the memory for sensitization can be trapped at a specific synaptic locus—the connections between identified mechanoreceptor sensory neurons and their follower cells—we have been able to analyze, in a set of identified neurons that are causally related to the behavior, the mechanisms underlying the acquisition and retention of a long-term memory trace. Central issues include the following: Can a long-term memory trace be specified in morphological terms? Can morphological approaches be used directly as probes for examining the mechanisms that underlie learning and memory? What is the time course of the structural synaptic changes? Which are necessary for the onset of the memory, and which are required for its maintenance?

Our results indicate that learning in *Aplysia* produces morphological as well as functional changes expressed at specific synaptic loci known to be critically involved in learning. Long-term memory (lasting several weeks) is accompanied by a profound degree of structural plasticity at the level of identified sensory neuron synapses. These structural changes occur at two different levels of synaptic organization: *(1)* remodeling of sensory neuron active zones—which for long-term sensitization is reflected by an increase in the number, size, and vesicle complement of these release sites—and *(2)* parallel but even more widespread changes involving modulation of the total number of presynaptic varicosities per sensory neuron. Quantitative analysis of the time course over which these anatomical changes occur has further demonstrated that only alterations in the number of sensory neuron synapses persist in parallel with the behavioral retention of the memory. These results directly link a change in synaptic structure to long-lasting behavioral memory and provide evidence for a fundamental idea—that varicosities and their active zones are plastic rather than immutable components of the nervous system. Such morphological changes could represent an anatomical substrate for memory consolidation.

The structural alterations exhibited by sensory neuron transmitter release sites following learning and memory are consistent in many respects with the alterations in active zone morphology reported at the neuromuscular junction following various forms of experimental manipulation (Atwood et al., 1989; Atwood and Govind, 1990; Atwood and Martin, 1983; Rheuben, 1985; Herrera et al., 1985; Walrond and Reese, 1985; Chiang and Govind, 1986). Correlative studies of both invertebrate and vertebrate neuromuscular junctions now seem to indicate that changes in specific aspects of active zone structure may be critical indicators of changes in synaptic efficacy (for reviews, see Atwood and Wojtowicz, 1986; Atwood and Lnenicka, 1986). Moreover, the changes in synapse number following long-term sensitization in *Aplysia* are remarkably similar to reports in the vertebrate CNS of alterations in the number and/or pattern of synaptic connections (for reviews, see Greenough, 1984; Greenough and Bailey, 1988; Bailey and Kandel, 1993).

What is the role of this structural plasticity during learning and memory? One important clue comes from the results of studies in both vertebrates and invertebrates that indicate that the consolidation of long-term memory is likely to depend on new protein and RNA synthesis (Davis and Squire, 1984; Montarolo et al., 1986). In *Aplysia* these studies indicate that long-term sensitization (lasting days to weeks) requires gene products that are not required for short-term sensitization (lasting minutes to hours). From a molecular perspective this means that the gene products required for short-term memory are either preexisting or else turned over slowly, whereas the gene products required for long-term memory must be newly synthesized.

In examining the possible role of these newly synthesized proteins, one is forced to consider the evidence that associates structural changes in synapses with behavioral training. In fact, the ample evidence that long-term memory involves a process of cell growth provides a rationale for thinking about the types of intracellular changes that protein synthesis might bring about. For example, in *Aplysia* at least some of the newly synthesized proteins induced during long-term sensitization training must lead not only to functional changes but must contribute as well to the potentially more enduring structural changes—growth of new synaptic contacts—that occur in the sensory neurons. One protein, whose expression increases 24 hours after long-term sensitization training in sensory neurons, is the *Aplysia* homologue of GRP78/BiP, which is thought to chaperone the correct folding and assembly of secretory and transmembrane proteins in the lumen of the endoplasmic reticulum (Kuhl et al., 1993). The specific increase in *Aplysia* BiP expression occurs 3 hours following 5-HT application and is coincident with the 3-hour increase in overall protein synthesis observed by Barzilai et al. (1989). This change in the specific expression of *Aplysia* BiP in sensory neurons suggests that BiP may serve as one of several rate-limiting steps in the assembly of protein necessary for the laying down of the structural changes characteristic of the long-term process.

Recent studies of the synaptic growth that accompanies long-term sensitization in *Aplysia* have begun to characterize further the subcellular and molecular events that might give rise to this learning-related structural change. This in turn has indicated that specific molecules and mechanisms important for development of the nervous system can be reutilized in the adult for the purposes of synaptic plasticity and memory storage.

For example, these studies indicate that the processing and storage of information in the nervous system may rely on the same cellular mechanisms utilized to regulate the trafficking of membrane seen during periods of cellular differentiation and growth. Indeed, an increasing body of evidence suggests that the growth changes accompanying the storage of long-term memory share features in common with the cascade of events that underlie synapse formation during development. In both cases, there is a requirement for new macromolecular synthesis. This increase in the production of protein and mRNA can be initiated in the long-term process by modulatory transmitters that, in this respect, appear to mimic the effects of growth factors and hormones during the cell cycle and differentiation. Thus, modulatory transmitters important for learning can activate a genomic cascade by which the transmitter can exert a long-term regulation over both the excitability and functional architecture of the neuron through changes in gene expression.

Studies in *Aplysia* have further demonstrated that the initial stages of long-term memory storage are associated with modulation of an immunoglobulin-related cell adhesion molecule homologous to NCAM. With the emergence of the nervous system, the *Aplysia* NCAM becomes expressed exclusively in neurons and is specifically enriched at synapses. These cell adhesion molecules are down-regulated by serotonin, a transmitter important for sensitization in *Aplysia* and cAMP, a second-messenger activated by serotonin. This down-regulation of preexisting cell adhesion molecules is achieved by a transient activation of the endocytic pathway leading to a protein synthesis-dependent internalization of apCAM. The clathrin-mediated internalization of apCAM may serve as a preliminary and perhaps even a permissive step for the growth of synaptic connections that accompanies the long-term process. Thus, a molecule utilized during the development of the nervous system for the purposes of cell adhesion and axonal outgrowth is retained into adulthood, at which point it seems to serve as an inhibitory constraint on growth until it is rapidly and transiently decreased at the cell surface by a modulatory transmitter important for learning. Surprisingly, in *Aplysia* 5-HT leads to the rapid internalization of only one isoform of apCAM (the transmembrane isoform) and not the others (the GPI-linked isoforms), raising the interesting possibility that learning-related synaptic growth in the adult may be initiated by an activity-dependent recruitment of specific isoforms of adhesion molecules, similar to the modulation of cell surface receptors during the fine tuning of synaptic connections in the developing nervous system.

Additional support for the idea that the nervous system may utilize similar cell biological mechanisms to achieve learning-related plasticity in the mature animal as it does for synapse formation during development comes from studies in the vertebrate brain where it has been shown that at critical developmental stages the refinement of synaptic connections is determined by an activity-dependent process that seems related to long-term potentiation in the hippocampus (Constantine-Paton et al., 1990; Goodman and Shatz, 1993 Antonini and Stryker, 1993). Thus, aspects of the mechanistic programs utilized for memory storage in the adult brain may eventually be understood in the context of the basic molecular logic that dctermines the rescaffolding of synaptic circuitry during the later stages of neuronal development.

References

Portions of the work reviewed in this chapter were supported by NIH grants MH37134 and GM32099 to C.H.B.

Alberini, C., Ghirardi, M., Metz, R., and Kandel, E. R. (1994). C/EBP is an immediate-early gene required for the consolidation of long-term facilitation in *Aplysia*. *Cell, 76,* 1099–1114.

Alkon, D. L. (1984). Calcium-mediated reduction of ionic currents: A biophysical memory trace. *Science, 226,* 1037–1045.

Antonini, A., and Stryker, M. P. (1993). Rapid remodeling of axonal arbors in the visual cortex. *Science, 260,* 1819–1821.

Atwood, H. L., Dixon, D., and Wojtowicz, J. H. (1989). Rapid introduction of long-lasting synaptic changes at crustacean neuromuscular junctions. *J. Neurobiol., 20,* 373–385.

Atwood, H. L., and Govind, C. K. (1990). Activity-dependent and age-dependent recruitment and regulation of synapses in identified crustacean neurons. *J. Exp. Biol., 153,* 105–127.

Atwood, H. L., and Lnenicka, G. A. (1986). Structure and function in synapses: Emerging correlations. *Trends Neurosci., 9,* 248–250.

Atwood, H. L., and Martin, L. (1983). Ultrastructure of synapses with different transmitter-releasing characteristics on motor axon terminals of a crab, *Hyas areaneas. Cell Tissue Res., 231,* 103–115.

Atwood, H. L., and Wojtowicz, J. M. (1986). Short-term and long-term plasticity and physiological differentiation of crustacean motor systems. *Int. Rev. Neurobiol., 28,* 275–362.

Bailey, C. H., Bartsch, D., and Kandel, E. R. (1996). Toward a molecular definition of long-term memory storage. *Proc. Natl. Acad. Sci. U.S.A., 93,* 13445–24452.

Bailey, C. H., and Chen, M. (1983). Morphological basis of long-term habituation and sensitization in *Aplysia. Science, 220,* 91–93.

Bailey, C. H., and Chen, M. (1988a). Long-term memory in *Aplysia* modulates the total number of varicosities of single identified sensory neurons. *Proc. Natl. Acad. Sci. U.S.A., 85,* 2373–2377.

Bailey, C. H., and Chen, M. (1988b). Long-term sensitization in *Aplysia* increases the number of presynaptic contacts onto the identified gill motor neuron L7. *Proc. Natl. Acad. Sci. U.S.A., 85,* 9356–9539.

Bailey, C. H., and Chen, M. (1989). Time course of structural changes at identified sensory neuron synapses during long-term sensitization in *Aplysia. J. Neurosci. 9,* 1774–1780.

Bailey, C. H., Chen, M., Keller, F., and Kandel, E. R. (1992a). Serotonin-mediated endocytosis of apCAM: An early step of learning-related synaptic growth in *Aplysia. Science, 256,* 645–649.

Bailey, C. H., Kaang, B.-K., Chen, M., Martin, K. C., Lim, C.-S., Casadio, A., and Kandel, E. R. (1997). Mutation in the phosphorylation sites of MAP kinase blocks learning-related internalization of apCAM in *Aplysia* sensory neurons. *Neuron, 18,* 913–924.

Bailey, C. H., and Kandel, E. R. (1985). Molecular approaches to the study of short- and long-term memory. In C. W. Coen (ed.): *Functions of the Brain*. New York: Clarendon Press, pp. 98–129.

Bailey, C. H., and Kandel, E. R. (1993). Structural changes accompanying memory storage. *Annu. Rev. Physiol., 55*, 397–426.

Bailey, C. H., Kandel, P., and Chen, M. (1981). The active zone at *Aplysia* synapses: Organization of presynaptic dense projection. *J. Neurophysiol., 46*, 356–368.

Bailey, C. H., Montarolo, P. G., Chen, M., Kandel, E. R., and Schacher, S. (1992b). Inhibitors of protein and RNA synthesis block the structural changes that accompany long-term heterosynaptic plasticity in the sensory neurons of *Aplysia. Neuron, 9*, 749–758.

Bailey, C. H., Thompson, E. B., Castellucci, V. F., and Kandel, E. R. (1979). Ultrastructure of the synapses of sensory neurons that mediate the gill-withdrawal reflex in *Aplysia. J. Neurocytol., 8*, 415–444.

Barzilai, A., Kennedy, T. E., Sweatt, J. D., and Kandel, E. R. (1989). 5-HT modulates protein synthesis and the expression of specific proteins during long-term facilitation in *Aplysia* sensory neurons. *Neuron, 2*, 1577–1586.

Bloom, F. E., and Aghajanian, G. K. (1968). Fine structural and cytochemical analysis of the staining of synaptic junctions with phosphotungstic acid. *J. Ultrastruct. Res., 22*, 361–375.

Bretscher, A. (1989). Rapid phosphorylation and reorganization of ezrin and spectrin accompany morphological changes induced in A-431 cells by epidermal growth factor. *J. Cell. Biol., 108*, 921–930.

Brodsky, F. M., Hill, B. L., Acton, S. L., Nathke, I., Wong, D. H., Ponnambalam, S., and Parham, P. (1991). Clathrin light chains: Arrays of protein motifs that regulate coated-vesicle dynamics. *Trends Biochem. Sci., 167*, 208–213.

Byrne, J. H. (1987). Cellular analysis of associative learning. *Physiol. Rev., 67*, 329–439.

Carew, T. J., and Sahley, C. L. (1986). Invertebrate learning and memory: From behavior to molecules. *Annu. Rev. Neurosci., 9*, 435–487.

Castellucci, F., Blumenfeld, H., Goelet, P., and Kandel, E. R. (1989). Inhibitor of protein synthesis blocks long-term behavioral sensitization in the isolated gill-withdrawal reflex of *Aplysia. J. Neurobiol., 20*, 1–9.

Chiang, R. G., and Govind, C. K. (1986). Reorganization of synaptic ultrastructure at facilitated lobster neuromuscular terminals. *J. Neurocytol., 15*, 63–74.

Connolly, J. L., Green, S. A., and Greene, L. A. (1984). Comparison of rapid changes in surface morphology and coated pit formation of PC12 cells in response to nerve growth factor, epidermal growth factor and dibutyryl cyclic AMP. *J. Cell Biol., 98*, 457–465.

Constantine-Paton, M., Cline, H. T., and Debski, E. (1990). Patterned activity, synaptic convergence, and the NMDA receptor in developing visual pathways. *Annu. Rev. Neurosci., 13*, 129–154.

Couteaux, R., and Pecot-Dechavassine, M. (1970). Vesicules synaptiques et poches au niveau des zones actives de la jonction neuromusculaire. *C. R. Acad. Sci., 271*, 2346–2349.

Dadabay, C. Y., Patton, E., Cooper, J. A., and Pike, L. J. (1991). Lack of correlation between changes in polyphosphoinositide levels and actin/gelsolin complexes in A431 cells treated with epidermal growth factor. *J. Cell Biol., 112*, 1151–1156.

Dale, N., Kandel, E. R., and Schacher S. (1987). Serotonin produces long-term changes in the excitability of *Aplysia* sensory neurons in culture that depend on new protein synthesis. *J. Neurosci., 7*, 2232–2238.

Dash, P. K., Hochner, B., and Kandel, E. R. (1990). Injection of the cAMP-responsive element into the nucleus of *Aplysia* sensory neurons blocks long-term facilitation. *Nature, 345,* 718–721.

Davis, G. W., Schuster, C. M., and Goodman, C. S. (1996). Genetic dissection of structural and functional components of synaptic plasticity: III. CREB is necessary for presynaptic functional plasticity. *Neuron, 17,* 669–679.

Davis, H. P., and Squire, L. R. (1984). Protein synthesis and memory: A review. *Psychol. Bull., 96,* 518–559.

Doherty, P., Fazelli, M. S., and Walsh, F. S. (1995). The neural cell adhesion molecule and synaptic plasticity. *J. Neurobiol., 26,* 437–446.

Fields, R. D., and Itoh, K. (1996). Neural cell adhesion molecules in activity-dependent development and synaptic plasticity. *Trends Neurosci., 19,* 473–480.

Frost, W. N., Castellucci, V. F., Hawkins, R. D., and Kandel, E. R. (1985). Monosynaptic connections made by the sensory neurons of the gill- and siphon-withdrawal reflex in *Aplysia* participate in the storage of long-term memory for sensitization. *Proc. Natl. Acad. Sci. U.S.A., 82,* 8266–8269.

Ghirardi, M., Braha, O., Hochner, B., Montarolo, P. G., Kandel, E. R., and Dale, N. (1992). Roles of PKA and PKC in facilitation of evoked and spontaneous transmitter release at depressed and nondepressed synapses in *Aplysia* sensory neurons. *Neuron, 9,* 479–489.

Glanzman, D. L., Kandel, E. R., and Schacher, S. (1989). Identified target motor neuron regulates neurite outgrowth and synapse formation of *Aplysia* sensory neurons *in vitro. Neuron, 3,* 441–450.

Glanzman, D. L., Kandel, E. R., and Schacher, S. (1990). Target-dependent structural changes accompanying long-term synaptic facilitation in *Aplysia* neurons. *Science, 249,* 799–802.

Goodman, C. S., and Shatz, C. J. (1993). Developmental mechanisms that generate precise patterns of neuronal connectivity. *Cell, 72,* 77–98.

Greenough, W. T. (1984). Structural correlates of information storage in the mammalian brain: A review and hypothesis. *Trends Neurosci., 7,* 229–233.

Greenough, W. T., and Bailey, C. H. (1988). The anatomy of memory: Convergence of results across a diversity of tests. *Trends Neurosci., 11,* 142–147.

Herrera, A. A., Grinnell, A. P., and Wolowske, B. (1985). Ultrastructural correlates of naturally occurring differences in transmitter release efficacy in frog motor nerve terminals. *J. Neurocytol., 14,* 193–202.

Heuser, J. E., Reese, T. S., Dennis, M. J., Jan, Y., Jan, L., and Evans, L. (1979). Synaptic vesicle exocytosis captured by quick freezing and correlated with quantal transmitter release. *J. Cell Biol., 81,* 275–300.

Hochner, B., Schacher, S., and Kandel, E. R. (1986). Action-potential duration and the modulation of transmitter release from the sensory neurons of *Aplysia* in presynaptic facilitation and behavioral sensitization. *Proc. Natl. Acad. Sci. U.S.A., 83,* 8410–8414.

Hu, Y., Barzilai, A., Chen, M., Bailey, C. H., and Kandel, E. R. (1993). 5-HT and cAMP induce the formation of coated pits and vesicles and increase the expression of clathrin light chains in sensory neurons of *Aplysia. Neuron, 10,* 921–929.

Kaang, B. K., Kandel, E. R., and Grant, S. G. N. (1993). Activation of cAMP-responsive genes by stimuli that produce long-term facilitation in *Aplysia* sensory neurons. *Neuron, 10,* 427–435.

Kaang, B.-K., Pfaffinger, P. J., Grant, S. G. N., Kandel, E. R., and Furukawa, Y. (1992). Overexpression of an *Aplysia* shaker K+ channel gene modifies the electrical properties and synaptic efficacy of identified *Aplysia* neurons. *Proc. Natl. Acad. Sci. U.S.A., 89,* 1133–1137.

Kandel, E. R. (1976). *Cellular Basis of Behavior: An Introduction to Behavioral Neurobiology.* San Francisco: CA: W. H. Freeman and Company.

Kandel, E. R., and Schwartz, J. H. (1982). Molecular biology of an elementary form of learning: Modulation of transmitter release by cyclic AMP. *Science, 218,* 433–443.

Keller, F., and Schacher, S. (1990). Neuron-specific membrane glycoproteins promoting neurite fasciculation in *Aplysia californica. J. Cell Biol., 111,* 2637–2650.

Klein, M., and Kandel, E. R. (1980). Mechanisms of calcium current modulation underlying presynaptic facilitation and behavioral sensitization in *Aplysia. Proc. Natl. Acad. Sci. U.S.A., 77,* 6912–6916.

Kuhl, D., Kennedy, T. E., Barzilai, A., and Kandel, E. R. (1993). Long-term sensitization training in *Aplysia* leads to an increase in the expression of BiP, the major protein chaperon of the endoplasmic reticulum. *J. Cell Biol., 119,* 1069–1076.

Landis, D. M. D., Hall, A. K., Weinstein, L. A., and Reese, T. S. (1988). The organization of cytoplasm at the presynaptic active zone of a central nervous system synapse. *Neuron, 1,* 201–209.

Martin, K. C., and Kandel, E. R. (1996). Cell adhesion molecules, CREB, and the formation of new synaptic connections during development and learning. *Neuron, 17,* 567–570.

Martin, K. C., Michael, D., Roe, J. C., Barad, M., Casadio, A., Zhu, H., and Kandel, E. R. (1997). MAP kinase translocates into the nucleus of the presynaptic cell and is required for long-term facilitation in *Aplysia. Neuron, 18,* 899–912.

Mayford, M., Barzilai, A., Keller, F., Schacher, S., and Kandel, E. R. (1992). Modulation of and NCAM-related adhesion molecule with long-term synaptic plasticity in *Aplysia. Science, 256,* 638–644.

Montarolo, P. G., Goelet, P., Castellucci, V. F., Morgan, J., Kandel, E. R., and Schacher, S. (1986). A critical period for macromolecular synthesis in long-term heterosynaptic facilitation in *Aplysia. Science, 234,* 1249–1254.

Nazif, F. A., Byrne, J. H., Cleary, L. J. (1991). cAMP induces long-term morphological changes in sensory neurons of *Aplysia. Brain Res, 539,* 324–327.

Pinsker, H. M., Hening, W. A., Carew, T. J., and Kandel, E. R. (1973). Long-term sensitization of a defensive withdrawal reflex in *Aplysia. Science, 182,* 1039–1042.

Pinsker, H. M., Kupfermann, I., Castellucci, V. F., and Kandel, E. R. (1970). Habituation and dishabituation of the gill-withdrawal reflex in *Aplysia. Science, 167,* 1740–1742.

Rayport, S. G., and Schacher, S. (1986). Synaptic plasticity *in vitro:* Cell culture of identified *Aplysia* neurons mediating short-term habituation and sensitization. *J. Neurosci., 6,* 759–763.

Rheuben, M. D. (1985). Quantitative comparison of the structural features of slow and fast neuromuscular junctions in *Manduca. J. Neurosci., 5,* 1704–1716.

Schacher, S., Castellucci, V. F., and Kandel, E. R. (1988). cAMP evokes long-term facilitation in *Aplysia* sensory neurons that requires new protein synthesis. *Science, 240,* 1667–1669.

Scholz, K. P., and Byrne, J. H. (1987). Long-term sensitization in *Aplysia*: Biophysical correlates in tail sensory neurons. *Science, 235,* 685–687.

Schwartz, J. H., Castellucci, V. F., and Kandel, E. R. (1971). Functions of identified neurons and synapses in abdominal ganglion of *Aplysia* in absence of protein synthesis. *J. Neurophysiol., 34,* 939–953.

Schuster, C. M., Davis, G. W., Fetter, R. D., and Goodman, C. S. (1996a). Genetic dissection of structural and functional components of synaptic plasticity: I. Fasciclin II controls synaptic stabilization and growth. *Neuron 17,* 641–654.

Schuster, C. M., Davis, G. W., Fetter, R. D., and Goodman, C. S. (1996b). Genetic dissection of structural and functional components of synaptic plasticity: II. Fasciclin II controls presynaptic structural plasticity. *Neuron, 17,* 655–667.

Thorpe, W. H. (1956). *Learning and instincts in animals.* Cambridge, MA: Harvard University Press.

Walrond, J. P., and Reese, T. S. (1985). Structure of axon terminals and active zones at synapses on lizard twitch and tonic muscle fibers. *J. Neurosci., 5,* 1118–1131.

5

Role of Intrinsic Circuitry in Motor Cortex Plasticity

ASAF KELLER

Recent anatomical and electrophysiological studies have provided data that are beginning to unravel the controversies surrounding the functional organization of the motor cortex. Many of these advances are derived from studies of intracortical connections, which, despite their numerical prominence and postulated roles in motor cortical function, have only recently been studied systematically. The role of intracortical synaptic interactions in shaping the functional organization of the motor cortex and the role of intracortical interactions in modulating this organization in response to neurological deficits and during motor skill acquisition are discussed in this chapter.

The motor cortex contains gross somatotopic representations of the major subdivision of the body musculature. Within each of these somatotopic maps there are multiple, noncontiguous, and overlapping representations of particular movement patterns. Intracortical, horizontal connections link neurons located within different representation zones, which may be located several millimeters from each other. These excitatory connections link representation zones related to different aspects of the same voluntary movement, thereby forming a substrate for the temporal coordination of movement segments required for the execution of multi-jointed movements. Other excitatory connections link representation of functionally unrelated movements, such as those of the facial and forelimb musculature. These heterotypical intrinsic connections are normally masked by intrinsic, inhibitory synaptic influences. Modulation of the intrinsic excitatory and inhibitory synapses are responsible for the pliability of representation maps in the motor cortex. These changes may underly plasticity in movement representations that occurs in response to neurological insults or during the acquisition of novel motor skills.

Functional Organization of the Motor Cortex

At least since the sixteenth century it has been recognized that the cerebral cortex is involved in the control of voluntary movements (for historical reviews, see Asanuma, 1989; Finger, 1994). The pioneering studies of Fritsch and Hitzig (1870) and Ferrier (1873) established that voluntary motor functions are localized within specific regions of the cerebral cortex, particularly within what was later defined as Brodman's area 4—the primary motor cortex. Subsequent research efforts were aimed primarily at revealing the somatotopic organization of this area (see Asanuma, 1989; Humphrey, 1986; Lemon, 1990) or deciphering the movement parameters coded by the activity of single motor cortical neurons (e.g., Evarts, 1986; Fetz, 1992). These studies established three major characteristics of the functional organization of the motor cortex: *(1)* At a macroscopic level, there are gross somatotopic representations of individual body parts within the primary motor cortex; *(2)* within these representations, there are multiple, overlapping regions representing individual movements; and *(3)* these movement representations can be continuously modified in response to behavioral experience. These features of the functional organization of the motor cortex are discussed below.

Gross Somatotopic Organization

Studies related to the somatotopic organization of the motor cortex aim to identify regions in the motor cortex that contain cells responsible for activation of individual muscles or movements. Earlier studies were performed with the use of macroelectrodes to electrically stimulate the surface of the motor cortex while monitoring muscle contractions evoked by stimulation at different sites (e.g., Penfield and Boldrey, 1937; Woolsey, 1964). This approach was refined by Asanuma and collaborators, who developed the intracortical microstimulation techniques (ICMS) (Asanuma, 1959, 1981). In this technique, movement representations are defined as the cortical loci from which movements about individual joints, or electromyographic activity in specific muscle groups, can be evoked. This is done by stimulating the cortex with microelectrodes placed in the deep cortical layers, where the somata of corticospinal cells reside. Because ICMS results in the activation of relatively small groups of corticospinal cells, this approach allows detailed analyses of the functional relationship between cortical loci and specific motoneuron pools.

The use of ICMS revealed similar features in the functional organization of the motor cortex in several mammalian species, including humans (reviewed by Keller, 1993a, 1996). Within the motor cortex of all mammalian species examined there is a gross somatotopic representation of the major divisions of the body, such as hindlimb, forelimb, and face. This gross somatotopy is generally similar in members of the same species such that a particular body part is usually represented within the same region of the motor cortex in all individuals. For example, in the rat motor cortex, representations of whisker movements are located medial to the forelimb representation, and hindlimb movements are posterior to both whisker and forelimb areas (see Fig. 5-1).

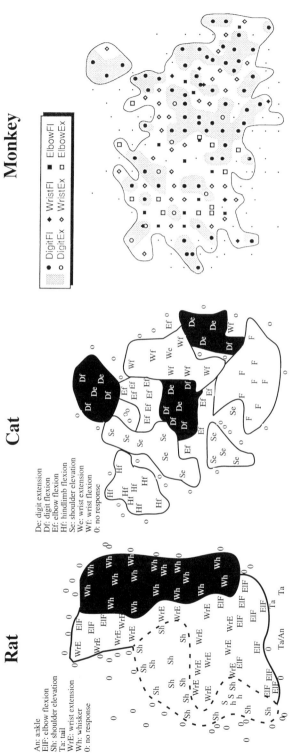

Figure 5-1. Movement representation maps obtained with the use of the intracortical microstimulation (ICMS) technique. All maps depict a dorsal view of the motor cortex. Letters and symbols indicate sites of microelectrode penetrations. *Rat:* Representations of the same movement are grouped within a common border. (Modified from Keller et al., 1996.) *Cat:* Movement representations related to the same joint are grouped within a common border; representations of digit movements are shown in black. (Modified from Keller, 1993b.) *Monkey:* Open symbols represent extensor actions, and solid symbols indicate flexor actions. Shading encloses digit representations. (From Donoghue et al., 1992.)

Distributed Nature of the Functional Organization

The second organizational feature of the motor cortex pertains to the representations of *individual* movements or muscle groups. Within each gross representation of a body part, there are multiple, noncontiguous, and overlapping representations of individual movement patterns (Fig. 5-1). For example, digit movements can be evoked by stimulating several noncontiguous sites in the cat motor cortex (Fig. 5-1), and ICMS of these sites may also evoke movements about other forelimb joints. This organizational feature has been described for several mammalian species, including the mouse (Li and Waters, 1991), rat (Weiss and Keller, 1994), cat (Keller, 1993b), and nonhuman primates (Donoghue et al., 1992; Waters et al., 1990). That the motor cortex contains overlapping and distributed movement representations is also supported by studies on the activities of individual motor cortical neurons during voluntary movements (Fetz, 1992; Schieber and Hibbard, 1993) and by data demonstrating that individual corticospinal axons provide input to several motoneuron pools in the spinal cord (Jankowska et al., 1975; Shinoda et al., 1976).

More recently, the functional organization of the human motor cortex has been studied with the use of approaches that are less invasive than the ICMS technique. These approaches include transcranial magnetic stimulation, positron emission tomography (PET), and functional magnetic resonance imaging (fMRI). Studies employing these approaches reveal that the human motor cortex, like that of other species, contains multiple, overlapping representations of movement patterns (Burke et al., 1992; Sanes et al., 1995; Shibasaki et al., 1993; Wassermann et al., 1992).

It appears, therefore, that the primary motor cortex is not somatotopically organized in the conventional sense (for a comprehensive discussion of this issue, see Sanes and Donoghue, 1997). This contrasts with the cortical organization of other modalities, such as vision and somasthesia, where discrete regions of the peripheral receptive sheet (retina and skin) are represented in discrete loci in the cerebral cortex. Rather, the distributed and overlapping nature of movement representations suggests that a particular group of cells in the motor cortex may participate in generating different types of movements and that execution of a particular movement requires the activation of multiple, noncontiguous groups of motor cortical neurons (see Keller, 1993a; Sanes and Donoghue, 1997; Schieber and Hibbard, 1993).

Role of Intracortical Connections

The spatial separation of representation zones related to the same movement pattern suggests that a mechanism exists by which these zones interact for the activation of their related muscles. This mechanism is likely to involve synaptic interactions among cells in different representation zones, mediated by intracortical axon collaterals.

A striking feature of the intracortical axon collaterals of motor cortical neurons are their long, horizontal projections within the motor cortex. Pyramidal tract neurons in layer V have horizontal axon collaterals that project to a distance of more than 2 mm within layers V and VI (Ghosh et al., 1988; Landry et al., 1980). The horizontal axon collaterals belonging to pyramidal neurons in layers II–III also project for long distances and commonly form clusters of axon terminals (Keller and Asanuma, 1993; Landry et al., 1980). Other studies analyzing the distribution of intrinsic axon terminals in the motor cortex labeled by lesion-induced degeneration (Gatter and Powell, 1978) or by the application of neuroanatomical tracers (DeFelipe et al., 1986; Jones et al., 1978) have also provided evidence for long-range horizontal connections within the motor cortex.

The existence of long, horizontal intracortical connections in the motor cortex was also revealed with the use of electrophysiological approaches in the *in vitro* slice preparation (Aroniadou and Keller, 1993; Hess et al., 1994). In addition to demonstrating long-range horizontal and oblique functional connections within the motor cortex, these studies revealed that these connections mediate excitatory synaptic interactions involving activation of both *N*-methyl-D-aspartate (NMDA) and kainate/α-amino-3-hydroxy-5-methyl-ioxyzole-4-propionic acid (AMPA) glutamate receptors.

Insight into the functional role of intrinsic connections in the motor cortex is derived from studies in which patterns of intrinsic connections were correlated with maps of movement representations. These studies were performed in the motor cortex of the monkey (Huntley and Jones, 1991), cat (Keller, 1993b), and rat (Weiss and Keller, 1994). In each of these studies, ICMS was used to map the representations of different parts of the body musculature (e.g., forearm, face, hindlimb), and neuroanatomical tracers were then used to demarcate the patterns of intracortical axon collaterals that link these representation zones. This approach yielded similar results in the three species examined: Injections of either antrograde or retrograde anatomical tracers revealed a profuse network of long, intrinsic connections that link representation zones within the same body part (Fig. 5-2). Thus, for example, cells in the forelimb representations (digits, elbow, wrist) of the monkey motor cortex are reciprocally connected via intrinsic axon collaterals, but have virtually no intrinsic connections with neurons in the face area (Huntley and Jones, 1991). Similarly, profuse intrinsic connections link neurons in the forelimb representation zones of the cat motor cortex, but only sparse connections are found with the hindlimb or the face representation (Keller, 1993b). In the rat motor cortex (Weiss and Keller, 1994), injections of anterograde tracers in the whisker representation zone result in dense axonal labeling restricted largely to the whisker zone. Similarly, injections in the forelimb representation produce labeling primarily restricted to the forelimb zone (Fig. 5-2). In summary, in the rat, cat, and monkey motor cortex, intrinsic connections are specific in that they preferentially link neurons within representation zones involved in movements of the same body part.

Although these studies reveal patterns of connections among gross somatotopic representations, they provide no information on the types of intracortical interactions among individual motor cortical neurons. We have recently addressed

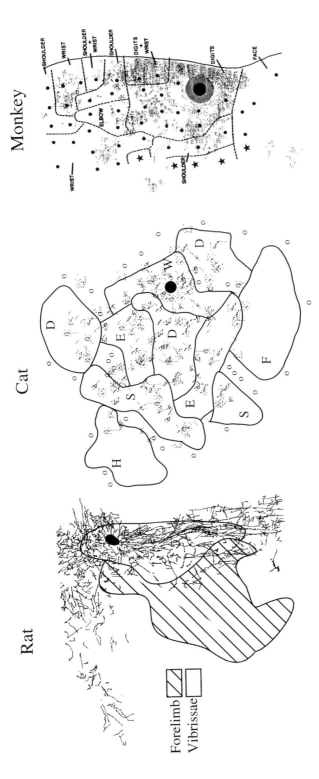

Figure 5-2. Patterns of intracortical connections within the motor cortex. Movement representations maps were obtained using procedures described in Figure 5-1 and the text. *Rat:* Injection of an anterograde tracer into the whisker representation labels intracortical axons that terminate preferentially in that region. Modified from Weiss and Keller (1994). *Cat:* Tracer injection into the wrist (W) representation reveals dense, clustered connections among the different representations of forelimb movements. Note the sparse connections formed with representations of facial (F) and hindlimb (H) movements representations. D, digits; S, shoulder; E, elbow. (Modified from Keller, 1993b.) *Monkey:* Tracer injection into a digit representation zone reveals terminal fiber labeling throughout the forelimb movement representations, with sparse labeling in the face area. (From Huntley and Jones, 1991.)

this issue by examining the patterns of connections formed by individual, identified pyramidal tract neurons in the cat motor cortex. Three pyramidal tract neurons were labeled with biocytin by intracellular injections *in vivo.* ICMS was used to delineate the movement representations occupied by the parent somata and the axon collaterals of the labeled cells. The somata of two of these cells were within a wrist-extension zone, and the soma of the third neuron was in a wrist-flexion zone. Detailed reconstructions of the intracortical axonal projections of these neurons revealed that they formed both *local* axon collaterals, arborizing within the immediate vicinity of the parent soma, and one or more long, *horizontal* axonal projections. These patterns of axonal projections are similar to those of layers II–III neurons in the cat motor cortex (Keller and Asanuma, 1993). The *local* axons of all three neurons terminated within the same representation zone as their parent soma, and electron microscopical analysis revealed that these axons provide input preferentially (78%–85% of the synapses) to excitatory cells. These synaptic patterns could result in feed-forward activation of additional excitatory neural components in the same representation zone. In contrast, the synaptic targets of the *horizontal* axons differed according to the representation zone they innervated. Axons projecting to a representation of a movement *agonist* to that represented at the locus of their parent soma provided inputs preferentially (69%–92% of the synapses) to other excitatory neurons. These synaptic interactions are likely to result in feed-forward excitation of neurons located in spatially segregated, but functionally related, representation zones. In contrast, horizontal axons projecting to representation zones of movements *antagonist* to that of the parent soma provided input preferentially (72%–83% of the synapses) to inhibitory cells, which presumably contain γ-aminobutyric acid (GABA). The horizontal axon collaterals of pyramidal cells synapsing with inhibitory neurons may form a basis for lateral inhibition between representation zones related to the activation of antagonist movement patterns. The synaptic patterns revealed by analysis of this small sample of pyramidal tract neurons could result in a recruitment of groups of cells related to a particular movement and a concurrent suppression of cells related to antagonistic movements. Pertinent to this hypothesis are findings that intrinsic excitatory interactions in the motor cortex occur preferentially among neurons related to the activation of a single or neighboring joints (Kwan et al., 1987; Murphy et al., 1985). The role of GABA-mediated inhibition in shaping movement representation maps is supported by findings that GABA receptor antagonists can alter these maps (Jacobs and Donoghue, 1991). Furthermore, suppression of GABAergic inhibition in the motor cortex results in disruptions to the spatiotemporal sequences of movement patterns (Matsumura et al., 1991). Removal of GABAergic inhibition also results in the appearance of task-related activity in neurons that were previously inactive during the execution of a motor task (Matsumura et al., 1991).

Thus, intracortical synaptic interactions within the motor cortex may constitute a substrate for spatiotemporal coordination of distributed neuronal groups that are co-activated during motor acts. As discussed below, these intrinsic interactions may also be involved in the pliability of movement representation maps.

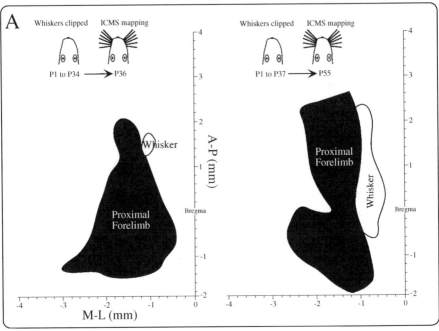

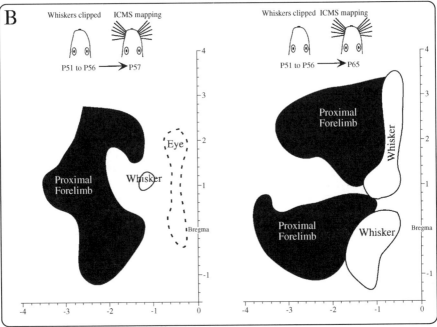

Figure 5-3. Maps of cortical representation zones in the rat motor cortex following whisker trimming. Maps were constructed as described in Figure 5-1. The schematic above each map denotes the period of whisker clipping and the age at which the map was obtained. *A,*

Pliability of Movement Representations

The third feature of the functional organization of the motor cortex is the pliability of movement representations. Early cartographers of the motor cortex noted that movement representation maps obtained from different subjects are often dissimilar and that maps obtained from the same subject may shift with time (Brown and Sherrington, 1912; Lashley, 1923). One possibility is that this variability in movement representations reflects differences in the history of behavioral experience. Support for this hypothesis was obtained relatively recently, following the seminal works of Donoghue, Nudo, and their collaborators (see, e.g., Nudo et al., 1996a; Sanes et al., 1992).

Several approaches have been used to demonstrate that the representations of movements in the motor cortex can be dynamically modulated. These motor maps can be modulated in response to repetitive cortical stimulation (Nudo et al., 1990) and following motor nerve lesions (Donoghue et al., 1990) and intracortical application of pharmacological agents (Jacobs and Donoghue, 1991). Relatively innocuous manipulations that affect sensorimotor experience also result in dramatic changes in movement representations. For example, reversibly restraining a rat's limb results in both immediate ($\leq$15 minutes) and late shifts in the borders between movement representation zones (Sanes et al., 1992). Similar changes in movement representations can be produced by clipping the whiskers on a rat's snout; this procedure results in the expansion of the forelimb representation at the expense of regions normally representing whisker movements (Fig. 5-3) (Keller et al., 1996). Allowing the whiskers to re-grow and normal whisking activity to resume results in a shift in the motor representations to their "normal" configuration (Fig. 5-3) (Keller et al., 1996).

Of particular interest are studies demonstrating the pliability of movement representations associated with training in a motor task (Donoghue and Sanes, 1991; Milliken et al., 1992; Nudo et al., 1996a; Woody and Black-Cleworth, 1973). Also pertinent are recent findings in nonhuman primates demonstrating that functional recovery from cortical infarcts, induced by rehabilitative training, is associated with shifts in movement representation maps (Nudo and Milliken, 1996; Nudo et al., 1996b).

The recent application of neuroimaging and transcranial magnetic stimulation techniques to studies of motor cortical organization in humans has also provided evidence for use-dependent pliability of movement representation maps. Anes-

---

left: Whisker clipping from the day of birth until P34 results in an expansion of the forelimb representation, at the expense of the whisker representation. *A, right:* In rats subjected to the same whisker clipping paradigm, but whose whiskers were allowed to regrow and resume normal whisking activity for at least 72 hours, the maps shift to their normal configuration (cf. Fig. 5-1). *B:* Maps of cortical representation zones in the motor cortex of *adult rats* following whisker trimming. The whisker representation is significantly reduced in size and surrounded by regions from which no movements could be evoked. (Modified from Keller et al., 1996.)

thetic block of peripheral nerves produces a rapid reorganization of movement representations, which reverses rapidly following cessation of the anesthesia (Brasil-Neto et al., 1992, 1993). Similar reversible changes can be produced by limb immobilization (Liepert et al., 1995). Substantial reorganization of movement representations occurs in amputees (Hall et al., 1990; Ojemann and Silbergeld, 1995; Pascual-Leone et al., 1996) and following brain injury during the perinatal period (Cao et al., 1994) and during adulthood (Seitz et al., 1995). Particularly pertinent are findings that, during the acquisition of a motor task, the cortical representations of movements involved in the task are increased and return to their baseline topography following skill acquisition (Pascual-Leone et al., 1994).

In proficient Braille readers, the cortical representation of the first dorsal interosseous muscle (FDI; the muscle responsible for the reading task) is significantly larger in the hemisphere contralateral to the reading hand compared with the ipsilateral FDI representation, whereas no such interhemispheric differences occur in nonproficient Braille readers (Pascual-Leone et al., 1993, 1995). Furthermore, the representation of FDI in the reading hand of proficient Braille readers becomes significantly larger after 6 hours of Braille reading compared with its size following a 2-day rest period (Pascual-Leone et al., 1995). Thus, these data demonstrate that movement representations in the human motor cortex, like those in other mammalian species, may be continuously subject to dramatic, and reversible, use-dependent changes.

Role of Intracortical Connection in Motor Cortex Plasticity

Use-dependent pliability of functional representations has been studied extensively in sensory areas of the cerebral cortex (see Merzenich et al., 1988). In both the visual cortex and somatosensory cortex, this plasticity is mediated, at least in part, by changes in intracortical synaptic interactions (e.g., Das and Gilbert, 1995; Fox, 1994). It is reasonable, therefore, to predict that intracortical interactions are involved also in use-dependent plasticity in the motor cortex. Several lines of evidence support this hypothesis.

Analyses of the arborization patterns of intracortical axons reveal that they form a potential anatomical substrate for synaptic plasticity. For example, although most intracortical axons originating from the whisker region of the rat motor cortex terminate within that region, some axons "invade" the immediately adjacent forelimb representation (Fig. 5-2). Huntley (1997) recently demonstrated that the extent to which the border between the whisker and forelimb regions may shift (following peripheral nerve lesions) correlates with—and is presumably constrained by—the extent of horizontal axons traversing the border between these representations zones. The existence of such "heterotypical" connections suggests that the synapses they form are normally inoperative, or "silent" (e.g., Isaac et al., 1995). Were they not "silent," ICMS in the whisker region would result in postsynaptic activation of cells in the forelimb region, producing combined forelimb and whisker movements (a rare phenomenon). If the efficacy of these "silent" synapses is enhanced, regions that normally represent whisker movements could immediately shift to become forelimb representations. This may occur in response to changes in sensorimotor activity related to a particular movement pattern, such as that occurring following whisker clipping, limb immobilization, or motor learning, as described above.

A critical requisite for the hypothesis described above is the existence of a mechanism by which the efficacy of intracortical synaptic interactions can be enhanced. Several plausible mechanisms have been identified in the motor cortex. The first is related to the induction of long-term potentiation (LTP), a use-dependent increase in synaptic efficacy (Cruikshank and Weinberger, 1996). Several studies have demonstrated that "Hebbian"* activation of synapses in the motor cortex results in a long-lasting enhancement of synaptic efficacies (Baranyi and Fehér, 1981; Baranyi et al., 1991; Iriki et al., 1989; Keller et al., 1990b, 1991). Most significantly, repetitive activation of intracortical, horizontal connections within the motor cortex can induce LTP of synaptic interactions mediated by these pathways (Aroniadou and Keller, 1995; Castro-Alamancos et al., 1995; Hess et al., 1996; Hess and Donoghue, 1996b). A persistent *decrease* in synaptic efficacy—long-term depression (LTD)—can also be induced in these intracortical pathways (Hess and Donoghue, 1996a, b). Thus, LTP and LTD, by modulating the efficacies of intracortical synaptic interactions, may be involved in shaping movement representations in the motor cortex.

Another potential mechanism for the pliability of motor maps is the modulation of GABA-mediated inhibition. Jacobs and Donoghue (1991) demonstrated that suppressing cortical GABAergic inhibition results in immediate shifts in the borders between movement representation zones. This suggests that GABAergic inhibition normally masks excitatory interactions between "inappropriate" representation zones (Jacobs et al., 1991; Jacobs and Donoghue, 1991). Modulation of this GABA-mediated process may result in rapid reorganization of movement representations.

Thus, enhancement of synaptic efficacies of specific intracortical pathways—by either Hebbian plasticity or modulation of inhibition—may reinforce interactions among neurons within cortical modules involved in different aspects of the same movement pattern. This process may be involved in establishing an engram for motor learning by shaping the temporal interactions between cortical modules related to different movement components of a learned motor skill. Similar processes may also be involved in mediating the recovery from neurological deficits related to voluntary movements.

Synaptogenesis in the Motor Cortex

An important mechanism postulated to mediate learning and memory processes in general (Cajal, 1911), and motor learning in particular (Anderson et al., 1996; Asanuma and Keller, 1991a, b), is the *de novo* formation of synapses. The hy-

---

*Donald Hebb, in his treatise *The Organization of Behavior* (1949), suggested that use-dependent synaptic modifications are involved in learning. In its simplest form, Hebb's synaptic modification rule states that the efficacy of a synapse would be enhanced when there is simultaneous activity in its pre- and postsynaptic elements.

pothesis that experience-mediated synaptic proliferation is a mechanism for in-formation storage is particularly attractive for motor learning because new motor skills—once acquired—are known to persist for remarkably long periods of time. Such a long-lasting engram is likely to involve persistent structural changes in the functional organization of the relevant brain structures. Similarly, the persistence of functional changes associated with the recovery from neurological deficits in motor functions, and the relatively slow onset of these changes (e.g., Pascual-Leone et al., 1996), suggest a role for synaptogenesis in this recovery process.

The capacity of the central nervous system of adult mammals to undergo synap-tic remodeling has been demonstrated repeatedly (see Flohr, 1988; Greenough and Chang, 1988; Weiler et al., 1995). Synaptogenesis in the mature brain has been demonstrated most conclusively in response to lesions of direct, as well as indirect, afferents to various brain regions (Ichikawa et al., 1987; Lund and Lund, 1971; Raisman, 1969; Vaughan and Peters, 1985). For example, lesions of the deep cere-bellar nuclei in adult cats result in sprouting of corticocortical inputs from the so-matosensory to the motor cortex (Keller et al., 1990a). These new synapses may be involved in the functional recovery from cerebellar ataxia induced by these le-sions because lesions of the somatosensory cortex—subsequent to the recovery from the ataxic symptoms—cause the neurological deficits to reappear (Keller et al., 1990a; see also Bornschlegl and Asanuma, 1987). Synaptogenesis can also oc-cur in the absence of neurological damage; several studies have demonstrated synaptogenesis in the mature brain following enhanced synaptic activation, evoked by repetitive electrical stimulation or training paradigms (see Weiler et al., 1995).

Greenough and collaborators have shown that acquisition of motor skills by adult rats is associated with the formation of new synapses in both the motor cor-tex and the cerebellum (see Anderson et al., 1996; Kleim et al., 1996, 1997). We demonstrated that 4 days of patterned stimulation of corticocortical afferents to the motor cortex of adult cats results in a significant increase in the number of syn-apses in the motor cortex (Keller et al., 1992).

Data demonstrating use-dependent synaptic proliferation in the mature motor cortex provide support for the postulate that rearrangement of synaptic circuitry plays an important role in normal motor function. These findings suggest that neur-al circuits within the motor cortex can be dynamically rewired in response to chang-ing experiences. Thus, repeated practice of particular motor acts may produce changes in synaptic patterns within the motor cortex, and these structural changes may be responsible for the ability to store motor engrams for practically indefinite periods. Similar mechanisms are likely involved in the recovery from motor deficits.

References

This work was supported by PHS:NINDS grants NS31078 and NS35360.

Anderson, B. J., Alcantara, A. A., and Greenough, W. T. (1996). Motor-skill learning: Changes in synaptic organization of the rat cerebellar cortex. *Neurobiol. Learn. Mem-ory, 66,* 221–229.

Aroniadou, V. A., and Keller, A. (1993). The patterns and synaptic properties of horizontal intracortical connections in the rat motor cortex. *J. Neurophysiol., 70,* 1493–1553.

Aroniadou, V. A., and Keller, A. (1995). Mechanisms of LTP induction in rat motor cortex *in vitro. Cereb. Cortex, 5,* 353–362.

Asanuma, H. (1959). Microelectrode studies on the evoked activity of a single pyramidal tract cell in the somatosensory cortex. *Jpn. J. Physiol., 9,* 94–105.

Asanuma, H. (1981). Microstimulation technique. In M. M. Patterson and R. P. Kesner (eds.) *Electrical Stimulation Research Techniques.* New York: Academic Press, pp. 61–70.

Asanuma, H. (1989). *The Motor Cortex.* New York: Raven Press.

Asanuma, H., and Keller, A. (1991a). Neural mechanisms of motor learning in mammals. *NeuroReport, 2,* 217–224.

Asanuma, H., and Keller, A. (1991b). Neurobiological basis of motor learning and memory. *Concepts Neurosci., 2,* 1–30.

Baranyi, A., and Fehér, O. (1981). Intracellular studies of cortical synaptic plasticity. Conditioning effects of antidromic activation on test-EPSPs. *Exp. Brain Res., 41,* 124–134.

Baranyi, A., Szente, M. B., and Woody, C. D. (1991). Properties of associative long-lasting potentiation induced by cellular conditioning in the motor cortex of conscious cats. *Neuroscience, 42,* 321–334.

Bornschlegl, M., and Asanuma, H. (1987). Importance of the projection from the sensory to the motor cortex for the recovery of motor function in the monkey. *Brain Res., 437,* 121–130.

Brasil-Neto, J. P., Cohen, L. G., Pascual-Leone, A., Jabir, F. K., Wall, R. T., and Hallett, M. (1992). Rapid reversible modulation of human motor outputs after transient deafferentation of the forearm: A study with transcranial magnetic stimulation. *Neurology, 42,* 1302–1306.

Brasil-Neto, J. P., Vallssole, J., Pascual-Leone, A., Cammarota, A., Amassian, V. E., Cracco, R., Maccabee, P., Cracco, J., Hallett, M., and Cohen, L. G. (1993). Rapid modulation of human cortical motor outputs following ischaemic nerve block. *Brain, 116,* 511–525.

Brown, T. G., and Sherrington, C. S. (1912). On the instability of a cortical point. *Proc. R. Soc. Lond. Biol., 85,* 250–277.

Burke, D., Hicks, R., and Stephen, J. (1992). Anodal and cathodal stimulation of the upper-limb area of the human motor cortex. *Brain, 115,* 1497–1508.

Cajal, S. (1911). Anatomicophysiological considerations on the cerebrum. In J. DeFelipe and E. G. Jones (eds.): *Cajal on the Cerebral Cortex. An Annotated Translation of the Complete Writings.* New York: Oxford University Press, pp. 465–490.

Cao, Y., Vikingstad, E. M., Huttenlocher, P. R., Towle, V. L., and Levin, D. N. (1994). Functional magnetic resonance studies of the reorganization of the human hand sensorimotor area after unilateral brain injury in the perinatal period. *Proc. Natl. Acad. Sci. U.S.A., 91,* 9612–9616.

Castro-Alamancos, M. A., Donoghue, J. P., and Connors, B. W. (1995). Different forms of synaptic plasticity in somatosensory and motor areas of the neocortex. *J. Neurosci., 15,* 5324–5333.

Cruikshank, S. J., and Weinberger, N. M. (1996). Evidence for the Hebbian hypothesis in experience-dependent physiological plasticity of neocortex: A critical review. *Brain Res. Rev., 22,* 191–228.

Das, A., and Gilbert, C. D. (1995). Long-range horizontal connections and their role in cortical reorganization revealed by optical recording of cat primary visual cortex. *Nature, 375,* 780–784.

DeFelipe, J., Conley, J., and Jones, E. G. (1986). Long-range focal collateralization of axons arising from corticocortical cells in monkey sensory-motor cortex. *J. Neurosci., 6,* 3749–3766.

Donoghue, J. P., Leibovic, S., and Sanes, J. N. (1992). Organization of the forelimb area in squirrel monkey motor cortex: Representation of digit, wrist, and elbow muscles. *Exp. Brain Res., 89,* 1–19.

Donoghue, J. P., and Sanes, J. (1991). Dynamic modulation of primate motor cortex output during movement. *Soc. Neurosci. Abstr., 21,* 1022.

Donoghue, J. P., Suner, S., and Sanes, J. N. (1990). Dynamic organization of primary motor cortex output to target muscles in adult rats. II. Rapid reorganization following motor nerve lesions. *Exp. Brain Res., 79,* 492–503.

Evarts, E. V. (1986). Motor cortex output in primates. In E. G. Jones and A. Peters (eds.): *Cerebral Cortex, vol. 5: Sensory Motor Areas and Aspects of Cortical Connectivity.* New York: Plenum Press, pp. 217–241.

Ferrier, D. (1873). Experimental researches in cerebral physiology and pathology. *West Riding Lunatic Asylum Rep., 3,* 1–50.

Fetz, E. E. (1992). Are movement parameters recognizably coded in the activity of single neurons? *Behav. Brain. Sci., 15,* 679–690.

Finger, S. (1994). *Origin of Neuroscience: A History of Explorations into Brain Function.* New York: Oxford University Press.

Flohr, H. (1988). *Post-Lesion Neural Plasticity.* Berlin: Springer-Verlag.

Fox, K. (1994). The cortical component of experience-dependent synaptic plasticity in the rat barrel cortex. *J. Neurosci., 14,* 7665–7679.

Fritsch, G., and Hitzig, E. (1870). Über die elektrische Erregbarkeit des Grosshirns. *Arch. Anat. Physiol. Wissen. Med., 37,* 300–332.

Gatter, K. C., and Powell, T. P. S. (1978). The intrinsic connections of the cortex of area 4 of the monkey. *Brain, 101,* 513–541.

Ghosh, S., Fyffe, R. E. W., and Porter, R. (1988). Morphology of neurons in area 4γ of the cat's cortex studied with intracellular injection of HRP. *J. Comp. Neurol., 269,* 290–312.

Greenough, W. T., and Chang, F. F. (1988). Plasticity of synapse structure and pattern in the cerebral cortex. In A. Peters and E. G. Jones (eds.): *Cerebral Cortex, vol. 7. Development and Maturation of Cerebral Cortex.* New York: Plenum Press.

Hall, E. J., Flament, D., Fraser, C., and Lemon, R. N. (1990). Non-invasive brain stimulation reveals reorganised cortical outputs in amputees. *Neurosci. Lett., 116,* 379–386.

Hebb, D. O. (1949). *The Organization of Behavior: A Neuropsychological Theory.* New York: John Wiley and Sons.

Hess, G., Aizenman, C. D., and Donoghue, J. P. (1996). Conditions for the induction of long-term potentiation in layer II/III horizontal connections of the rat motor cortex. *J. Neurophysiol., 75,* 1765–1778.

Hess, G., and Donoghue, J. P. (1996a). Long-term depression of horizontal connections in rat motor cortex. *Eur. J. Neurosci., 8,* 658–665.

Hess, G., and Donoghue, J. P. (1996b). Long-term potentiation and long-term depression of horizontal connections in rat motor cortex. *Acta Neurobiol. Exp., 56,* 397–405.

Hess, G., Jacobs, K. M., and Donoghue, J. P. (1994). N-methyl-D-aspartate receptor mediated component of field potentials evoked in horizontal pathways of rat motor cortex. *Neurosci., 61,* 225–235.

Humphrey, D. R. (1986). Representation of movements and muscles within the primate precentral motor cortex: Historical and current perspectives. *Fed. Proc., 45,* 2687–2699.

Huntley, G. W. (1997). Correlation between patterns of horizontal connectivity and the extent of short-term representational plasticity in rat motor cortex. *Cereb. Cortex, 7,* 143–156.

Huntley, G. W., and Jones, E. G. (1991). Relationship of intrinsic connections to forelimb movement representations in monkey motor cortex: A correlative anatomic and physiological study. *J. Neurophysiol., 66,* 390–413.

Ichikawa, M., Arissian, K., and Asanuma, H. (1987). Reorganization of the projection from the sensory cortex to the motor cortex following elimination of the thalamic projection to the motor cortex in cats: Golgi, electron microscope and degeneration study. *Brain Res., 437,* 131–141.

Iriki, A., Pavlides, C., Keller, A., and Asanuma, H. (1989). Long term potentiation in the motor cortex. *Science, 245,* 1385–1387.

Isaac, J. T. R., Nicoll, R. A., and Malenka, R. C. (1995). Evidence for silent synapses—Implications for the expression of LTP. *Neuron, 15,* 427–434.

Jacobs, K. M., Connors, B. W., and Donoghue, J. P. (1991). Layer V contains a substrate for reorganization of motor cortex maps. *Soc. Neurosci. Abstr., 17,* 311.

Jacobs, K. M., and Donoghue, J. P. (1991). Reshaping the cortical motor map by unmasking latent intracortical connections. *Science, 251,* 944–947.

Jankowska, E., Padel, Y., and Tanaka, R. (1975). Projections of pyramidal tract cells to alpha-motoneurons innervating hindlimb muscles in the monkey. *J. Physiol. (Lond.), 249,* 637–669.

Jones, E. G., Coulter, J. D., and Hendry, S. H. C. (1978). Intracortical connectivity of architectonic fields in the somatic sensory, motor and parietal cortex of monkeys. *J. Comp. Neurol., 181,* 291–348.

Keller, A. (1993a). Intrinsic synaptic organization of the motor cortex. *Cereb. Cortex, 3,* 430–441.

Keller, A. (1993b). Patterns of intrinsic connections between motor representation zones in the cat motor cortex. *NeuroReport, 4,* 515–518.

Keller, A. (1996). Exploring the functions of the motor cortex: Hiroshi Asanuma's legacy. *NeuroReport, 7,* 2253–2260.

Keller, A., Arissian, K., and Asanuma, H. (1990a). Formation of new synapses in the cat motor cortex following lesions of the deep cerebellar nuclei. *Exp. Brain Res., 80,* 23–33.

Keller, A., Arissian, K., and Asanuma, H. (1992). Synaptic proliferation in the motor cortex of adult cats following long-term thalamic stimulation. *J. Neurophysiol., 68,* 295–308.

Keller, A., and Asanuma, H. (1993). Synaptic relationships involving local axon collaterals of pyramidal neurons in the cat motor cortex. *J. Comp. Neurol., 336,* 229–242.

Keller, A., Iriki, A., and Asanuma, H. (1990b). Identification of neurons producing LTP in the cat motor cortex: Intracellular recordings and labeling. *J. Comp. Neurol., 300,* 47–60.

Keller, A., Miyashita, E., and Asanuma, H. (1991). Minimal stimulus parameters and the effects of hyperpolarization on the induction of long-term potentiation in the cat motor cortex. *Exp. Brain Res., 87,* 295–302.

Keller, A., Weintraub, N. D., and Miyashita, E. (1996). Tactile experience determines the organization of movement representations in rat motor cortex. *NeuroReport, 7,* 2373–2378.

Kleim, J. A., Lussnig, E., Schwarz, E. R., Comery, T. A., and Greenough, W. T. (1996). Synaptogenesis and FOS expression in the motor cortex of the adult rat after motor skill learning. *J. Neurosci., 16,* 4529–4535.

Kleim, J. A., Vij, K., Ballard, D. H., and Greenough, W. T. (1997). Learning-dependent synaptic modifications in the cerebellar cortex of the adult rat persist for at least four weeks. *J. Neurosci., 17,* 717–721.

Kwan, H. C., Murphy, J. T., and Wong, Y. C. (1987). Interaction between neurons in the precentral cortical zones controlling different joints. *Brain Res., 400,* 259–269.

Landry, P., Labelle, A., and Deschênes, M. (1980). Intracortical distribution of axonal collaterals of pyramidal tract cells in the cat motor cortex. *Brain Res., 191,* 327–336.

Lashley, K. S. (1923). Temporal variations in the function of the gyrus precentralis in primates. *Am. J. Physiol., 65,* 585–602.

Lemon, R. N. (1990). Mapping the output functions of the motor cortex. In G. M. Edelman, W. E. Gall, and W. M. Cowan (eds.): *Signal and Sense.* New York: Wiley-Liss, pp. 315–355.

Li, C.-S., and Waters, R. S. (1991). Organization of the mouse motor cortex studies by retrograde tracing and intracortical microstimulation (ICMS) mapping. *Can. J. Neurol. Sci., 18,* 28–38.

Liepert, J., Tegenthoff, M., and Malin, J.-P. (1995). Changes of cortical motor area size during immobilization. *Electromyogr. Motor Control, 97,* 382–386.

Lund, R. D., and Lund, J. S. (1971). Modification of synaptic patterns in the superior colliculus of the rat during development and following deafferentation. *Vis. Res., Suppl., No. 3,* 281–298.

Matsumura, M., Sawaguchi, T., Oishi, T., Ueki, K., and Kubota, K. (1991). Behavioral deficits induced by local injection of bicuculline and muscimol into the primate motor and premotor cortex. *J. Neurophysiol., 65,* 1542–1553.

Merzenich, M. M., Recanzone, G., Jenkins, W. M., Allard, T. T., and Nudo, R. J. (1988). Cortical representational plasticity. In P. Rakic and W. Singer (eds.): *Neurobiology of Neocortex.* New York: Wiley, pp. 41–67.

Milliken, G. W., Nudo, R. J., Grenda, R., Jenkins, W. M., and Merzenich, M. M. (1992). Expansion of distal forelimb representations in primary motor cortex of adult squirrel monkeys following motor training. *Soc. Neurosci. Abstr.,* 8:506.

Murphy, J. T., Kwan, H. C., and Wong, Y. C. (1985). Cross correlation studies in primate motor cortex: Synaptic interactions and shared input. *Can. J. Sci. Neurol. Sci., 12,* 11–23.

Nudo, R. J., Jenkins, W. M., and Merzenich, M. M. (1990). Repetitive microstimulation alters the cortical representation of movements in adult rats. *Somatosens. Motor Res., 7,* 463–483.

Nudo, R. J., and Milliken, G. W. (1996). Reorganization of movement representations in primary motor cortex following focal ischemic infarcts in adult squirrel monkeys. *J. Neurophysiol., 75,* 2144–2149.

Nudo, R. J., Milliken, G. W., Jenkins, W. M., and Merzenich, M. M. (1996a). Use-dependent alterations of movement representations in primary motor cortex of adult squirrel monkeys. *J. Neurosci., 16,* 785–807.

Nudo, R. J., Wise, B. M., Sifuentes, F., and Milliken, G. W. (1996b). Neural substrates for the effects of rehabilitative training on motor recovery after ischemic infarct. *Science, 272,* 1791–1794.

Ojemann, J. G., and Silbergeld, D. L. (1995). Cortical stimulation mapping of phantom limb Rolandic cortex—Case report. *J. Neurosurg., 82,* 641–644.

Pascual-Leone, A., Cammarota, W., Wassermann, E. M., Brasil-Neto, J. P., Cohen, L. G., and Hallett, M. (1993). Modulation of motor cortical outputs to the reading hand of braille readers. *Ann. Neurol., 34,* 33–37.

Pascual-Leone, A., Grafman, J., and Hallett, M. (1994). Modulation of cortical motor output maps during development of implicit and explicit knowledge. *Science, 263,* 1287–1289.

Pascual-Leone, A., Peris, M., Tormos, J. M., Pascual-Leone Pascual, A., and Catalá, M. D. (1996). Reorganization of human cortical motor output maps following traumatic forearm amputation. *NeuroReport, 7,* 2068–2070.

Pascual-Leone, A., Wassermann, E. M., Sadato, N., and Hallett, M. (1995). The role of reading activity on the modulation of motor cortical outputs to the reading hand in braille readers. *Ann. Neurol., 38,* 910–915.

Penfield, W., and Boldrey, E. (1937). Somatic motor and sensory representation in the cerebral cortex of man as studied by electrical stimulation. *Brain, 60,* 389–443.

Raisman, G. (1969). Neuronal plasticity in the septal nuclei of the adult rat. *Brain Res., 14,* 25–48.

Sanes, J. N., Wang, J., and Donoghue, J. P. (1992). Immediate and delayed changes of rat motor cortical output representation with new forelimb configurations. *Cereb. Cortex, 2,* 141–152.

Sanes, J. S., and Donoghue, J. P. (1997). Static and dynamic organization of motor cortex. In H.-J. Freund, B. A. Sabel, and O. W. Witte (eds.): *Brain Plasticity, Advances in Neurology, Vol. 73.* Philadelphia: Lippincott-Raven, pp. 277–296.

Sanes, J. S., Donoghue, J. P., Thangaraj, V., Edelman, R. R., and Warach, S. (1995). Shared neural substrates controlling hand movements in human motor cortex. *Science, 268,* 1775–1777.

Schieber, M. H., and Hibbard, L. S. (1993). How somatotopic is the motor cortex hand area? *Science, 261,* 489–492.

Seitz, R. J., Huang, Y. X., Knorr, U., Tellmann, L., Herzog, H., and Freund, H.-J. (1995). Large-scale plasticity of the human motor cortex. *NeuroReport, 6,* 742–744.

Shibasaki, H., Sadato, N., Lyshkow, H., Yonekura, Y., Honda, M., Nagamine, T., Suwazono, S., Magata, Y., Ikeda, A., Miyazaki, M., Fukuyama, H., Asato, R., and Konishi, J. (1993). Both primary motor cortex and supplementary motor area play an important role in complex finger movement. *Brain, 116,* 1387–1398.

Shinoda, Y., Arnold, A. P., and Asanuma, H. (1976). Spinal branching of corticospinal axons in the cat. *Exp. Brain Res., 26,* 215–234.

Vaughan, D. W., and Peters, A. (1985). Proliferation of thalamic afferents in cerebral cortex altered by callosal deafferentation. *J. Neurocytol., 14,* 705–716.

Wassermann, E. M., Mcshane, L. M., Hallett, M., and Cohen, L. G. (1992). Noninvasive mapping of muscle representations in human motor cortex. *Electroencephalogr. Clin. Neurol., 85,* 1–8.

Waters, R. S., Samulack, D. D., Dykes, R. W., and Mckinley, P. A. (1990). Topographic organization of baboon primary motor cortex: Face, hand, forelimb, and shoulder representation. *Somatosens. Motor Res., 7,* 485–514.

Weiler, I. J., Hawrylak, N., and Greenough, W. T. (1995). Morphogenesis in memory formation: Synaptic and cellular mechanisms. *Behav. Brain Res., 66,* 1–6.

Weiss, D. S., and Keller, A. (1994). Specific patterns of intrinsic connections between representation zones in the rat motor cortex. *Cerebr. Cortex, 4,* 205–214.

Woody, C. D., and Black-Cleworth, P. (1973). Differences in excitability of cortical neurons as a function of motor projection in conditioned cats. *J. Neurophysiol., 36,* 1104–1116.

Woolsey, C. N. (1964). Cortical localization as defined by evoked potentials and electrical stimulation studies. In G. Schaltembrand and C. N. Woolsey (eds.): *Cerebral Localization and Organization.* Madison: University of Wisconsin Press.

6

Immature Visual Cortex Lesions: Global Rewiring, Neural Adaptations, and Behavioral Sparing

BERTRAM R. PAYNE

Little is known about either the multiple repercussions of focal cerebral cortical lesions in young brains or the role that neuroplasticity plays in ameliorating the potentially devastating aftereffects. Besides comparisons of the behaviors and brain images of normal children and those who have either incurred some form of damage or experienced some form of maldevelopment of brain structures, little progress in our understanding can be made without resorting to studies of the repercussions of lesions incurred early in life by animals. Such studies both permit specific, circumscribed, and highly reproducible lesions to be made and allow for accurate assessments and linkages to be established between the repercussions of the lesions on anatomy of brain connections, physiological properties and responsiveness of neurons, and, the final expression of brain connections and neural function, behavior. It is our goal to establish these linkages between anatomy, physiology, and behavior in cats, which sustained removal of primary visual cortex either shortly after birth or at 1 month of age, as a model for understanding the repercussions of focal lesions in fetal and perinatal human infants. As can be readily appreciated from this book, detailed knowledge on the repercussions of focal lesions in human fetuses, infants, and children is limited.

At the outset it is important to recognize that in the system we are studying many of the anatomical rewirings following focal lesions are *specific* and *ordered* and that they contribute to both neuronal compensations and spared, ordered behaviors. Thus, following the lesion, the connections and function of pathways and circuits are shaped into new, useful forms and channeled into new, useful functions both of which are retained into adult life. These new forms and functions make both the brain and the individual more fit for existence and optimize the individual's useful interactions with the environment under the new conditions. In this

114

way, and because the pathways and circuits have changed in a positive useful way, the rewirings can be considered *adaptive*. Such positive features are a distinguishing characteristic of the *plastic* capacities of the brain that operate to ameliorate the otherwise debilitating effects of lesions. This is an important point because nonspecific and disordered alterations in pathways and function can also be induced by lesions. However, alterations in this negative, nonbeneficial direction are maladaptive, impair neural function, and do not contribute to organized behavior. Thus, demonstration of highly specific alterations in neuronal connectivity coupled with evidence of both neuronal compensations and effective ordered behaviors following lesions incurred early in life argues forcefully for a *substantial latent flexibility* of the immature brain to overcome major challenges to its normal development. This flexibility does not appear to be a major feature of either nonfocal lesions or multifactorial maldevelopment. In these instances the immature brain appears to be largely incapable of overcoming the widespread impairments, and many aspects of organized complex cerebral- and cerebellar-based behaviors are absent.

It is likely that individuals with focal lesions fare better because systemwide adjustments can occur between components within a highly interconnected neural system, or network, in some reasonable and coherent way. In contrast, nonfocal lesions and multifactorial maldevelopment act simultaneously on multiple neural systems. Accordingly potential coherence of neural compensations within individual neural systems may be masked or counteracted by interactions at network nodes where systems intersect. Such masking or counteractions preclude the establishing of ordered connections, development of neural compensations, and organized behaviors.

The information we have obtained on the plasticity of neural connections and repercussions of early focal lesions in the visual cortex of cats is significant in its own right and for understanding the consequences of circumscribed lesions elsewhere in the cortex and in other animals including humans. Many of our current thoughts on this topic and their relevance to both spared visual capacities and humans have been published recently (Payne et al., 1996b). Moreover, complementary evidence from other animal studies has appeared in recent years (Bachevalier and Mishkin, 1994; Bachevalier et al., 1990; Bertolino et al., 1997; Màlkovà et al., 1995; Moore et al., 1996; Webster et al., 1991b). These studies foster general conclusions similar to those we have reached on neuroplasticity in the visual system of the cat brain.

It is reasonable to ask: Why study the visual system, and why study the cat? It is sagacious to acknowledge that of all neural systems, the visual system is the best understood, and many of the general principles we have learned from it have proved applicable to other neural systems, at least those associated with the cerebral cortex. For studies on the visual system, the cat is an extremely good model animal because in broad terms there are many aspects of visual system connections, layout, and function that are similar to those of monkeys and, by extension, humans (Payne, 1993; Payne et al., 1996b). In the context of the current topic this similarity is attested to by limited evidence that indicates that surgical removals of visual cortex from young monkeys (Moore et al., 1996) and accidental and traumatic damage of visual cortex in infant humans and children (Barbur et al., 1993, 1994; Blythe et al., 1987) afford greater visual capacities than equivalent damage incurred by adults. Moreover, anatomical repercussions so far identified, and the factors influencing them, of early lesions in humans and monkeys are broadly similar to those identified for the cat (reviewed by Payne et al., 1996b). Nonetheless, it is important to affirm that details, magnitude, and complexity of monkey and human visual systems exceed those of the cat.

Also of great importance for valid transfer of knowledge between cats and primates is the great similarity in the developmental programs of the visual system that the species share (Payne et al., 1988; Rakic, 1977; Williams et al., 1989). However, it is important to recognize that the tempo of brain and visual system development in the cat is considerably faster than that of both monkeys and humans, and cats reach maturity well in advance of monkeys and humans. This greater tempo has distinct advantages for scientific investigations because it means that the broad group of studies we are carrying out on neuroplasticity in the cat visual system can be carried out over a reasonable period of years rather than over the period of decades that it would take to investigate the broad long-term consequences of early lesions in monkeys or human infants and children. Consequently, studies in the cat are likely to continue at a pace substantially faster than those of either monkeys or humans. In the next section I summarize the status of our knowledge of the sparing of visually guided behaviors following lesions of visual cortical areas 17 and 18 shortly after birth.

Sparing of Visually Guided Behaviors

What are the consequences of the early lesion of areas 17 and 18 on behavior? We have examined both cognitive and reflexive capacities mediated by cerebral cortex. Overall, many of the behaviors of cats with lesions incurred within a few days of birth are superior to the behaviors of cats with similar lesions incurred in adulthood. This higher level of performance is termed *sparing,* and it has been demonstrated for both learned and natural, or reflexive, visually guided behaviors. For example, cats with early lesions of areas 17 and 18 (Figs. 6-1 and 6-2) learn to discriminate an outline *I* shape from an outline *O* shape in substantially fewer trial errors than do cats with late lesions. In addition, under some conditions, cats with early lesions of areas 17 and 18 are able to learn complex-pattern discriminations involving a simple shape overlain with a grid masking pattern, as readily as intact cats, and much more adeptly than cats with equivalent lesions incurred in adulthood (P180; Figs. 6-3 and 6-4). One condition that allows complete, or almost complete, sparing on this task employs a procedure of increasing the complexity of the masking in a series of small steps, insuring that at each step the animal has mastered that level before progressing to the next (Cornwell et al., 1989). The performance of cats with lesions incurred in adulthood benefits from this ascending staircase procedure, but even with this assistance cats with lesions made in adulthood fail to acquire the series of discriminations as readily as the controls or the cats with lesions incurred in infancy. Sparing on this set of pattern of discriminations with overlain grids is also complete, or almost complete, if the lesions incurred in infancy are made in two stages with 3 days between operations (Cornwell and Payne, 1989). No special behavioral shaping procedures are needed to reveal the sparing if the lesions are made in two stages during the first 2 weeks of life (Cornwell and Payne, 1989).

Clearly, not all complex-pattern discrimination learning is spared after lesions of areas 17 and 18 incurred in infancy, at least if the lesions are made in one stage. When a simple shape is surrounded by a peripheral mask, cats with early lesions of areas 17 and 18 perform as poorly as cats with later lesions (Cornwell et al., 1989; Cornwell and Payne, 1989). No information is available on whether a method of increasing the peripheral masks in gradual steps would occasion relatively more sparing by cats with lesions made in infancy than by those with similar damage incurred in adulthood. It is clear, however, that cats with lesions incurred in two stages during infancy perform as well as unoperated cats on these complex discriminations and that an interoperative interval of only 3 days is sufficient to allow such complete sparing (Fig. 6-3) (Cornwell and Payne, 1989). These differences in levels of performance show that in adult cats areas 17 and 18 are critical for proficient performance on these pattern discrimination tasks. In the absence of these two areas performance is markedly depressed. In contrast, in cats with early lesions, proficiency is high and, relative to the data from the cats with the lesions incurred in adulthood, provides strong evidence for some kind of *neural compensation* somewhere in the cat's brain to *support* the highly proficient, *spared* behavioral *capacities.*

Similar conclusions have been reached for the partial or almost complete sparing of a number of reflexive visually guided behaviors modulated or guided by the cerebral cortex. The spared behaviors include orienting to novel stimuli introduced into the periphery of the visual field, monocular optokinetic nystagmus, and depth judgments as assessed on the visual cliff (Shupert et al., 1993). For example, in intact cats, detecting and orienting toward stimuli introduced at a variety of positions in the visual field is almost perfect within 60° of the visual field midline (Fig. 6-5, left), and it decreases toward the field periphery. In contrast, lesions of areas 17 and 18 incurred in adulthood severely impair performance on this task, which hovers about the 50% level of performance in the binocular part of the visual field, and much lower performance at the periphery. This difference between the intact and adult-lesioned cats shows that areas 17 and 18 are critical for proficient orienting in all parts of the visual field. In contrast, performance of cats with early lesions of areas 17 and 18 is far superior and approaches normal performance toward the center of the visual field and falls to a level of only ~75% on the fringes of the binocular field (Fig. 6-5, left) (Shupert et al., 1993). We conclude from the difference between the performance levels of the adult- and early-lesioned cats that the early lesions substantially spare detection and orienting behavior. Again, this sparing argues strongly for neural compensations somewhere in the cat's brain.

Suprasylvian cortex contributes importantly to behavioral competence on the re-

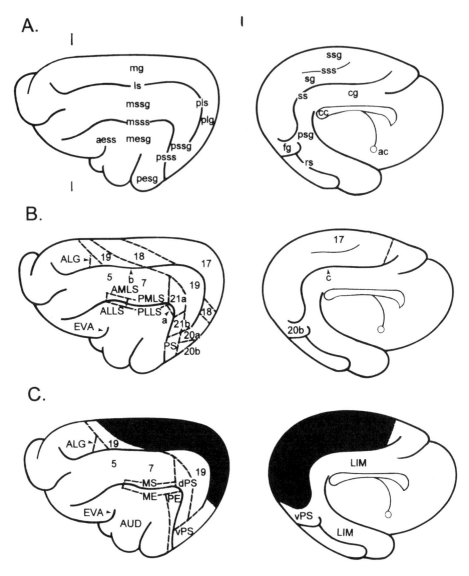

A.

B.

C.

Figure 6-1. *(A)* Dorsolateral (left) and medial (right) views of the left hemisphere of the cat illustrating gyri, sulci, and other pertinent structures. *(B)* The physiologically defined visual cortical areas of Kalia and Whitteridge (1973), Marcotte and Updyke (1982), Olson and Graybiel (1987), Tusa et al. (1981), and Updyke (1986). Arrowheads indicate cortical areas buried within sulci. a, dorsal and ventral lateral suprasylvian areas within the junction of the middle and posterior suprasylvian sulci (Tusa et al., 1981); b, area described by Marcotte and Updyke (1982) on the lateral bank of the lateral sulcus; c, splenial visual area on the upper bank close to the fundus of the cingular sulcus (Kalia and Whitteridge, 1973). *(C)* Anatomically defined cortical regions. Blackened region represents areas 17 and 18 and the cortical lesion. ac, anterior commissure; aess, anterior ectosylvian sulcus; ALG, anterolat-

flexive tasks because extension of the early cortical lesion beyond areas 17 and 18 to include area 19 and the middle and posterior suprasylvian regions reduces visually guided behaviors to levels determined for cats with lesions of areas 17 and 18 incurred in adulthood (Shupert et al., 1993). This can be seen clearly for cats tested for their ability to detect and orient to visual stimuli (cf. Fig. 6-5, left and right). We suspect that the sparing of behavioral capacities is importantly related to specific pathway expansions we have identified into and out of thalamus, extrastriate cortex, and midbrain that characterize the response of the brain to early lesions of areas 17 and 18. Moreover, the sparing is accompanied paradoxically with the death of specific neuronal populations in the visual system. In the next section I summarize both visual system connections in the intact cat and, following lesions of areas 17 and 18, the neuron degenerations and pathway expansions, the factors influencing these anatomical repercussions, and the evidence for neural compensations.

Global Rewiring of the Visual System

The major visual pathway originates in the retina and passes bilaterally through the magnocellular layers of the dorsal lateral geniculate nucleus (dLGN) to primary visual cortex, which is designated areas 17 and 18 in the cat, and then onto the supra- and ectosylvian extrastriate cortices (color plate I, A and B). In addition, there are two supplementary pathways that bypass primary visual cortex to reach supra- and ectosylvian cortices of which, for simplicity, we have selected one region for inclusion in the circuitry shown in color plate I (middle suprasylvian cortex [MS]). One of these pathways is minor and includes the parvocellular layers of dLGN, the medial interlaminar nucleus (MIN), and the retinal recipient zone of the pulvinar, and it projects directly to MS cortex. The second is more substantial and involves both superior colliculus and the lateral posterior complex. In addition, both primary and extrastriate cortex project to a number of subcortical structures, of which I depict the superior colliculus as a representative. In the superior

---

eral gyrus visual area; ALLS, anterior lateral lateral suprasylvian visual area; AMLS, anterior medial lateral suprasylvian visual area; AUD, auditory region; cc, corpus callosum; cg cingulate gyrus; DLS, dorsal lateral suprasylvian visual area; EVA, ectosylvian visual area; fg, fusiform gyrus; LIM, limbic cortex; ls, lateral sulcus; ME, middle ectosylvian region; mesg, middle ectosylvian gyrus; mg, marginal gyrus; MS, middle suprasylvian region; mssg, middle supraslyvian gyrus; msss, middle suprasylvian sulcus; MU, visual area of Marcotte and Updyke (1982); PE, posterior ectosylvian region; pesg, posterior ectosylvian gyrus; plg, posterolateral gyrus; PLLS, posterior lateral lateral suprasylvian visual area; pls, posterolateral sulcus; PMLS, posterior medial lateral suprasylvian visual area; PS (v, d), posterior suprasylvian region (ventral and dorsal divisions); psg, postsplenial gyrus; pssg, posterior suprasylvian gyrus; psss, posterior suprasylvian sulcus; rs, rhinal sulcus; ss, splenial sulcus; ssg, suprasplenail gyrus; sss, suprasplenial sulcus; VLS, ventral lateral suprasylvian visual area; 5, area 5; 7, area 7; 17, area 17; 18, area 18; 19, area 19; 20 (a, b), area 20 (subdivisions a and b); 21 (a, b), area 21 (subdivisions a and b).

a. Intact

b. P180

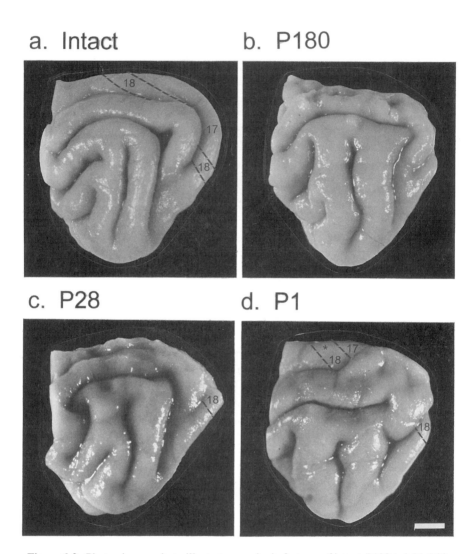

c. P28

d. P1

Figure 6-2. Photomicrographs to illustrate gross brain features of intact, P180 (adult), P28 (1 month of age), and P1 (day of birth) lesion cats. Note absence of significant distortion following lesions. Areas 17 and 18 in intact brains and fragments of same areas in lesioned brains are identified. See Figure 6-1 for identification of regions. *(A–C)* Lateral views. *(D)* Dorsolateral view. Bar = 5 mm.

colliculus, projections from areas 17 and 18 terminate heavily in the superficial layers, and projections from the MS cortex terminate more deeply, primarily in the stratum opticum.

The direct effect of lesions of primary visual cortex in adulthood is to remove the marginal and posterolateral gyri to expose the cingulate gyrus and spare the

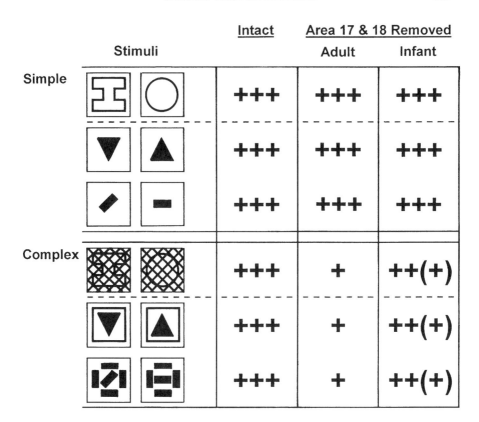

	Stimuli		Intact	Area 17 & 18 Removed	
				Adult	Infant
Simple			+++	+++	+++
			+++	+++	+++
			+++	+++	+++
Complex			+++	+	++(+)
			+++	+	++(+)
			+++	+	++(+)

Figure 6-3. Summary of visual capacities and defects for learned pattern discriminations. Relative performance of intact cats and cats that sustained lesions of areas 17 and 18 in adulthood or within a few days of birth. Simple stimuli: All cats can learn simple pattern discriminations and do not require the presence of primary visual cortex. Even so, the ease of learning by the cats with damage incurred in adulthood is less than for intact cats or cats with early damage. Complex stimuli: Adult-damaged cats have great difficulty learning the simple pattern discrimination when the patterns are either obscured by grid masks or surrounded by a peripheral border. Infant-damaged cats have less difficulty learning the same discriminations providing the level of masking is increased gradually or when lesions are incurred in two stages. This difference in levels of performance between cats with infant and with adult lesions argues for a neural compensation somewhere in the cat's brain to support the spared behavior. Data drawn from Cornwell et al. (1989) and Cornwell and Payne (1989). (Payne et al., 1996b)

supra- and ectosylvian regions (Fig. 6-2B). The net effect of this lesion is to disconnect suprasylvian cortex from the massive volume of signals passing through the magnocellular layers of LGN and to eliminate much of the cortical input from the superficial layers of superior colliculus (color plate I,B). However, the bypass pathways remain intact, and they support residual visual activity in some parts of suprasylvian cortex and superior colliculus, but the residual activity is markedly

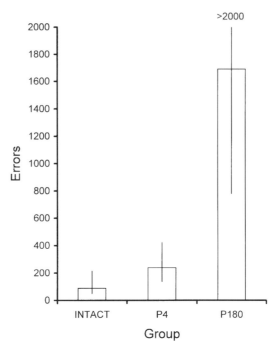

Figure 6-4. Comparison of number of errors made in the staircase acquisition of a 10-line masked outline I and O figures by intact cats and P4 and P180 ablation cats. Data on P4 and P180 cats are from Cornwell et al. (1989) and show median and first and third quartile values. P180 third quartile is more than 2,000 errors. I and O patterns with 10 masking lines across the patterns are shown in row 4 of Figure 6-3.

depressed, receptive field properties are less sophisticated than normal (Mendola and Payne, 1993; Guido et al., 1990b; Michalski et al., 1993; Spear and Baumann, 1979), and performance on many cerebrally linked, visually guided tasks is poor (for reviews, see Payne, 1993; Payne et al., 1996b).

Primary visual cortex lesions incurred during the first month after birth (Figs. 6-2C,D) also remove the marginal and posterolateral gyri, spare the supra- and ectosylvian regions, and disconnect suprasylvian regions from the major pathway emanating from the magnocellular layers of dLGN. In addition, there are constellations of *secondary specific regressive and progressive repercussions* that reverberate through the visual system to involve several regions distant from the focal damage. These distant, systemwide repercussions are understandable because the visual system is both a highly distributed and a highly interconnected network. The regressive repercussions include the death of specific neurons in dLGN, retina, and suprasylvian cortex and the progressive repercussions involving expansion and increased coupling between limbs of numerous pathways, identified with red in color plate I, that bypass damaged and degenerated regions. Together, the repercussions involve all major visual system structures. However, it is pertinent to note

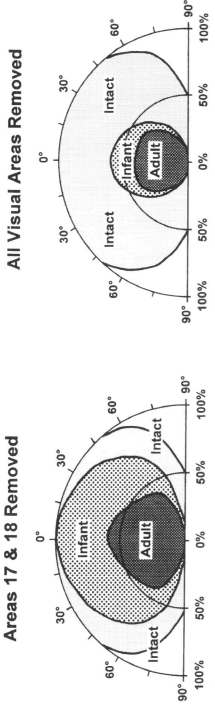

Areas 17 & 18 Removed

All Visual Areas Removed

Figure 6-5. Performances of intact cats and cats that incurred damage of primary visual cortex, either during infancy or adulthood, on a visual detection and orienting task. Binocular viewing condition. In this task the cat attends to a stimulus (the cynosure) introduced at 0° azimuth, and a second high incentive stimulus is introduced at one of the peripheral locations. If the cat orients strongly and promptly to the second stimulus the trial is scored as correct. For intact cats (light stipple), performance is virtually perfect 60° either side of the midline, and it drops off further toward the field periphery. (*Left*) Following damage of areas 17 and 18 incurred in adulthood, performance is poor at ~50% in the binocular field and lower at more peripheral locations (dense stipple). Equivalent damage incurred in infancy results in competent performance (≥75% for positions 60° either side of the midline; intermediate stipple). This level of performance compared with the poor performance of the adult lesioned cats is strong evidence for substantial sparing of orienting behavior. (*Right*) Same data from intact cats and data from cats that sustained removal of all contiguous visual areas of the middle and posterior suprasylvian regions in addition to areas 17 and 18. Removals were made either in adulthood or in infancy. Same stipple conventions apply. Note markedly inferior performance of infant-damaged cats compared with left side and the similarity with data on performance following later removal of areas 17 and 18 (left). This similarity reveals the contribution suprasylvian cortex makes to residual and spared behaviors and argues for functional compensations by neurons in the region or by neurons in associated circuits. Data drawn from Shupert et al. (1993). Figure reproduced from Payne et al., 1996b.

that the constellation of repercussions in cats that sustained lesions at 1 month of age differs from the constellation of effects in cats that incurred equivalent lesions within days of birth. These differences are likely linked in important ways to differences in maturational status of structures and levels of interconnectivity at the times the lesions are sustained. Even so, at both ages the rewirings are so extensive that the early-lesioned cats have a visual system, and indeed a brain, that is very different from either intact cats or cats that incurred equivalent lesions in adulthood. The repercussions of the early lesions identified so far are summarized below.

Regressive: Death of specific neurons

1. Specific death of neurons in extrastriate cortex highly connected with areas 17 and 18 (Payne et al., 1991).
2. Specific death of types II and III neurons in dLGN and their functional counterparts, β ganglion cells, in retina (Ault et al., 1993; Callahan et al., 1984; Kalil, 1984; MacNeil et al., 1997; Payne et al., 1984; Payne and Lomber, 1998; Pearson et al., 1981; Rowe, 1990; Tong et al., 1982; Tumosa et al., 1989). These neurons are normally highly connected with areas 17 and 18. The net result of these degenerations is to largely eliminate X* visual signals from the brain.

Progressive: Expansion of specific pathways

1. Expansion and increased coupling in the ascending retino-geniculo-MS pathway (Kalil and Behan, 1987; Kalil et al., 1991; Lomber et al., 1993, 1995; MacNeil et al., 1997; Tong et al., 1984; Payne and Lomber, 1998).
2. Expansion of the ascending retino-lateral posterior/pulvinar-MS projections (Labar et al., 1981; Lomber et al., 1995; Payne et al., 1993).
3. Expansion of the transcortical projection from the ventral posterior suprasylvian region (vPS) cortex to the MS cortex (MacNeil et al., 1996).
4. Expansion of the descending projection from MS cortex to stratum opticum

---

X signals arise from β retinal ganglion cells that have small receptive fields and high sensitivity to low contrasts. They extend visual capabilities into fine spatial and the low contrast domains, and they likely contribute greatly to dynamic range of contrast sensitivity, high spatial frequency cut-off and visual acuity; and they are implicated in local aspects of vision. Y signals arise from α retinal ganglion cells that have larger receptive fields and poor sensitivity to low contrasts. They extend visual capabilities into the high temporal domain, and they likely contribute to detection and temporal aspects of vision; and they are implicated in coarse and more global aspects of spatial vision. Both X and Y signals are brisk, and, up to the limit of α-cell acuity, α-cell activity dominates β-cell activity and α cells are superior to β cells at stimulus detection (Hughes et al., 1984; Kimchi, 1992; Robertson and Lamb, 1991; Shapley and Perry, 1986; Shulman and Wilson, 1987; Wässle and Boycott, 1991). W signals arise from γ retinal ganglion cells. They are a rather heterogeneous group primarily concerned with peripheral ambient vision, and they are rather sluggish and have rather poorly defined functions (Stone, 1983). Under most circumstances and under high contrast conditions, Y signals are dominant, whereas X signals introduce acuity into the visual system. Under conditions of low spatial contrast, signals from β cells become increasingly important for form vision.

throughout the thickness of the superficial layers of the superior colliculus (Sun et al., 1994).

5. The net result of all of these pathway expansions is to increase the traffic throughout the remaining visual circuits of W and Y signals that originate from α and γ ganglion cells (Lomber et al., 1993, 1995; MacNeil et al., 1997; Payne et al., 1996b; Payne and Lomber, 1998).

Progressive: Neural compensations

The increased traffic of W and Y signals results in neural compensations in

1. C complex of LGN (Payne and Lomber, 1996)
2. MS cortex (Guido et al., 1992; Long et al., 1996; Spear et al., 1980; Tong et al., 1984)
3. Superior colliculus (Berman and Cynader, 1976; Mendola and Payne, 1993; Mize and Murphy, 1976; Stein and Magalhaes-Castro, 1975).

Degeneration of specific neurons

Patterns of connections and maturational status are two factors that influence the survival and death of neurons following lesions of primary visual cortex. Neurons normally highly connected with areas 17 and 18 are very vulnerable, whereas neurons only weakly or not connected at all with areas 17 and 18 are not. Following lesions of areas 17 and 18 shortly after birth the dLGN is only a fraction of its normal size, magnocellular layers are reduced to mere ghosts, whereas the parvocellular C complex is obvious (cf. Figs. 6-6A and 6-6B). In the magnocellular layers virtually every neuron dies, whereas numerous neurons survive in the parvocellular C complex (Fig. 6-6A). This differential pattern of death and survival is linked to the normally massive and sole projections of magnocellular neurons to areas 17 and 18 and the dispersed projections of parvocellular neurons across cortex from areas 17 and 18 to supra- and ectosylvian regions (e.g., Rosenquist, 1985; Sherman, 1985). The lesion axotomizes virtually all magnocellular neurons and large numbers die, whereas many parvocellular neurons projecting to nondamaged cortex survive or have the capacity to redirect damaged axons there. Note that a small number of magnocellular neurons are protected in some way from the damaging effects of the lesion, and they survive and establish permanent projections to extrastriate cortex.

The sensitivity of neurons to visual cortex damage in young cats is not confined to dLGN, but extends trans-synaptically out to the eye (Pearson et al., 1981) where the vast majority of β, and possibly a small number of γ, retinal ganglion cells also die (Fig. 6-7) (Payne et al., 1984; Payne and Lomber, 1998; Rowe, 1990; Tong et al., 1982). The degeneration of β retinal ganglion cells is matched by a massive withdrawal of retinal fibers from the degenerated magnocellular layers of dLGN (Figs. 6-6D and 6-7C) (Lomber et al., 1993; Payne et al., 1984). As in dLGN, the selective loss and survival of ganglion cells is linked to normal patterns of connections (Payne et al., 1984; Payne and Cornwell, 1994).

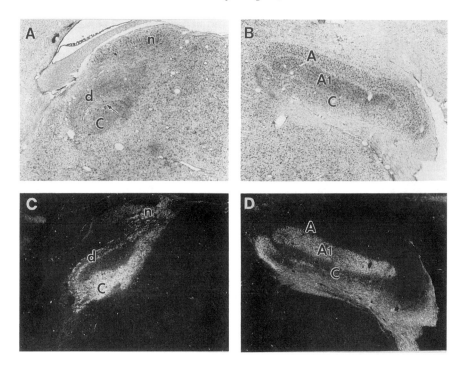

Figure 6-6. *(A, B)* Light field photomicrographs of dLGN in an adult cat after unilateral ablation of primary visual cortical areas 17 and 18 on the day of birth (A, dLGN ipsilateral to cortical ablation; B, dLGN ipsilateral to intact cortex). *(C, D)* Darkfield photomicrographs of the same sections in A and B to show the distribution of tritiated amino acids that had been injected into the eye (C, contralateral projections; D, ipsilateral projections). Layers A and A1 and the C complex are indicated. In the intact dLGN note dominant retinal projections to magnocellular layer A1 and very weak retinal projections to parvocellular C layers. In the degenerated dLGN note the reverse: greatly reduced projections to the severely degenerated ghost magnocellular layers and a massive increase in projections to the residual neurons in the C complex. Note that residual C neurons (A, arrow) are large and hypertrophied. d, Severely degenerated magnocellular layers A and A1; n, normal tail of dLGN that is connected to an intact, caudal portion of areas 17 and 18 in this instance. (Modified from Payne et al., 1984.)

Maturational status is also a factor linked to dLGN and ganglion cell survival following damage of primary visual cortex. For example, there is evidence of much less neuron death in the magnocellular layers of dLGN and little or no neuron death in retina following lesions of primary visual cortex sustained in adulthood (Color Plate IB) (Kalil, 1984; Tong et al., 1982; Callahan et al., 1984). Similar conclusions have also been reached about the role patterns of connectivity and maturational status play in the survival and death of extrastriate neurons highly or poorly connected with areas 17 and 18 (Payne et al., 1991). However, it is worth noting that under certain circumstances *mature* neurons and ganglion cells can be induced to die when

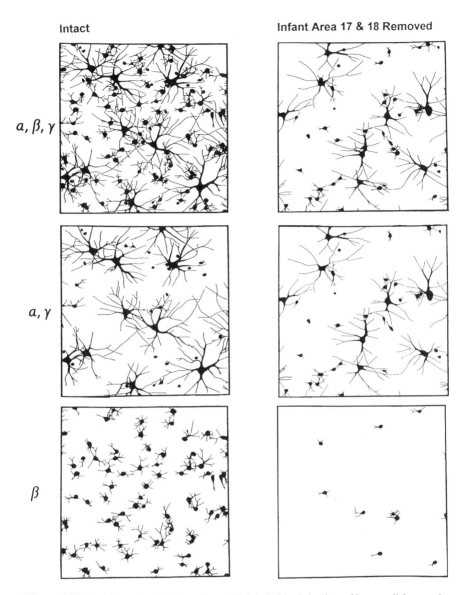

Figure 6-7. Drawings of retinal ganglion cells labeled by injection of horseradish peroxidase into an intact dLGN *(left)* and a dLGN of a cat that sustained a complete lesion of areas 17 and 18 shortly after birth *(right)*. Top row, α, β, and γ cells; middle row, α and γ cells; bottom row, β cells. Note: 1, In intact cats β cells are the most abundant cell type, being about 3 times as common as γ cells and about 10 times as common as α cells. 2, After the early lesion approximately 90% of β cells have been eliminated, yet all α and γ cells remain. 3, Some α cells are smaller than normal, and some γ cells are larger than normal. (From Payne et al., 1984.)

their sole or principal target neurons are eliminated rapidly by either ablation (e.g., dLGN, see above) or the application of neurotoxins (retinal ganglion cells) (Pearson and Stoffler, 1992; Pearson and Thompson 1993; Pearson et al., 1992).

Expansion of specific pathways

Even though there are many fewer neurons in the brains of early lesioned cats, many of those that remain *expand* their *projections* to bypass damaged or degenerated regions (color plate I, D and Figs. 6-8 and 6-9). Moreover, neuronal *coupling* in these pathways *increases* (Payne and Lomber, 1998). The pathway expansions induced include intraretinal circuits (not shown), projections arising from α and γ retinal ganglion cells to thalamus, ascending thalamic projections to cortex, transcortical projections, and descending cortical projections to the superior colliculus (see Progressive: Expansion of specific pathways for citation). It is not known if retinal projections into the superior colliculus or pretectum, or projections from these midbrain structures to the lateral-posterior/pulvinar complex, are modified by early cortical lesions in cats. However, it is known that lesions of primary visual cortex in adult monkeys modifies retinal projections to the pretectum (Dineen et al., 1982).

It is important to note that the anatomical repercussions of lesions incurred at the end of the first postnatal month differ from those incurred within days of birth (cf. Color Plate I, C and D). For example, coupling between retinal axons and dLGN neurons and the expansion of the projection from dLGN to MS cortex are both greater following lesions incurred at 1 month compared with on the day of birth (Lomber et al., 1995; Payne and Lomber, 1998). In contrast, the magnitude of the expanded MS cortical projection into the stratum griseum superficiale of the superior colliculus is more limited (Sun et al., 1994), and no expansions can be identified for projections from either the medial part of the lateral posterior nucleus or vPS cortex to MS cortex (Lomber et al., 1995; MacNeil et al., 1996). Expansions in these projections are considerable following lesions incurred on the day of birth (Lomber et al., 1995; MacNeil et al., 1996). These differences are understandable because the maturational status of a 1-month-old cat brain differs from that of a newborn (Payne et al., 1988, 1996b). In any event, whatever expansions that do occur following lesions at 1 month of age they too are likely to increase the brain traffic in Y- and W-based visual signals and possibly include a number of X signals because approximately 40% of β retinal ganglion cells survive area 17/18 lesions at that age (Callahan et al., 1984; Payne and Lomber, 1998).

We also suspect that other subcortical and transcortical pathways also expand to innervate structures deafferented by the early lesions of primary visual cortex and that they may do so differentially following lesions incurred at different developmental stages. But these suspicions need to be confirmed in future studies. If confirmed they too will likely implicate increased traffic in Y- and W-based visual signals in the rewired brains. Lastly, it is important to acknowledge that none of the adjustments in pathways described above accompany equivalent lesions in fully mature cats (Lomber et al., 1993, 1995; MacNeil et al., 1996; Payne and Cornwell, 1994; Payne and Lomber, 1998; Sun et al., 1994; Tong et al., 1984).

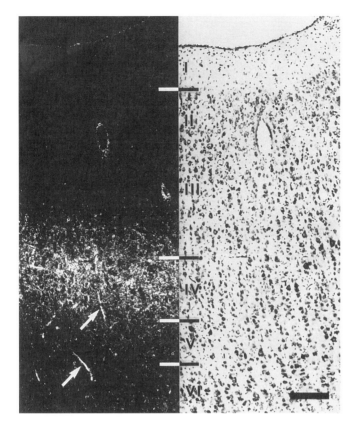

Figure 6-8. Darkfield photomicrograph to show the distribution of label transported from the eye via dLGN to MS cortex in a cat that sustained a lesion of areas 17 and 18 on the day of birth. High density label both corroborates the expanded retino-MS pathway and establishes the high degree of coupling between retinal axons and dLGN neurons. Presence of expanded projection and high degree of coupling have been verified with retrograde tracers (Payne and Lomber, 1998). Arrows indicate labeled axons. Equivalent data have been collected from cats that incurred like lesions at 1 month of age. No labeling is detected in MS cortex of intact cats or cats that sustained lesions of areas 17 and 18 in adulthood (Payne and Lomber, 1998). Bar = 200 μm. From Payne et al., 1996b.

Adjustments in Neural Activity and
Functional Compensations by Neurons

Following early lesions, pathways expand by the addition of extra neurons and by the enlargement of dendritic arbors and axonal fields, all of which are likely to contribute in a substantial way to increased coupling between neurons and to functional compensations. The addition of neurons to pathways increases the number of signals that are transmitted, while the enlargement of dendritic and axon arbors permits greater convergence of signals at the input to the neuron and greater di-

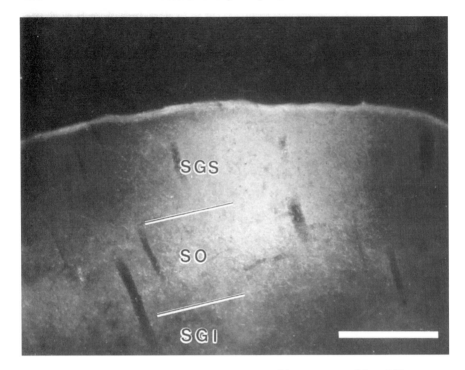

Figure 6-9. Wheatgerm agglutinin–horseradish peroxidase transported from MS cortex to the superior colliculus in a cat that sustained a bilateral removal of areas 17 and 18 on the day of birth. Note dense label throughout both stratum griseum superficiale (SGS) and stratum opticum (SO). This pattern of label is unusual because MS cortex in normal cats projects most densely into SO and the deep one third of SGS (Harting et al., 1992; Sun et al., 1994). This pattern of labeling shows that the MS projection has expanded to innervate the full thickness of SGS and physically substitute for the fibers from areas 17 and 18 that terminate in the upper two thirds of SGS. SGI, stratum griseum intermediale. Bar = 500 μm. Reproduced from Payne et al., 1996b.

vergence at the output. Together, the expansions and increased coupling between neurons also increase brain traffic of Y and W signals, likely raise signal transmission and transfer levels through the remains of the visual system, and contribute to functional compensations and to spared behavioral capacities. Evidence for functional compensation is provided by the near-normal levels of metabolic activity in dLGN and MS cortex of early lesioned cats as demonstrated by the cytochrome oxidase method (Long et al., 1996; Payne and Lomber, 1996) and by direct electrophysiological measurements taken from dLGN (Murphy and Kalil, 1979), MS, and posterior suprasylvian cortices (Cornwell et al., 1978; Doty, 1961; Guido et al., 1990a,b, 1992) and the superior colliculus (Berman and Cynader, 1976; Mendola and Payne, 1993; Mize and Murphy, 1976; Stein and Magalhaes-Castro, 1975). It is straightforward to understand how pathway expansions are adaptive and contribute to the neural compensations, but not the death of neurons and elimination of circuits. We interpret the deaths as purging the brain of poorly connected neurons, thereby eliminating unnecessary and inefficient computations, spurious signals, and erroneous damping of useful signals. The net outcome is a more efficient and accurate processing of signals in the remaining circuits, which we speculate is a prerequisite for near-normal neuronal processing and accurate performance on a number of perceptual and cognitive functions by cats with early lesions (Cornwell et al., 1989; Cornwell and Payne, 1989; Guido et al., 1990a, 1992; Mendola and Payne, 1993; Shupert et al., 1993).

This speculation is borne out by the substantial functional compensation neurons in MS cortex undergo following the lesion of areas 17 and 18 incurred on the day of birth. In MS cortex neurons develop receptive field properties that are largely indistinguishable from those in MS cortex of intact cats (Guido et al., 1990a, 1992; Spear et al., 1980; Tong et al., 1984) and quite different from the abnormal properties in MS cortex of cats that incurred lesions of areas 17 and 18 in adulthood (Guido et al., 1990b; Spear and Baumann, 1979). In both the early postnatal- and adult-lesioned cats, the visual signals driving neurons and guiding behavior are derived primarily from α (Y) and γ (W) ganglion cells. However, there is one important difference; the traffic in Y and W signals is considerably greater following lesions sustained early in life. This greater traffic likely has a major influence on the composition of neuronal receptive fields of cats with early-sustained lesions and on levels of neuronal activity. Even so, a major point to bear in mind is that in the same cats the composition of the retinal inner plexiform layer (IPL) is likely to be fundamentally different from that of the IPL of normal cats (Rowe, 1988). The implication is that the visual signals sent to the brain may differ fundamentally from those in normal cats, and this difference is likely to have a substantial impact on the subsequent processing of visual signals in all visual centers in the brain. However, even with that caveat we can still reach secure conclusions that lesions of areas 17 and 18 sustained early in life result in systemwide rewirings involving all major visual system structures and that these rewirings are accompanied by neural compensations and the sparing of visually guided behaviors. These repercussions are understandable because the visual system is a highly interconnected network.

Future Work on Cats

As is quite evident from the preceding sections, considerable progress has been made identifying in cats the systemwide anatomical repercussions of visual cortex lesions incurred early in postnatal life, and some progress has been made identifying neural compensations and spared visually guided behaviors. But where to go from here with the work on the repercussions of early lesions of areas 17 and 18?

In future studies it will be profitable to identify other behaviors that are spared by the lesions and start identifying behaviors that are impaired. We can certainly speculate that functions based on β retinal ganglion cells and X signals are likely severely impaired. These functions likely include detection and processing based on low contrasts, detection of high spatial frequencies, or both; and fine-grained segmentation and analyses of fine textures. We can also speculate that functions largely dominated by α and γ retinal ganglion cells and, respectively, Y and W signals will be spared. These functions likely include detection, temporal and coarse aspects of form vision, or both; and analyses of coarse textures.

In preliminary experiments we have obtained evidence that the sparing of pattern vision described earlier is limited to high contrast stimuli in P1 cats (Table 6-1). Intact cats are highly proficient at masked pattern discriminations at both high and intermediate contrast levels and only start to show a slightly attenuated performance when contrast levels are very low (Michaelson contrast of 0.26). In contrast, performance of two cats with lesions of areas 17 and 18 incurred at 6 months of age (P180) shows poorer performance at intermediate (0.8) or even higher (0.9) contrast levels, and when contrast levels are low performance declines to chance levels. Likewise, cats with equivalent lesions incurred on P1 have performance levels that are equally poor for the same range of contrasts. These preliminary data are in accord with the data of Mitchell (1990). He showed that the maximum visual grating acuity of both groups of cats was in the range of 2–3 cyc/deg and far below the 7–9 cyc/deg range of intact cats.

However, we know that the learning of high-contrast, masked pattern discriminations is spared in P1 cats as it is in cats that sustained lesions on P4 (Fig. 6-10) (Cornwell et al., 1989). The difference between the P1 and P180 cats is that in P180 cats β (X) ganglion cells, the origin of low spatial contrast signals, are present in retina but they are not materially connected to central processing structures, whereas in P1 cats this retinal substrate for low spatial contrast vision is essentially absent because the majority of β (X) ganglion cells have died (Payne et al., 1984; Payne and Lomber, 1998; Tong et al., 1982). Presumably, the sparing under high contrast conditions in P1 cats is linked to signals emanating from α (Y) retinal ganglion cells that survive and retain significant connections with central processing structures (Payne et al., 1984; Payne and Lomber, 1998).

In future studies it will also be profitable to investigate the behavioral capaci-

Table 6-1. Masking and contrast pattern discrimination: Combined test for neural compensations and β (X) signals

		Percent Errors						
		Intact		P28		P1		P180	
Michaelson Ratio	Contrast	Cat A	Cat B	Cat A	Cat B	Cat A	Cat B	Cat A	Cat B
---	---	---	---	---	---	---	---	---	---
0.9	High	0	0	0	2.4	2.5	4.8	10	14
0.8		0	0	0.8	4.8	17	27	21	28
0.66		0	0.8	1.7	7.2	31.1	40	36	42
0.44		0.8	1.7	17	21	37.5	42	46	40
0.26	Low	13.3	24.3	35	37.5	38.3	42	42	45

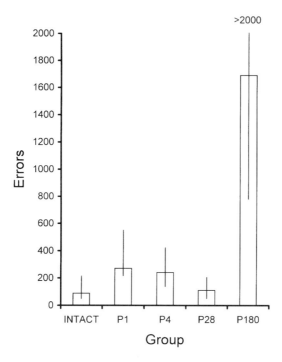

Figure 6-10. Comparison of number of errors made in the staircase acquisition of a 10-line masked outline I and O figures by intact cats and P1, P4, P28, and P180 ablation cats. Data from P1 and P28 cats show mean and range of values. For the remainder, median and first and third quartile values are given. Data for intact, P4, and P180 cats are shown in Figure 6-4. P180 third quartile is more than 2,000 errors. I and O patterns with 10 masking lines across the patterns are shown in row 4 of Figure 6-3. Note that performance by P1 cats is indistinguishable from that of P4 cats. P28 cats make fewer errors than either P1 or P4 cats, and performance is in the normal range.

ties of cats that incurred cortical lesions at other stages of development, when we know the final outcome of pathway development and the types of signals circulating in the brain are quite different. For them we can predict a broader repertoire of perceptual capacities. This broader repertoire likely involves functions based on β (X), as well as α (Y), signals and includes functions normally associated with areas 17 and 18. This suspicion is supported by the greater visual grating acuity of P28 cats, which is close to the normal range at 6–8 cyc/deg (Mitchell, 1990), and by the fact that significant numbers of MS neurons are selective for stimulus orientation (Tong et al., 1984); frank orientation selectivity is normally a property of areas 17 and 18 and not MS cortex (Orban, 1984). Also, preliminary evidence suggests that fewer errors in the learning of the high contrast masked pattern discriminations are made by cats with lesions of areas 17 and 18 incurred on P28 than by cats with equivalent lesions incurred on either P1 or P4, and performance is in the normal range (Fig. 6-10).

Moreover, testing of the same pattern discriminations with various levels of reduced contrast suggest that P28 lesions spare pattern vision at both high and intermediate contrast levels (Table 6-1). This sparing is understandable because approximately 40% of β (X) retinal ganglion cells survive the ablation of areas 17 and 18 (Payne and Lomber, 1998; Callahan et al., 1984), and many are highly connected to extrastriate cortex (Payne and Lomber, 1998). However, whatever compensations have occurred they are incomplete because performance at the lower contrast levels by the P28 cat does not differ from either P1 or P180 cats and is lower than that of intact cats (Fig. 6-10). This result suggests that a more complete population, and/or greater connectivity of the surviving population, of β (X) cells is required to ensure normal levels of performance at the lower contrast levels and to bring visual grating acuity to the highest levels. The same conclusion can be extended to greater levels of masking, because performance by cats with lesions of areas 17 and 18 sustained on P1, P28, or P180 is always inferior to that of intact cats at intermediate and low contrast levels.

In future studies it will also be highly profitable to ascertain the specific contributions various extrastriate regions make to the spared behaviors. One possible important outcome of the extensive rewiring across broad regions of cortex is that functions normally localized to one region become dispersed. For example, two major systems that contribute to the redistribution of signals are the expanded projection from vPS cortex to MS cortex (Fig. 6-6D) (MacNeil et al., 1996) and the expanded projection from MS cortex that reaches vPS cortex via the superior colliculus and medial division of the lateral posterior nucleus (Fig. 6-6D) (Lomber et al., 1995). The presence of these relays suggests that the processing of signals in vPS cortex is altered in significant ways by the signals arriving from MS cortex and vice versa. Moreover, it suggests that functions normally associated with one region of cortex may be weakened by diluting signals arriving from atypical sources. Accordingly, it seems that the redistribution may be accompanied by a "price," and some functions normally associated with MS and vPS cortices may be displaced, or "crowded out," as the regions acquire or emphasize functions normally only weakly represented, if at all (Teuber, 1975). It will be possible to test for this possibility by comparing the spectrum of deficits induced on a battery of tasks by temporarily cooling and deactivating MS and vPS cortices, in turn, and comparing behavioral deficits in P1 and P28 cats with those induced in intact cats.

To this end, Stephen Lomber and I have refined the reversible, cooling deactivation technique to probe the visual functions of extrastriate cortex (Lomber et al., 1996a,b; Lomber and Payne, 1998; Payne et al., 1996) and have reached a number of conclusions about both the technique and visual processing in intact cat extrastriate cortex.

1. Behavioral, electrophysiological, and histological measures show that there are no deleterious effects of the surgical procedures to permanently implant the cooling probes or maintaining and operating them over long periods of time.
2. Limited regions of cortex can be selectively and reversibly deactivated in

a controlled and reproducible way, and baseline and experimental measurements can be made virtually concurrently (within minutes).

3. Repeated coolings over months and years (currently at 3.2 years) produce stable, reversible deficits with no evidence of attenuation or exaggeration across testing sessions.

4. Repeated coolings induce neither local nor distant degenerations that might compromise conclusions.

5. The cooling does not permit the cat to practice for extended periods of time with the secondary cooling-induced defect because it is only temporary and of short duration. Consequently, alternative circuits do not have an opportunity to strengthen and compromise interpretation of data.

6. Compared with ablation studies, many fewer animals are needed because sensitive within-animal comparisons and double dissociations are possible, permitting large volumes of high quality data to be acquired from each animal.

Thus, the technique is extremely useful and powerful for deciphering the contributions MS and posterior suprasylvian cortices make to the spared functions. In intact cats we have already dissociated the learning, recall, and form processing functions of posterior suprasylvian cortex from the motion and orienting functions of MS cortex (Lomber et al., 1996a,b; Payne et al., 1996a,c) and anterior MS cortex from posterior MS cortex (Lomber et al., 1996b; Payne et al., 1996a) and have even identified the different laminar contributions to visually guided behavior by deactivating superficial versus all layers of a cortical region (Lomber and Payne, 1999). Thus, the technique has great promise for probing the contributions to visual processing of suprasylvian cortices in cats with early lesions of areas 17 and 18.

Also, in future studies it will be profitable to test for spared functions normally associated with areas 17 and 18, to ascertain with the cooling technique whether extrastriate regions can adopt functions normally associated with areas 17 and 18, and to identify subclasses of tasks dominated by signals derived from α (Y) and β (X) retinal ganglion cells.

Finally, it will be highly useful to develop ways to investigate the functional impact of one brain region on others in the rewired brains. Advances in this direction have already been made for the intact cat brain by us and our Belgian colleagues by combining our localized cooling method with reduced uptake of deoxyglucose at distant sites (Payne and Lomber, 1999; Vanduffel et al., 1997, 1998).

Parallel Sequelae of Primary Visual Cortex Damage in Monkeys and Humans

There are a number of parallel sequelae in the repercussions of primary visual cortex lesions in cats, monkeys, and humans. These parallels are greatest for the induced degenerations, there being virtually no information on pathway expansions in either monkeys or humans.

Monkeys

As in the cat, both patterns of connections and maturational status govern survival and death of neurons after early lesions of monkey primary visual cortex. For example, neurons projecting solely to primary visual cortex die following its removal, whereas neurons projecting to extrastriate cortices survive (Cowey and Stoerig, 1989; Kisvarday et al., 1991; Yukie and Iwai, 1981). Also, the vast majority of monkey β retinal ganglion cells are vulnerable to the cortical lesion, yet α and γ ganglion cells, because of their maintained projections to central structures, are protected (Cowey, 1974; Cowey et al., 1989). Moreover, the rapidity of the β-cell degenerative response is graded in an age-dependent way and is characterized by a marked attenuation in both sensitivity and rapidity with advancing age at the time the lesion is incurred (Dineen and Hendrickson, 1981; Weller and Kaas, 1989).

Even though no information is available for pathway expansions there is evidence that monkeys with early lesions can navigate and retrieve and manipulate objects (Humphrey, 1970, 1972, 1974; Humphrey and Weiskrantz, 1967), make eye movements to stimuli presented in the "cortical scotoma," and discriminate between different directions of motion (Moore et al., 1995, 1996) more accurately than monkeys with equivalent lesions incurred in adulthood. These results suggest that one or more pathways have expanded in response to the early lesion. If so, they likely transmit signals derived from the surviving α (Y) and γ (W) ganglion cells. Whatever adaptions are based on these signals, they are counterbalanced by the large loss of β ganglion cells and the X signals, which greatly attenuate other visual functions such as discrimination of fine details and reduced contrast sensitivity (Miller et al., 1980) and chromatic signals (Schilder et al., 1972).

Humans

To our knowledge, there is no information on differences in the structure of the visual system of human subjects who incurred damage of primary visual cortex early in life compared with later in life. However, the patterns of degeneration induced by lesions incurred in adulthood resemble closely those identified following damage in monkeys of equivalent maturational status and, by extension, the cat (Haddock and Berlin, 1950; Van Buren, 1963a,b; Walsh, 1947). Also, there are virtually no systematic data comparing the visual functions in patients with earlier versus later damage of primary visual cortex, although there are some suggestions that visual capacities may be greater following earlier lesions (for discussion, see Payne et al., 1996b). To give one example, a patient who sustained bilateral damage of visual cortex at birth could avoid obstacles while navigating new ground (Rizzo and Hurtig, 1989), and, in broad terms, his visual capacities resemble those of the monkey with early bilateral lesion of striate cortex studied by Humphrey (1970, 1972, 1974). Moreover, the patient could detect motion and make moder-

Color Plate I. (See Chapter 6.) Diagrams to summarize the major visual circuits in intact cats *(A)* and changes in connections of middle suprasylvian region (MS) cortex induced by damage of primary visual cortical areas 17 and 18 incurred in adulthood *(B)*, at 1 month of age *(C)*, or on the day of birth *(D)*. Width of arrows indicates approximate magnitude of projections. Blue indicates normal connections, red indicates increased connections, and green indicates no information on pathway changes available (primarily circuits related to superior colliculus [SC]). For clarity, several pathways have been omitted. These pathways include those involving the pretectum and many extrastriate regions other than MS, dorsal posterior suprasylvian region (dPS), and ventral posterior suprasylvian region (vPS) cortices that either do not change following lesions of areas 17 and 18 or for which no information is available. Also note that dPS and vPS cortices receive substantial projections from visual thalamic nuclei and, either directly or indirectly, from areas 17 and 18. These latter connections are not well understood even in the intact brain. They have been omitted in the interests of simplicity of the presentation of known lesion-induced repercussions and major pathways. Pul, pulvinar nucleus. Reproduced from Payne et al., 1996b.

Notes for A: 1, Note progressive amplification of visual signals transmitted through the lateral geniculate nucleus, dorsal division (dLGN), to primary visual cortex (Peters and Payne, 1993). 2, X and Y signals (see footnote on page 124) reach extrastriate cortex via the magnocellular (M) layers of dLGN and primary visual cortex (Sherman, 1985). 3, Y signals also reach extrastriate cortex via the medial interlaminar nucleus (MIN) and via the superior colliculus and the lateral posterior complex (Sherman, 1985). 4, W signals (see footnote) reach extrastriate cortex via the parvocellular (P) layers of dLGN, MIN, and via the superior colliculus and the lateral posterior complex (Sherman, 1985). 5, W, X, and Y signals reach the superior colliculus either directly or via primary and extrastriate cortex (Berson, 1988; Sherman, 1985). 6, Visual signals reach MS cortex via dPS and vPS cortices, which receive substantial visual inputs via the lateral posterior (LP) nucleus (m, medial division; l, lateral division) (Rosenquist, 1985).

Notes for B: 1, Partial shrinkage of magnocellular layers due to death of neurons (Lomber et al., 1993; Spear et al., 1980). Dense retinal projection maintained to all dLGN compartments (Lomber et al., 1993). 2, Following the damage of primary visual cortex, X signal transmission to extrastriate cortex is interrupted and Y signal transmission is greatly reduced. 3, In some cats, direct retinal projections to LP nucleus appear following lesions of areas 17 and 18 incurred early in adult life (Payne et al., 1993). 4, No X signals reach the superior colliculus, and no Y signals are relayed to the superior colliculus through primary visual cortex (Berson, 1988). 5, W and Y signal transmission to the superior colliculus and through MIN to extrastriate cortex is unaffected by the lesion (Lomber et al., 1995). The one caveat to this statement is that signal transmission through the connected layers of dLGN and superior colliculus may be severely compromised by the absence of facilitatory signals descending from areas 17 and 18. 6, Neuronal activity is depressed and receptive field properties in extrastriate cortex and superior colliculus disrupted (Berman and Cynader, 1976; Guido et al., 1992; Mendola and Payne, 1993; Spear and Baumann, 1979). Behavioral performance on many cerebrally based tasks is poor.

Notes for C: 1, Retention of substantial retinal projections to dLGN, even though magnocellular layers of dLGN have partially degenerated (Payne and Lomber, 1998; Lomber et al., 1993). Note survival of ~40% of β (X) retinal ganglion cells in addition to α (Y) and γ (W) cells (Payne and Lomber, 1998). 2, Expansion of retinal projections into LP (Payne et al., 1993). 3, Massive expansion of projections from the parvocellular layers of dLGN to MS cortex and the rescue and recruitment of neurons in magnocellular layers of dLGN to the projection (Payne and Lomber, 1998; Lomber et al., 1995). Expansion of MS cortical projection in superior colliculus (Sun et al., 1994). 4, Increased traffic of W and Y signals (Payne and Lomber, 1998; Lomber et al., 1993, 1995; Payne et al., 1996). Some traffic in X signals (Payne and Lomber, 1998).

Notes for D: 1, Note virtually complete elimination of X signals from the brain due to death of massive numbers of β retinal ganglion cells and types II and III dLGN neurons (Ault et al., 1993; Callahan et al., 1984; Kalil, 1984; MacNeil et al., 1997; Payne and Lomber, 1998; Payne et al., 1984; Pearson et al., 1981; Rowe, 1990b; Tong et al., 1982). 2, Very few neurons survive in the magnocellular layers of dLGN (Kalil, 1984; Labar et al., 1981; MacNeil et al., 1997; Murphy and Kalil, 1979; Payne et al., 1984; Spear et al., 1980; Tumosa et al., 1989). 3, Increased W and Y signal transmission to MS cortex and superior colliculus via expansions and increased coupling between ascending pathways through both parvocellular layers of dLGN and LPm to MS cortex and descending projections to the superior colliculus (Kalil and Behan, 1987; Kalil et al., 1991; Labar et al., 1981; Lomber et al., 1993, 1995; MacNeil et al., 1997; Payne and Lomber, 1998; Payne et al., 1984, 1993; Sun et al., 1994; Tong et al., 1984). 4, Massive amplification in projections from vPS cortex to MS cortex (MacNeil et al., 1996). 5, Increased traffic of W and Y signals linked to neural compensation in parvocellular complex of dLGN, MS, and vPS cortices and superior colliculus (Berman and Cynader, 1972; Cornwell et al., 1978; Doty, 1961; Guido et al., 1990a,b, 1992; Long et al., 1996; Mendola and Payne, 1973; Mize and Murphy, 1976; Payne and Lomber, 1996; Spear et al., 1980; Stein and Magalhaes-Castro, 1975; Tong et al., 1984).

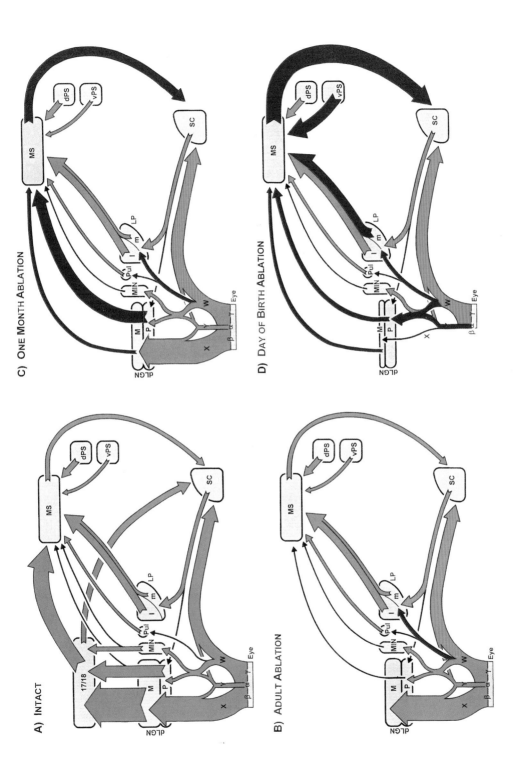

A) INTACT

B) ADULT ABLATION

C) ONE MONTH ABLATION

D) DAY OF BIRTH ABLATION

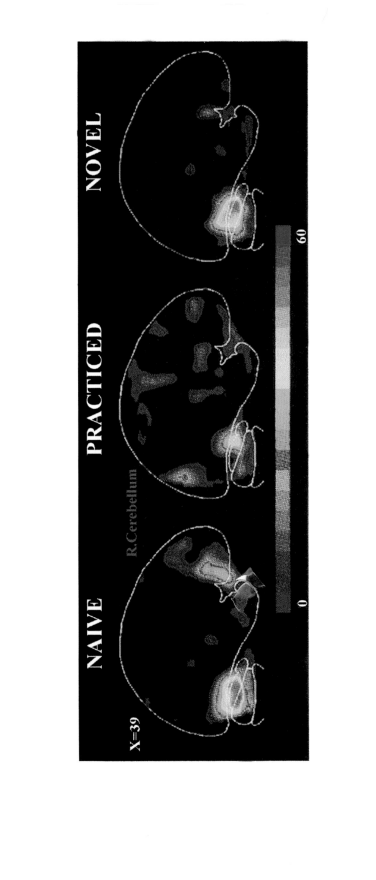

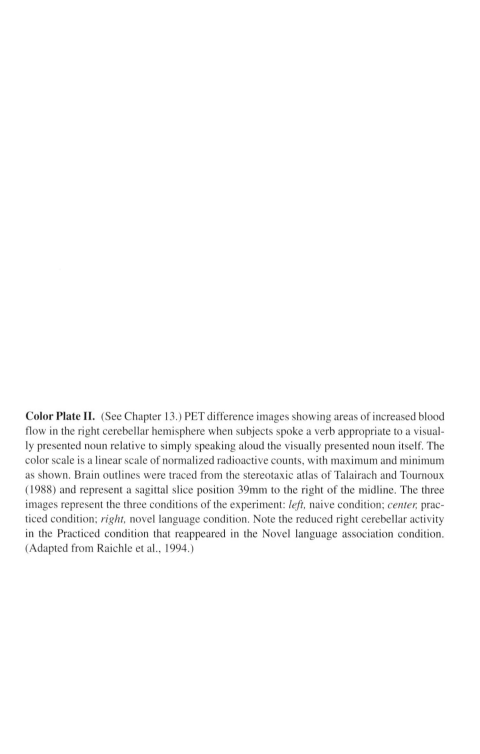

Color Plate II. (See Chapter 13.) PET difference images showing areas of increased blood flow in the right cerebellar hemisphere when subjects spoke a verb appropriate to a visually presented noun relative to simply speaking aloud the visually presented noun itself. The color scale is a linear scale of normalized radioactive counts, with maximum and minimum as shown. Brain outlines were traced from the stereotaxic atlas of Talairach and Tournoux (1988) and represent a sagittal slice position 39mm to the right of the midline. The three images represent the three conditions of the experiment: *left,* naive condition; *center,* practiced condition; *right,* novel language condition. Note the reduced right cerebellar activity in the Practiced condition that reappeared in the Novel language association condition. (Adapted from Raichle et al., 1994.)

ately accurate saccades, which suggests some sparing of perceptual and cerebral-ly mediated detection and eye movement functions.

Future Work on Monkeys and Humans

We recognize that it is risky to speculate about the details of monkey and human brains and their response to injury based on work carried out on the cat. Howev-er, we think it appropriate to speculate in broad terms because, as outlined earlier, there are broad and substantial similarities in the organization, function, and de-velopment of the visual system of cats and monkeys and, by extension, humans. Moreover, there are several similarities in the systemwide anatomical repercus-sions that result from primary visual cortex damage in young and adult cats and monkeys so that we are secure in our prediction that commensurate systemwide repercussions follow primary visual cortex damage in infant and adult humans. Furthermore, we suspect that the repercussions of early lesions in monkeys and humans will spare similar classes of behavior to those already described for the cat. Indeed, studies carried out so far support this idea, for we know that visuo-spatial tasks are performed more adroitly by monkeys and humans with early com-pared to late lesions of primary visual cortex (Blythe et al., 1987; Moore et al., 1996).

Our suspicions are borne out further by results obtained from one human sub-ject who sustained damage of primary visual cortex in childhood and who shows strong neural activity, as revealed by regional cerebral blood flow measurements, in both the area V3 and area V5 complexes (Barbur et al., 1993). In cats, the par-alogue of the V5 complex is considered to be MS cortex (Payne, 1993; Payne et al., 1996b), and this cortex is a major site for pathway rewiring and substantial neuronal compensations, and the same may be true of the paralogue of the V3 com-plex (area 19 and adjoining cortices) (Payne, 1993). The V3 complex is implicat-ed in pattern vision (Payne, 1993; Zeki and Lamb, 1994), and some aspects of com-plex-pattern vision are spared by early lesions of primary visual cortex in cats (Cornwell et al., 1978, 1989; Cornwell and Payne, 1989). It may be that visual pathways reaching these regions expand, or are at least strengthened, as they are in the cat following early lesions of primary visual cortex. Moreover, increased connections and traffic in signals between occipitoparietal into occipitotemporal cortices, akin to MS ↔ PS connections in cats, may lead to awareness and experi-ence of stimuli (Weiskrantz et al., 1995; Sahraie et al., 1997).

We also suspect that many of the widespread physiological and anatomical repercussions of early lesions identified in cats likely occur in humans and mon-keys following equivalent damage. Moreover, the techniques are now available to examine some of these repercussions. For instance, activity changes in area V5 can be examined noninvasively in monkeys or humans with early or late lesions of the visual cortex using evoked potentials or functional magnetic resonance imaging. In humans such analyses may provide evidence of differences between blindsight (e.g., Weiskrantz, 1996; Stoerig and Cowey, 1997) in the more normal unconscious mode and that in the rarer conscious mode (Weiskrantz et al., 1995; Sahraie et al., 1997). Methods are also available for studying, with intracellular injection, the possibility of detailed anatomical changes in fixed postmortem tissue as it becomes available from cases of early or late damage of the visual cortex (Einstein, 1988; MacNeil et al., 1997). One good place to initiate these anatomical investigations is in the retina, where β ganglion cells are likely depleted and α and γ ganglion cell morphologies are likely to be modified by transneuronally mediated effects of early cortical lesions, which are known to have significant repercussions even on the inner plexiform layer in cats (Rowe, 1988).

One further, extremely important avenue to pursue is to identify differences in visual capacities of monkeys and people who incurred lesions of primary visual cortex at different ages. Particularly important are subjects who sustained lesions very early in postnatal life, in infancy, to ascertain whether their visual capacities are greater than, or of a different type from, those presented by subjects with lesions incurred later. If the sparing is greater or of a different type, it will be a potent example of how experimental investigations on laboratory animals can guide investigations of the human brain and the repercussions of early focal lesions. Such studies are likely to be highly valuable for interpreting the repercussions of cerebral lesions sustained early in life in other regions of the cerebral cortex.

Epilogue

Finally, I hope that future studies will recognize the plastic capacities of immature human brain that permit it to overcome major challenges to its normal development. I am optimistic about this possibility because a limited number of studies on humans (e.g., Craft et al., 1994; Milner, 1974; Rudel et al., 1974; Stiles and Nass, 1991; Woods, 1981) and animals (e.g., Goldman-Rakic et al., 1983; Kolb, 1995; Payne et al., 1996b; Schneider, 1979) foster the idea that immature brains exhibit great developmental flexibility that supports neuroplastic and adaptive responses by young neurons that result in rewired pathways, neural compensations, and the sparing of behaviors. Once plastic capacities of the human brain are identified, I anticipate that enriched environments and training strategies, as documented elsewhere in this book, may be usefully employed to potentiate the natural capacity of the brain to overcome the challenges and contribute to considerable neural compensations and sparing of neural functions to result in organized behaviors. Furthermore, medicinal or pharmaceutical treatments may one day be used to extend the therapeutic strategies further. There is much that needs to be done.

References

I acknowledge the National Institute of Neurological Disorders and Stroke and the National Institute of Mental Health for their financial support of my research endeavors.

Ault, S. J., Thompson, K. G., Zhou, Y., and Leventhal, A. G. (1993). Selective depletion of beta cells affects development of alpha cells in cat retina. *Vis. Neurosci., 10,* 237–245.

Bachevalier, J., Brickson, M., Hagger, C., and Mishkin, M. (1990). Age and sex differences in the effects of selective temporal lobe lesions on the formation of visual discrimination habits in rhesus monkeys. *Behav. Neurosci., 104,* 885–889.

Bachevalier, J., and Mishkin, M. (1994). Effects of selective neonatal temporal lobe lesions on visual recognition memory in rhesus monkeys. *J. Neurosci., 14,* 2128–2139.

Barbur, J. L., Harlow, A., and Weiskrantz, L. (1994). Spatial and temporal response properties of residual vision in a case of hemianopia. *Philos. Trans. R. Soc. Ser. B, 343,* 157–166.

Barbur, J. L., Watson, J. D. G., Frackowiak, R. S. J., and Zeki, S. (1993). Conscious visual perception without V1. *Brain, 116,* 1293–1302.

Berman, N., and Cynader, M. (1976). Early versus late visual cortex lesions: Effects on receptive fields in cat superior colliculus. *Exp. Brain Res., 25,* 131–137.

Berson, D. M. (1988). Retinal and cortical inputs to cat superior colliculus: Composition, convergence and laminar specificity. *Prog. Brain Res., 75,* 17–26.

Bertolino, A., Saunders, R. C., Mattay, V. S., Bachevalier, J., Frank, J. A., and Weinberger, D. R. (1997). Altered development of prefrontal neurons in rhesus monkeys with neonatal temporo-limbic lesions: A proton magnetic resonance imaging study. *Cereb. Cortex, 7,* 740–748.

Blythe, I. M., Kennard, C., and Ruddock, K. H. (1987). Residual vision in patients with retrogeniculate lesions of visual pathways. *Brain 110,* 887–905.

Callahan, E. C., Tong, L., and Spear, P. D. (1984). Critical period for the loss of retinal X-cells following visual cortex damage in cats. *Brain Res., 323,* 302–306.

Cornwell, P., Herbein, S., Corso, C., Eskew, R., Warren, J. M., and Payne, B. R. (1989). Selective sparing after lesions of visual cortex in newborn cats. *Behav. Neurosci., 103,* 1176–1190.

Cornwell, P., Overman, W. H., and Ross, C. (1978). Extent of recovery from neonatal damage to the cortical visual system in cats. *J. Comp. Physiol. Psychol., 92,* 255–270.

Cornwell, P., and Payne, B. R. (1989). Visual discrimination by cats with adult or one- or two-stage neonatal lesions of visual cortex. *Behav. Neurosci., 103,* 1191–1199.

Cowey, A. (1974). Atrophy of retinal ganglion cells after removal of striate cortex in a rhesus monkey. *Perception, 3,* 257–260.

Cowey, A., and Stoerig, P. (1989). Projection patterns of surviving neurons in the dorsal lateral geniculate nucleus following discrete lesions of striate cortex. *Exp. Brain Res., 75,* 631–638.

Cowey, A., Stoerig, P., and Perry, V. H. (1989). Transneuronal retrograde degeneration of retinal ganglion cells after damage of striate cortex in macaque monkeys: Selective loss of Pβ cells. *Neuroscience, 29,* 65–80.

Craft, S., White, D. A., Park, T. S., and Figial, G. (1994). Visual attention in children with perinatal brain injury: Asymmetric effects of bilateral lesions. *J. Cog. Neurosci., 6,* 165–173.

Dineen, J. T., and Hendrickson, A. E. (1981). Age-correlated differences in the amount of retinal degeneration after striate cortical lesions in monkeys. *Invest. Ophthalmol. Vis. Sci., 21,* 749–752.

Dineen, J. T., Hendrickson, A. E., and Keating, E. G. (1982). Alterations in retinal inputs following striate cortex removal in adult monkey. *Exp. Brain Res., 47,* 446–456.

Doty, R. W. (1961). Functional significance of the topographical aspects of the retinocortical projection. In R. Jung and H. Kornhuber (eds.): *The Visual System: Neurophysiology and Psychophysics.* Berlin: Springer Verlag, pp. 228–247.

Einstein, G. E. (1988). Intracellular injection of lucifer yellow into cortical neurons lightly fixed sections and its application to human autopsy material. *J. Neurosci. Methods, 26,* 95–103.

Goldman-Rakic, P. S., Isseroff, A., Schwartz, M. L., and Bugbee, N. M. (1983). The neurobiology of cognitive development. In P. Mussen (ed.): *Handbook of Child Psychology: Infancy and Developmental Psychobiology.* New York: Wiley, pp. 281–344.

Guido, W., Spear, P. D., and Tong, L. (1990a). Functional compensation in the lateral suprasylvian visual area following bilateral visual cortex damage in kittens. *Exp. Brain Res., 83,* 219–224.

Guido, W., Spear, P. D., and Tong, L. (1992). How complete is the physiological compensation in extrastriate cortex after visual cortex damage in kittens? *Exp. Brain Res., 91,* 455–466.

Guido, W., Tong, L., and Spear, P. D. (1990b). Afferent bases of spatial- and temporal-frequency processing by neurons in the cat's posteromedial lateral suprasylvian cortex: Effects of removing areas 17, 18, and 19. *J. Neurophysiol., 64,* 1636–1651.

Haddock, J. N., and Berlin, L. (1950). Transsynaptic degeneration in the visual system. *Arch. Neurol. (Chicago), 64,* 66–73.

Harting, J. K., Updyke, B. V., and van Lieshout, D. P. (1992). Corticotectal projections in the cat: Anterograde transport studies in twenty-five cortical areas. *J. Comp. Neurol., 324,* 379–414.

Hughes, H. C., Layton, W. M., Baird, J. C., and Lester, L. S. (1984). Global precedence in visual pattern recognition. *Percep. Psychophys., 35,* 361–371.

Humphrey, N. K. (1970). What the frog's eye tells the monkey's brain. *Brain Behav. Evol., 3,* 324–337.

Humphrey, N. K. (1972). Seeing and nothingness. *New Scientist, 53,* 682–684.

Humphrey, N. K. (1974). Vision in a monkey without striate cortex: A case study. *Perception, 3,* 241–255.

Humphrey, N. K., and Weiskrantz, L. (1967). Vision in monkeys after removal of striate cortex. *Nature, 215,* 595–597.

Kalia, M., and Whitteridge, D. (1973). The visual areas in the splenial sulcus of the cat. *J. Physiol. (Lond.), 232,* 275–283.

Kalil, R. E. (1984). Removal of visual cortex in the cat: Effects on the morphological development of the retino-geniculo-cortical pathway. In J. Stone, B. Dreher, and D. H. Rapaport (eds.). *Development of Visual Pathways in Mammals.* New York: Alan R. Liss, pp. 257–274.

Kalil, R. E., and Behan, M. (1987). Synaptic reorganization in the dorsal lateral geniculate nucleus following damage to visual cortex in newborn or adult cats. *J. Comp Neurol., 257,* 216–236.

Kalil, R. E., Tong, L. L., and Spear, P. D. (1991). Thalamic projections to the lateral suprasylvian visual area in cats with neonatal or adult visual cortex damage. *J. Comp Neurol., 314,* 512–525.

Kimchi, R. (1992). Primacy of wholistic processing and global/local paradigm: A critical review. *Psychol. Bull., 112,* 24–38.

Kisvarday, Z. F., Cowey, A., Stoerig, P., and Somogyi, P. (1991). Direct and indirect retinal input into degenerated dorsal lateral geniculate nucleus after striate cortical removal in monkey: Implications for residual vision. *Exp. Brain Res., 86,* 271–292.

Kolb, B. (1995). *Brain Plasticity & Development*. Mahwah, NJ: Lawrence Erlbaum.

Labar, D. R., Berman, N. E., and Murphy, E. H. (1981). Short- and long-term effects of neonatal and adult visual cortex lesions on the retinal projection to the pulvinar. *J. Comp. Neurol., 197,* 639–659.

Lomber, S. G., MacNeil, M. A., and Payne, B. R. (1995). Amplification of thalamic projections to middle suprasylvian cortex following ablation of immature primary visual cortex in the cat. *Cereb. Cortex, 5,* 166–191.

Lomber, S. G., and Payne, B. R. (1999). Evidence for different laminar contributions to visually guided behaviors revealed by limited cerebral cooling deactivation. *Cereb. Cortex,* submitted for publication.

Lomber, S. G., Payne, B. R., and Cornwell, P. (1996a). Learning and recall of form discriminations during reversible cooling deactivation of ventral-posterior suprasylvian cortex in the behaving cat. *Proc. Natl. Acad. Sci. U.S.A., 93,* 1654–1658.

Lomber, S. G., Payne, B. R., Cornwell, P., and Long, K. D. (1996b). Perceptual and cognitive visual functions of parietal and temporal cortices of the cat. *Cereb. Cortex, 6,* 673–695.

Lomber, S. G., Payne, B. R., Cornwell, P., and Pearson, H. E. (1993). Capacity of the retinogeniculate pathway to reorganize following ablation of visual cortical areas in developing and mature cats. *J. Comp. Neurol., 338,* 432–457.

Long, K. D., Lomber, S. G., and Payne, B. R. (1996). Increased oxidative metabolism in middle suprasylvian cortex following removal of areas 17 and 18 from newborn cats. *Exp. Brain Res., 110,* 335–346.

MacNeil, M. A., Einstein, G. E., and Payne, B. R. (1997). Transgeniculate signal transmission to middle suprasylvian extrastriate cortex in intact cats and following early removal of areas 17 and 18: A morphological study. *Exp. Brain Res., 114,* 11–23.

MacNeil, M. A., Lomber, S. G., and Payne, B. R. (1996). Rewiring of transcortical projections to middle suprasylvian cortex following early removal of cat areas 17 and 18. *Cereb. Cortex, 6,* 362–376.

Màlkovà, L., Mishkin, M., and Bachevalier, J. (1995). Long-term effects of selective neonatal temporal lobe lesions on learning and memory in monkeys. *Behav. Neurosci., 109,* 212–226.

Marcotte, R. R., and Updyke, B. V. (1982). Thalamocortical relations of a visual area on the lateral bank of the lateral sulcus of the cat. *Neurosci. Abstr., 8,* 810.

Mendola, J. D., and Payne, B. R. (1993). Direction selectivity and physiological compensation in the superior colliculus following removal of areas 17 and 18. *Vis. Neurosci., 10,* 1019–1026.

Michalski, A., Wimborne, B. M., and Henry, G. H. (1993). The effect of reversible cooling of cat's primary visual cortex on the responses of area 21 neurons. *J. Physiol. (Lond.), 466,* 133–156.

Miller, M., Pasik, P., and Pasik, T. (1980). Extrageniculostriate vision in the monkey, VII. Contrast sensitivity function. *J. Neurophysiol., 43,* 1510–1526.

Milner, B. (1974). Sparing of language function after unilateral brain damage. *Neurosci. Res., Prog. Bull., 2,* 213–217.

Mitchell, D. E. (1990). Sensitive periods in visual development: Insights gained from studies of recovery of function in cats following early monocular deprivation or cortical lesions. In C. Blakemore (ed.): *Vision: Coding and Efficiency*. Cambridge: Cambridge University Press, pp. 234–246.

Mize, R. R., and Murphy, E. H. (1976). Alterations of receptive field properties of superior colliculus cells produced by visual cortex ablation in infant and adult cats. *J. Comp. Neurol., 168,* 393–424.

Moore, T., Repp, A. B., Rodman, H. R., and Gross, C. G. (1995). Preserved motion discrimination in monkeys with early lesions of striate cortex. *Neurosci. Abstr., 21,* 1651.

Moore, T., Rodman, H. R., Repp, A. B., Gross, C. G., and Mezrich, R. S. (1996). Greater residual vision in monkeys after striate cortex damage in infancy. *J. Neurophysiol., 76,* 3928–3933.

Murphy, E. H., and Kalil, R. E. (1979). Functional organization of lateral geniculate cells following removal of visual cortex in the newborn kitten. *Science 206,* 713–716.

Orban, G. A. (1984). *Neuronal Operations in Visual Cortex.* New York: Springer-Verlag.

Olson, C. R., and Graybiel, A. M. (1987). Ectosylvian visual areas of the cat: Location, organization and connections. *J. Comp. Neurol., 261,* 277–294.

Payne, B. R. (1993). Feature article: Evidence for visual cortical area homologues in cat and macaque monkey. *Cereb. Cortex 3,* 1–25.

Payne, B. R., Connors, C., and Cornwell, P. (1991). Survival and death of neurons in cortical area PMLS after removal of areas 17, 18 and 19 from cats and kittens. *Cereb. Cortex 1,* 469–491.

Payne, B. R., and Cornwell, P. (1994). System-wide repercussions of damage to the immature visual cortex. *Trends Neurosci., 17,* 126–130.

Payne, B. R., Foley, H., and Lomber, S. G. (1993). Visual cortex damage-induced growth of retinal axons into the lateral posterior nucleus of the cat. *Vis. Neurosci., 10,* 747–752.

Payne, B. R., and Lomber, S. G. (1996). Age dependent modification of cytochrome oxidase activity in the cat dorsal lateral geniculate nucleus following removal of primary visual cortex. *Vis. Neurosci., 13,* 805–816.

Payne, B. R., and Lomber, S. G. (1998). Neuroplasticity in the cat's visual system: Origin, termination, expansion and increased coupling in the retino-geniculo-middle suprasylvian visual pathway following early lesions of areas 17 and 18. *Exp. Brain Res., 121,* 334–349.

Payne, B. R., and Lomber, S. G. (1999). A method to assess the functional impact of cerebral connections on target populations of neurons. *J. Neurosci. Methods* (in press).

Payne, B. R., Lomber, S. G., Geeraerts, S., Van der Gucht, E., and Vandenbussche, E. (1996a). Reversible visual hemineglect. *Proc. Natl. Acad. Sci. U.S.A., 93,* 290–294.

Payne, B. R., Lomber, S. G., MacNeil, M. A., and Cornwell, P. (1996b). Perspective: Evidence for greater sight in blindsight following damage of primary visual cortex early in life. *Neuropsychologia, 34,* 741–774.

Payne, B. R., Lomber, S. G., Villa, A. E., and Bullier, J. (1996c). Reversible deactivation of cerebral network components. *Trends Neurosci., 19,* 535–542.

Payne, B. R., Pearson, H. E., and Cornwell, P. (1984). Transneuronal degeneration of beta retinal ganglion cells in the cat. *Proc. R. Soc. Lond. Ser. B, 222,* 15–32.

Payne, B. R., Pearson, H. E., and Cornwell, P. (1988). Development of connections in cat visual and auditory cortex. In A. Peters and E. G. Jones (eds.): *Cerebral Cortex, vol. 7, Development and Maturation of Cerebral Cortex.* New York: Plenum Press, pp. 309–389.

Pearson, H. E., Labar, D. R., Payne, B. R., Cornwell, P., and Aggarwall, N. (1981). Transneuronal retrograde degeneration in the cat retina following neonatal ablation of visual cortex. *Brain Res., 212,* 470–475.

Pearson, H. E., and Stoffler, D. J. (1992). Retinal ganglion cell degeneration following loss of postsynaptic target neurons in the dorsal lateral geniculate nucleus of the adult cat. *Exp. Neurol., 116,* 163–171.

Pearson, H. E., Stoffler, D. J., and Sonnstein, W. J. (1992). Response of retinal terminals to loss of postsynaptic target neurons in the dorsal lateral geniculate nucleus of the adult cat. *J. Comp. Neurol., 315,* 333–343.

Pearson, H. E., and Thompson, T. P. (1993). Atrophy and degeneration of ganglion cells in central retina following loss of postsynaptic target neurons in the dorsal lateral geniculate nucleus of the adult cat. *Exp. Neurol., 119,* 113–119.

Peters, A., and Payne, B. R. (1993). Numerical relationships between geniculo-cortical afferents and pyramidal cell modules in cat primary visual cortex. *Cereb. Cortex 3,* 69–78.

Rakic, P. (1977). Prenatal development of the visual system in the rhesus monkey. *Philos. Trans. R. Soc. Lond. Ser. B, 278,* 245–260.

Rizzo, M., and Hurtig, R. (1989). The effect of bilateral visual cortex lesions on the development of eye movements and perception. *Neurology, 39,* 406–413.

Robertson, L. C., and Lamb, M. R. (1991). Neuropsychological contributions to theories of part/whole organization. *Cog. Psychol., 23,* 299–330.

Rosenquist, A. C. (1985). Connections of visual cortical areas in the cat. In A. Peters and E. G. Jones (eds.): *Cerebral Cortex, vol. 3, Visual Cortex.* New York: Plenum Press, pp. 81–117.

Rowe, M. H. (1988). Changes in inner plexiform layer thickness following neonatal visual cortical ablation in cats. *Brain Res., 439,* 345–349.

Rowe, M. H. (1990). Evidence for degeneration of retinal W cells following early visual cortex removal in cats. *Brain. Behav. Evol., 35,* 253–267.

Rudel, R. G., Teuber, H.-L., and Twitchell, T. E. (1974). Levels of impairment of sensorimotor functions in children with early brain damage. *Neuropsychologia 12,* 95–108.

Sahraie, A., Weiskrantz, L., Barbur, J. L., Simmons, A., Williams, S. C. R., and Brammer, M. J. (1997). Pattern of neuronal activity associated with conscious and unconscious processing of visual signals. *Proc. Natl. Acad. Sci. U.S.A., 94,* 9406–9411.

Schilder, P., Pasik, P., and Pasik, T. (1972). Extrageniculostriate vision in the monkey. III. Circle vs. triangle and "red vs. green" discrimination. *Exp. Brain Res., 14,* 436–448.

Schneider, G. E. (1979). Is it really better to have your brain lesion early? A revision of the "Kennard Principle." *Neuropsychologia 17,* 557–583.

Shapley, R., and Perry, V. H. (1986). Cat and monkey retinal ganglion cells and their visual functional roles. *Trends Neurosci., 9,* 229–235.

Sherman, S. M. (1985). Functional organization of the W-, X- and Y- cell pathways in the cat: a review and hypothesis. In J. M. Sprague and A. N. Epstein (eds.): *Progress in Psychobiology and Physiological Psychology,* vol. 11. New York: Academic Press, pp. 233–314.

Shulman, G. L., and Wilson, J. (1987). Spatial frequency and selective attention to local and global information. *Perception, 16,* 89–101.

Shupert, C., Cornwell, P., and Payne, B. R. (1993). Differential sparing of depth perception, orienting and optokinetic nystagmus after neonatal versus adult lesions of cortical areas 17, 18 and 19 in the cat. *Behav. Neurosci., 107,* 633–650.

Spear, P. D., and Baumann, T. P. (1979). Effects of visual cortex removal on the receptive field properties of neurons in lateral suprasylvian visual area of the cat. *J. Neurophysiol., 42,* 31–56.

Spear, P. D., Kalil, R. E., and Tong, L. (1980). Functional compensation in lateral suprasylvian visual area following neonatal visual cortex removal in cats. *J. Neurophysiol., 43,* 851–869.

Stein, B. E., and Magalhaes-Castro, B. E. (1975). Effects of neonatal cortical lesions upon the cat superior colliculus. *Brain Res., 83,* 480–485.

Stiles, J., and Nass, R. (1991). Spatial grouping activity in young children with congenital right or left hemisphere brain injury. *Brain Cog., 15,* 201–222.

Stoerig, P., and Cowey, A. (1997). Blindsight in man and monkey. *Brain, 120,* 535–539.

Stone, J. (1983). *Parallel Processing in the Visual System.* New York: Plenum.

Sun, J.-S., Lomber, S. G., and Payne, B. R. (1994). Expansion of suprasylvian cortex projections in the superficial layers of the superior colliculus following damage of areas 17 and 18 in developing cats. *Vis. Neurosci., 11,* 13–22.

Teuber, H.-L. (1975). Recovery of function after brain injury in man. In: *Outcome of severe damage to the nervous system.* Ciba Foundation Symposium 34. Amsterdam: Elsevier North-Holland.

Tong, L., Kalil, R. E., and Spear, P. D. (1984). Critical periods for functional and anatomical compensation in the lateral suprasylvian visual area following removal of visual cortex in cats. *J. Neurophysiol., 52,* 941–960.

Tong, L., Spear, P. D., Kalil, R. E., and Callahan, E. C. (1982). Loss of retinal X cells in cats with neonatal or adult visual cortex damage. *Science 217,* 72–75.

Tumosa, N., McCall, M. A., Guido, W., and Spear, P. D. (1989). Responses of lateral geniculate neurons that survive long-term visual cortex damage in kittens and adult cats. *J. Neurosci., 9,* 280–298.

Tusa, R. J., Rosenquist, A. C., and Palmer, L. A. (1981). Multiple cortical visual areas: Visual field topography in the cat. In C. N. Woolsey (ed.): *Cortical Sensory Organization: Multiple Visual Areas.* Clifton, NJ: Humana Press, pp. 1–31.

Updyke, B. V. (1986). Retinotopic organization within the cat's suprasylvian sulcus and gyrus. *J. Comp. Neurol., 246,* 265–280.

Van Buren, J. M. (1963a). Transsynaptic retrograde degeneration in the visual system of primates. *J. Neurol. Neurosurg. Psychiatry, 26,* 402–407.

Van Buren, J. M. (1963b). *The Retinal Ganglion Cell Layer.* Springfield, IL: CC Thomas.

Vanduffel, W., Orban, G. A., Lomber, S. G., and Payne, B. R. (1998). Functional impact of cerebral projection systems. *Mol. Psychol., 3,* 215–219.

Vanduffel, W., Payne, B. R., Lomber, S. G., and Orban, G. A. (1997). Functional impact of cerebral connections. *Proc. Natl. Acad. Sci. U.S.A., 94,* 7617–7620.

Walsh, F. B. (1947). *Clinical Neuro-Ophthalmology.* Baltimore: Williams & Wilkins.

Wässle, H., and Boycott, B. B. (1991). Functional architecture of the mammalian retina. *Physiol. Rev., 71,* 447–480.

Webster, M. J., Ungerleider, L. G., and Bachevalier, J. (1991). Lesions of inferior temporal area TE in infant monkeys alter cortico-amygdalar projections. *NeuroReport 2,* 769–772.

Weiskrantz, L. (1996). Blindsight revisited. *Curr. Opin. Neurobiol. 6,* 215–220.

Weiskrantz, L., Barbur, J. L., and Sahraie, A. (1995). Parameters affecting conscious versus unconscious visual discrimination with damage to the visual cortex (V1). *Proc. Natl. Acad. Sci. U.S.A., 92,* 6122–6126.

Weller, R. E., and Kaas, J. H. (1989). Parameters affecting the loss of ganglion cells of the retina following ablations of striate cortex in primates. *Vis. Neurosci., 3,* 327–349.

Williams, P. L., Warwick, R., Dyson, M., and Bannister, L. H. (1989). *Gray's Anatomy,* 37th ed. Edinburgh: Churchill-Livingstone.

Woods, B. T. (1981). The restricted effects of right-hemisphere lesions after age one: Wechsler test data. *Neuropsychologia 18,* 65–70.

Yukie, M., and Iwai, E. (1981). Direct projection from the dorsal lateral geniculate nucleus to the prestriate cortex in macaque monkeys. *J. Comp. Neurol., 201,* 181–197.

Zeki, S., and Lamb, M. (1994). Review article. The neurology of kinetic art. *Brain 117,* 607–636.

III

NEURODEVELOPMENTAL COURSE OF EARLY BRAIN DISORDERS

7

Role of the Corpus Callosum in the Cognitive Development of Children with Congenital Brain Malformations

H. JULIA HANNAY, JACK M. FLETCHER,
AND MICHAEL E. BRANDT

With the advent of magnetic resonance imaging (MRI) of the brain, it has become apparent that children with congenital brain malformations often have abnormalities of the corpus callosum. This observation is important for several reasons. The corpus callosum is the primary pathway for association fibers that connect the two hemispheres of the brain. In addition to providing connectivity of the two hemispheres, the development of the corpus callosum may also exert a facilitatory influence on neuronal responses in each of the two hemispheres. These neuronal responses participate in the cerebral specialization of cognitive functions that begins early in development. Early damage to the corpus callosum may interfere with the development of cognitive and motor functions. Moreover, in a child born with a brain insult, malformation or damage to the corpus callosum may compromise opportunities for restoration of function. A major mechanism of restoration is the opportunity for brain regions in one hemisphere to support a particular function usually subsumed by the brain regions in the opposite hemisphere. Early compromise of the corpus callosum may interfere with this type of functional substitution. Damage to the corpus callosum, therefore, may be a critical component of the degree of plasticity and recovery of function in children with congenital brain malformations.

The purpose of this chapter is to examine the role of the corpus callosum in the development of cognitive and motor skills for children with congenital brain malformations. We review the structure, development, and function of the corpus callosum. The early neuroembryogenesis of the corpus callosum and its implications for congenital brain disorders are discussed. Then a group of studies of the corpus callosum in children with congenital brain malformations that lead to early hydrocephalus follows. We conclude with a discussion of the role of the corpus callosum in the reorganization of cognitive and motor functions in children with congenital brain malformations.

Corpus Callosum: Structure, Development, and Function

Structure

The corpus callosum is the largest fiber tract connecting the left and right cerebral hemispheres. On the basis of experimental work with monkeys and clinical work with humans, the corpus callosum has been subdivided into several regions (Witelson, 1989) that includes the rostrum, genu, body (anterior midbody, posterior midbody, and isthmus), and splenium (see Fig. 7-1). In going from the posterior to the anterior aspect of the corpus callosum, the first region is the splenium, which connects occipital and inferior temporal cortical regions. In front of the splenium is the isthmus, which connects superior temporal and posterior parietal cortical regions. Then there is the posterior midbody, which connects somesthetic and posterior parietal cortical regions. This is followed by the anterior midbody, which

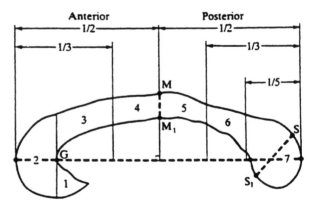

Region	Anatomical label	Cortical region
1	Rostrum	Caudal/orbital prefrontal, inferior premotor
2	Genu	Prefrontal
3	Rostral body	Premotor, supplementary motor
4	Anterior midbody	Motor
5	Posterior midbody	Somaesthetic, posterior parietal
6	Isthmus	Superior temporal, posterior parietal
7	Splenium	Occipital, inferior temporal.

Figure 7-1. Anatomy of the corpus callosum, including the seven regions defined by Witelson (1989).

connects the motor cortices. The genu connects the prefrontal cortical regions. Finally, the most anterior section of the corpus callosum—the rostrum—connects the caudal/orbital prefrontal and inferior premotor cortical regions. Each of these regions has a different developmental progression and, depending on the areas of the hemispheres connected by the region, may participate differently in cognitive functions.

Development

The development of the corpus callosum begins at about 7 weeks of age and continues through 20 weeks gestation. With the exception of the rostrum—the most anterior segment—the corpus callosum develops in an anteroposterior direction, from the genu to the splenium. At about 12 weeks gestation, the partially formed corpus callosum is clearly present and continues to fill out in a rostral (genu to splenium) direction. The rostrum develops between 18 and 20 weeks. Subsequent anatomical gestational development of the corpus callosum involves the extension of axons crossing contralaterally through the corpus callosum, which leads to increased thickening and the bulb-like appearance of the genu and splenium. During the remainder of gestation and after birth, the corpus callosum continues to thicken, but the essential appearance is usually present by 20 weeks gestation. Disturbance of this developmental process leads to a spectrum of callosal defects ranging from complete to partial agenesis and usually involving posterior aspects of the corpus callosum, depending on when development is disrupted (Barkovich, 1995).

Function

The role of the corpus callosum in integrating activity between and within the cerebral hemispheres has been the subject of much speculation over the years. One of the major controversies has been over its presumed inhibitory and facilitatory roles. Some investigators have theorized that the corpus callosum participates in cerebral lateralization by allowing each hemisphere to prevail for a given function (Corballis and Morgan, 1978; Jeeves, 1986; Moscovitch, 1977). In the context of development, Dennis (1976) contended that the corpus callosum has an *inhibitory* role by suppressing ipsilateral sensory and motor pathways. Contralateral pathway dominance is believed to be necessary for finely tuned sensation and motor control. Lassonde (1986) argued that there is little physiological evidence for an inhibitory function. Rather, the corpus callosum exerts a *facilitatory* influence on neural activity in each hemisphere that enhances communication between the hemispheres and promotes cerebral specialization (Lassonde, 1986; Payne, 1986). A variety of studies have addressed these hypotheses, including correlational studies in normal subjects and research on patients with congenital absence of the corpus callosum.

Cognitive Functions and the Corpus Callosum

Correlational studies

In several recent studies, researchers have correlated the size of the corpus callosum with behavioral measures in normal individuals. Some of the studies have used dichotic listening tasks in which verbal stimuli are presented simultaneously to the right and left ears. There appears to be inhibition of ipsilateral auditory pathways with this paradigm. Right ear stimuli are sent by contralateral pathways to the left hemisphere, which is usually specialized for language. Left ear stimuli are sent to the right hemisphere by contralateral pathways and are processed less efficiently in the right hemisphere or transferred callosally to the left hemisphere for processing with some degradation. Thus normal individuals generally identify more verbal stimuli from the right ear.

Theories of callosal functioning have led to specific predictions about the number of stimuli correctly identified from each ear (ear accuracy) and/or the magnitude of the difference in ear accuracy (ear advantage). Yazgan et al. (1995) reasoned that a *callosal inhibitory* model would predict that a larger corpus callosum would produce greater inhibitions so that cerebral functions should be more lateralized. More specifically, a larger corpus callosum would permit the left hemisphere to exert more of an inhibitory influence on the right hemisphere. A larger right ear advantage would result from a reduction of left ear accuracy. As the size of the corpus callosum increases, the right ear advantage should increase because of a decrease in the left ear accuracy. A *callosal facilitatory* model would predict that the larger the corpus callosum, the more activation of the hemisphere not thought to be specialized for language. This would result in a higher left ear accuracy and thus a smaller right ear advantage. As the size of the corpus callosum increases, the right ear advantage should increase because of an increase in the left ear accuracy. Yazgan et al. (1995) reported that the right ear advantage *decreased* as the cross-sectional area of the corpus callosum became larger, a finding that supports a facilitatory function for the corpus callosum.

In contrast to these findings, Clarke et al. (1993) did not find a significant relationship between a ratio of right ear and left ear responses and measures of the corpus callosum, including the posterior body. As the size of the corpus callosum and its regions increased, right ear accuracy decreased, a finding that does not fit the predictions from either model. With the inhibition model, left ear accuracy should decrease as the size of the corpus callosum increases. With the facilitatory model, left ear accuracy should increase as the corpus callosum enlarges.

In a study relating performance on cognitive tests to the size of the genu, isthmus, and splenium, Hines et al. (1992) found that verbal fluency (retrieving words from categories or with specific initial letters) was positively related to the size of the posterior corpus callosum, primarily the splenium, while language laterality was negatively related to the size of this region. This latter finding is again supportive of the facilitatory model of callosal functioning. Overall, the results of these three studies are somewhat inconclusive, but tend to support a facilitatory model of the corpus callosum.

Studies of acallosal patients

Much of the information on the function of the corpus callosum has been obtained through investigation of children and adults born with only partial development or complete agenesis of the corpus callosum. These studies are important because of the possibility that the acallosal brain has had the opportunity to compensate for the absent corpus callosum even before birth (Lassonde et al., 1988). Investigations of such cases has been carried out using methods from experimental psychology developed to study lateralization of function and information transfer across the hemispheres (Hannay, 1986a). The results are believed to reflect in part cerebral specialization for verbal (left hemisphere) and nonverbal (right hemisphere) material, although interpretations of performance that involves factors other than cerebral specialization have also been made. These studies have been completed in visual, auditory, and somesthetic modalities and for visuomotor skills.

Vision. Tachistoscopic studies of the perception of stimuli presented in the left or right visual field for a very brief duration in acallosal individuals have yielded useful information about the effects of congenital agenesis of the corpus callosum. For the most part, the tachistoscopic studies have produced similar visual field effects for acallosals and control subjects (Ettlinger et al., 1974; Karnath et al., 1991; Lassonde et al., 1988; Lehmann and Lampe, 1970).

One explanation for the apparent reorganization of function in the acallosal subject is increased use of the anterior commissure. One study addressed this explanation with MRI visualizations of both the corpus callosum and the anterior commissure of two children (Fischer et al., 1992). Both children had total agenesis of the corpus callosum. The right-handed boy with an absent or very small anterior commissure showed an abnormally large right visual field superiority in reaction time for naming drawings of common objects and words due to a much reduced ability to name the stimuli quickly when presented in the left visual field. This suggests that the stimuli were being degraded in their transfer from the right hemisphere to the language-dominant left hemisphere. The left-handed boy with an enlarged or hypertrophied anterior commissure showed a slight left visual field superiority in reaction time, which suggested that stimuli were being successfully transferred from the nondominant hemisphere. The fact that this child was left handed makes the interpretation of the results less clear because he might have bilateral representation of language. In any case, this research does suggest that investigators should determine the size and integrity of the anterior commissure in order to interpret findings for tasks requiring interhemispheric transmission of information. Of course, if only 10% of acallosals have an enlarged anterior commissure (Rauch and Jinkins, 1994), there are likely other explanations for their performance.

Audition. Dichotic listening studies of the perception of stimuli presented simultaneously to the right and left ears have also aided in our understanding of the effects of congenital agenesis of the corpus callosum on auditory interhemispheric transfer. Normal individuals usually show a right ear advantage for perception of verbal stimuli, but the findings for acallosal subjects are contradictory (Chiarello, 1980). Different studies report no ear advantage, a right ear advantage, and a left ear advantage (Chiarello, 1980; Lassonde et al., 1990). While most acallosals show a right ear advantage, there does appear to be a greater incidence of left ear advantage in that population than in the normal population (Chiarello, 1980; Lassonde et al., 1990). The lack of an ear effect could be due to bilateral representation of language, but this finding and the left ear advantage in some studies could result from the strengthening of ipsilateral pathways. It is interesting to note that studies in which both tachistoscopic and dichotic listening tasks are given to the same subjects have produced results that indicate that different mechanisms may be primarily responsible for compensation for a lack of callosal transfer of visual and auditory information (Fischer et al., 1992; Ettlinger et al., 1974). For example, the acallosal subject, who had an absent or very small anterior commissure, of Fischer et al. (1992), showed an exaggerated right visual field superiority for naming words and drawings of common objects, but a left ear advantage for the perception of words. Because tactile performance as well as tachistoscopic performance indicated that the subject was probably left hemisphere dominant for language, the authors suggest that there may be enhancement of ipsilateral auditory pathways and/or use of subcortical pathways.

Touch. Tactile naming of objects felt out of sight appears to be intact in both the left and right hands of acallosal subjects despite the fact that naming of objects felt by the left hand normally requires callosal transfer of information to the language-dominant left hemisphere (Lassonde et al., 1991; Ettlinger et al., 1974; Reynolds and Jeeves, 1977). However, tactile localization deficits and longer tactile naming times have been noted in acallosal children and adults with intact tactile naming and matching (Dennis, 1976; Geffen et al., 1994), which suggests that compensatory interhemisphere transfer of tactile information is incomplete (Dennis, 1976). Greater use of ipsilateral pathways and/or subcortical pathways has again been proposed (Dennis, 1976; Ettlinger et al., 1974; Jeeves, 1979; Lassonde et al., 1991).

Visuomotor tasks. A variety of visuomotor tasks that require coordination of the two hands have been given to acallosal patients. A deficit in bimanual coordination on simple tasks such as bead stringing under time stress (Jeeves, 1965; Jeeves and Rajalakshmi, 1964) appears to be a common problem for acallosals (Chiarello, 1980) that does not diminish with maturity (Jeeves, 1979). Difficulties have also been demonstrated on a more complex visuomotor task (Jeeves et al., 1988) requiring bimanual movement of a recorder along a diagonal line (Preilowski, 1972).

Interhemispheric transmission time (ITT) for visual information has also been measured with acallosals by presenting a simple stimulus in the left or right visual field and comparing the subject's reaction times for detecting the presence of the stimulus under different response conditions. When the subject responds with the hand ipsilateral to the field of stimulus presentation, the response does not require callosal transfer of information (uncrossed response). When the subject responds with the hand contralateral to the field of stimulus presentation, the response involves callosal transfer of information (crossed response). Crossed response reaction time should be longer. The crossed–uncrossed reaction time difference provides a measure of ITT. The ITT is normally about 2 to 6 msec (Bashore, 1981) and is usually much longer for acallosal subjects (Clarke and Zaidel, 1989; Di Stefano et al., 1992; Milner et al., 1985). Milner et al. (1985) have argued that the ITT task measures sensory and not motor pathway transmission. This is because the ITT is longer in acallosals than in normals when the intensity of the visual stimulus is reduced. Clarke and Ziedel (1989) have suggested that the anterior commissure might be involved in the transfer of the information because ITT appears to be a sensory task. Lassonde (1994) assessed the ITT in acallosals and a callosotomized patient with sparing of the splenium, and she found comparable ITTs of 51.3 and 58.3 msec, respectively. This comparability supports the idea that the response on the ITT task is conveyed by the motor components of the callosal pathway rather than the splenium. Thus, the performance of the acallosals probably involves strengthening of ipsilateral and/or subcortical motor pathways.

In summary, acallosal individuals do not show the signature disconnection syndrome of the adult split brain, but are less intact than neurologically normal age peers (Chiarello, 1980; Milner and Jeeves, 1979). They show a variety of sometimes subtle problems, such as slower reaction time for interhemispheric comparison of visual stimuli (Sauerwein et al., 1994), an atypical ear advantage for dichotic listening (Bryden and Zurif, 1970), difficulties in tactile localization (Dennis, 1976), and slower intermanual coordination (Jeeves, 1965). These reported difficulties vary across studies for reasons that are not always clearly apparent, including the methodological factors reviewed above and potential compensatory mechanisms.

Compensatory mechanisms

On the basis of these studies, a variety of compensatory mechanisms involving neural reorganization have been suggested. These mechanisms include bilateral representation of function, enhanced transmission by the anterior commissure, and ipsilateral and/or subcortical pathways (Jeeves, 1994). In a recent overview, Jeeves (1994) concluded that bilateral representation of function is probably not a compensatory neural mechanism in acallosals, although this mechanism has not been completely eliminated. As Jeeves (1994) pointed out, evidence from a variety of sources (see Jeeves and Milner, 1987; Sauerwein et al., 1994) suggests that there is some degree of hemispheric specialization in acallosals, but not to the same extent as normals. Acallosals appear to have a clear hand preference (Chiarello,

1980; Jeeves, 1986), and most are right handed. Paw preference also has been reported in a mouse model of early callosal defects (Schmidt, 1994). With no dominance for motor control, there should be a significant number of ambidextrous acallosals, but most do show hand preferences. Wada testing of eight acallosals has produced evidence of left hemisphere lateralization of speech in six of the cases; the two cases in which left hemisphere lateralization was not apparent were left handed (Sauerwein et al., 1994).

The anterior commissure has been suggested as the most likely compensatory mechanism for interhemispheric transfer of visual information, particularly patterned visual information, because it contains fibers connecting the visual association areas of the temporal lobes (Jeeves, 1994). Located slightly ventral to the rostrum, the anterior commissure is known to contain fibers connecting the olfactory nuclei of the two hemispheres in its anterior limb and fibers connecting the middle and inferior temporal gyri and the visual and auditory association areas in the temporal lobes (Fox and Schmitz, 1943; Klinger and Gloor, 1960; Pandya et al., 1971; Whitlock and Nauta, 1956; Zeke, 1973). There is some evidence of involvement of the anterior commisure in the transfer of visual, auditory, and olfactory information in patients with complete sectioning of the corpus callosum excluding the anterior commissure, although successful transfer in all three systems was not shown by all patients (Risse et al., 1978). Spatial integration may be mediated by the superior colliculus and the intertectal commissure rather than the anterior commissure (Milner, 1994). If the anterior commissure serves as a compensatory neural mechanism, it may do so for only a small proportion of the cases, and its absence or reduced size may further compromise interhemispheric transmission. Wahlsten and Ozaki (1994) did not find an expansion of the anterior commissure in mice with an absent or small corpus callosum. Rauch and Jinkins (1994) reported that the anterior commissure is enlarged in only 10% of the cases of callosal agenesis and appears to be absent or smaller in 10% of the cases. Loeser and Alvord (1968) found that the anterior commissure might be absent in about 20% of all agenesis patients.

Enhanced development of ipsilateral somatosensory and motor pathways with integration of information between crossed and uncrossed pathways within each hemisphere has been endorsed as a compensatory mechanism (Dennis, 1976). For instance, this mechanism has been used to explain atypical ear effects in dichotic listening and the fact that acallosal patients can successfully complete tactile discrimination and naming tasks but have difficulty with tactile integration, as discussed earlier.

These proposed mechanisms for neural reorganization are often viewed as competing explanations for interhemispheric transfer and the performance of cognitive tasks by individuals with agenesis and partial agenesis of the corpus callosum. All of these mechanisms may actually have some role in that one or more may be operating in a particular individual depending on the commissural anomalies present. Unfortunately, it is difficult to address this possibility because of the small number of acallosals in most studies as well as methodological factors that interfere with comparisons across studies.

Limitations of prior research

There is no standardized set of tasks for assessing interhemispheric transfer, and variations in methodology can certainly produce different findings. This may, in part, explain why the results of particular interhemispheric paradigms are not always in agreement. Some studies have included both patients with total and partial agenesis and have considered possible differences in their functioning (Ettlinger et al., 1974), while other studies have not made this important distinction (Lehmann and Lampe, 1970). Many of the studies are essentially case studies involving only one or two individuals (Bryden and Zurif, 1970; Dennis, 1976; Lassonde et al., 1981), and only rarely does the sample size approach 10 or more (Lehmann and Lampe, 1970). Only recently have callosal anomalies been documented by MRI, which is more sensitive to callosal dysmorphology than other imaging methods.

What is needed is a large sample of subjects to whom a single set of interhemispheric transfer tasks can be given. These subjects could be divided into subgroups on the basis of their callosal dysmorphology as determined by MRI, which can also be used to determine the size and integrity of the anterior commissure. It may be possible to obtain such samples in children with certain congenital brain malformations.

Callosal Defects in Children With Congenital Brain Malformations

Defects of the corpus callosum are common in children with congenital brain malformations. For example, in holoprosencephaly, where there is largely no development of the two hemispheres in the brain, portions of the corpus callosum simply fail to develop, reflecting very early gestational disruption (Norman et al., 1995). In an early MRI investigation, Barkovich and Norman (1988) examined callosal defects in children with other congenital anomalies of the brain. The conditions included the malformations of the cerebellum and hindbrain classified as the Arnold-Chiari malformations (I and II), the Dandy-Walker malformation (see Dennis et al., Chapter 8), neuronal migration disorders (e.g., lissencephaly, polymicrogria), and encephaloceles.

In the children with the less severe Arnold-Chiari I malformation, virtually all studied (22/24) had a normal corpus callosum. In contrast, virtually all (10/12) of the Arnold-Chiari II malformations were associated with partial agenesis of the corpus callosum. The degree to which the corpus callosum was formed did not relate to the degree of cerebellum/hindbrain malformation. Two cases with Dandy-Walker syndrome had a normal corpus callosum, while two had partial agenesis. Encephaloceles largely showed complete to partial agenesis of the corpus callosum. Other studies have shown complete (rare) and partial (common) agenesis of the corpus callosum, particularly in children with midline defects such as septo-optic dysplasia and aqueductal stenosis, a common etiology of early hydrocephalus (Barkovich, 1995).

The Arnold-Chiari II malformation is usually associated with meningomyelo-cele, a spinal dysraphism in children with spina bifida that is due to a failure of the caudal end of the neural tube to close during the first week of gestation. Because of the Arnold-Chiari II malformation, about 80%–90% of children with spina bifida meningomyelocele develop hydrocephalus that requires shunting (Reigel and Rotenstein, 1994). Although complete agenesis of the corpus callosum is rare, most children with spina bifida meningomyelocele have a corpus callosum defect in-volving partial agenesis and/or hypoplasia (thinning). The prevalence of spina bi-fida meningomyelocele, about 0.5–1.0 per 1,000 live births, makes it the most com-mon severely disabling birth defect in North America. Figure 7-2 shows midsagital

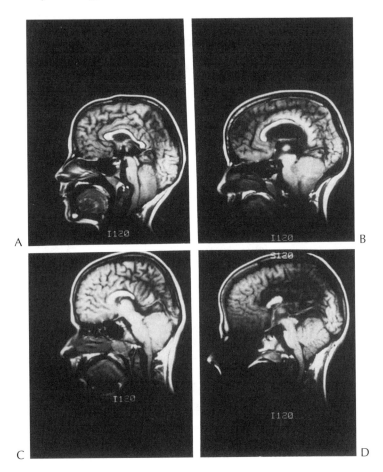

Figure 7-2. Midsagital magnetic resonance images of the brains of four children with spina bifida meningomyelocele. All four brains show the characteristic malformation of the cere-bellum and hindbrain (Arnold-Chiari II malformation) and dilation of the lateral ventricles representative of hydrocephalus. They vary in corpus callosum anomalies: intact corpus cal-losum (*A*), hypoplastic corpus callosum (*B*), and severe partial agenesis of the corpus cal-losum (*C, D*).

views of the brain from MRI in four children with spina bifida meningomyelocele. The malformed nature and downward extension of the cerebellum and varying degrees of partial agenesis and hypoplasia of corpus callosum are clearly shown.

The corpus callosum anomalies include partial agenesis and hypoplasia, potentially involving the rostrum, splenium, and various degrees of the posterior body. Agenesis occurs when callosal axons that cross the midline are absent or deficient (Norman et al., 1995). Hypoplasia is simply stretching and/or thinning of callosal fibers. Given the developmental progression of the corpus callosum, partial agenesis represents a disruption in neuroembryogenesis that extends through the first trimester and beyond the closure of the neural tube. These anomalies are not simply mechanical defects due to hydrocephalus. The destructive effects of hydrocephalus can be seen in thinning of the corpus callosum (hypoplasia) and loss of the genu, infrequent in spina bifida meningomyelocele, partly because of the early treatment of hydrocephalus. In children with spina bifida meningomyelocele, the fact that the ends of the corpus callosum are missing and the genu is usually present indicates that the agenesis is a product of a disturbance of the normal developmental process in the formation of the corpus callosum and not simply a secondary destructive effect of hydrocephalus (Barkovich, 1995). Hence, the corpus callosum is almost always abnormal, with partial agenesis in 65% of cases and hypoplasia in an additional 30% (Fletcher et al., 1959). In addition to congenital defects related to the fundamental defects in neuroembryogenesis, children with spina bifida meningomyelocele experience injury to the brain because of hydrocephalus and its treatment.

Other congenital brain malformations also lead to early hydrocephalus and are associated with partial agenesis of the corpus callosum. Aqueductal stenosis is a rare disorder involving congenital narrowing of the aqueduct of Sylvius, which invariably leads to hydrocephalus usually requiring shunting. The prevalence is about 1 per 17,000 births. Children with aqueductal stenosis also have corpus callosum defects, including partial agenesis and hypoplasia, but not at the same frequency as children with spina bifida meningomyelocele. Aqueductal stenosis occurs somewhat later in gestation than spina bifida meningomyelocele, which may be why these children tend to show a lower frequency of partial agenesis. Children with aqueductal stenosis develop hydrocephalus because of a congenital narrowing of the cerebral aqueduct (Barkovich, 1995). In contrast to spina bifida meningomyelocele and Dandy-Walker syndrome, the cerebellum is generally normal, although some downward extension of the cerebellum may be present because of pressure effects from hydrocephalus (Robertson et al., 1990).

Callosal defects are common in Dandy-Walker syndrome, which usually requires shunting for the fourth ventricle cyst characteristic of the malformation. Dandy-Walker syndrome is quite rare, occurring in about 1 per 30,000 live births. About 70%–80% of children with Dandy-Walker syndrome develop hydrocephalus. The primary defining characteristic is the presence of a large cystic fourth ventricle with partial to complete agenesis of the cerebellar vermis. The posterior fossa is enlarged with substantial dilation of the fourth ventricle. Partial agenesis of the corpus callosum is common (Chuang, 1986).

Septo-optic dysplasia is rare and most likely represents a heterogeneous group of disorders. It is characterized by optic atrophy and defects of the septum pellucidum. Shunting for hydrocephalus is rare. Callosal defects are common as part of the spectrum of midline defects characterizing this heterogeneous syndrome.

Hydrocephalus in these populations is caused by the congenital malformations of the brain, which obstruct the flow of cerebrospinal fluid and lead to ventricular enlargement often necessitating shunting. In spina bifida meningomyelocele, the spinal dysraphism present at birth usually indicates the presence of the brain malformation (Arnold-Chiari II) that causes obstruction of cerebrospinal fluid. Aqueductal stenosis and Dandy-Walker syndrome are usually detected because of rapid expansion of head size in infancy to accommodate the increases in cerebrospinal fluid, although some infants with Dandy-Walker syndrome also have problems with head control that lead to discovery of the cystic malformation of the cerebellum. Whenever significant hydrocephalus occurs, there is additional insult to the brain, including stretching of white matter fibers (Del Bigio, 1993). Oculomotor impairment may result from damage to the midbrain, cerebellum, and optic tracts. Long-term consequences of hydrocephalus can include disruption of the process of myelination, with reductions in thickness of the cortical mantle, reduced overall brain mass, and selective thinning of posterior brain regions.

Corpus Callosum Function in Children
With Congenital Brain Malformations

Children with spina bifida meningomyelocele, aqueductal stenosis, and Dandy-Walker syndrome have shared neurobehavioral deficits. In particular, many of these children have impairments of motor coordination and spatial cognition that are virtually ubiquitous in the first two conditions. Identification of neural correlates of these characteristic cognitive deficits has not been adequately pursued. It is common to simply attribute these deficits to the presence of hydrocephalus. Although the extent of posterior brain thinning does appear to be related to the extent of the deficits in motor skills and spatial functions (Dennis et al., 1981; Fletcher et al., 1996b), the relationships are relatively weak and there remains considerably variability not accounted for by hydrocephalus and its treatment.

Because children with spina bifida meningomyelocele and Dandy-Walker syndrome have cerebellum malformations, it may be that these malformations are responsible for the motor and spatial deficits. However, such deficits are also apparent in children with aqueductal stenosis, who typically have a normal cerebellum. Motor function differences are apparent on a qualitative basis, particularly when children with these three etiologies of early hydrocephalus are compared.

Another possibility is that the corpus callosum abnormalities characteristic of all three of these populations account for some of the variability apparent in motor and spatial skill outcomes. We have been investigating all three of these possible explanations in a series of studies using quantitative analysis of the MRI. The initial studies were primarily correlational, but a subsequent study involved the experimental paradigms used to study acallosal subjects in an attempt to evaluate callosal functions.

Correlational studies

Figure 7-3 displays the characteristic findings when measures of verbal and spatial functions in children with spina bifida meningomyelocele and aqueductal stenosis are compared. As Figure 7-3 shows, children with different etiologies of hydrocephalus have, on average, significantly lower scores on spatial measures relative to their verbal scores. It is well known that children with early hydrocephalus have problems with visuomotor and spatial abilities (Dennis et al., 1981; Fletcher et al., 1992b, 1995; Wills, 1993). These problems are apparent on tasks involving fine motor and perceptual-motor skills, as well as on motor-free tests that require spatial perception but no constructional performance. Etiological differences are not readily apparent. Hence, spatial and motor skills are certainly impaired in children with early hydrocephalus, but there is no evidence that these impairments vary across etiologies. Most children with hydrocephalus show pre-

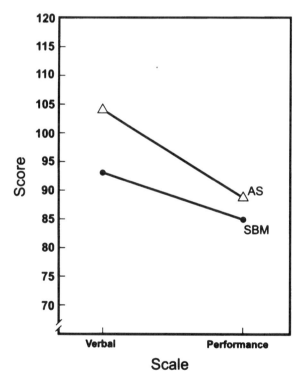

Figure 7-3. Verbal and Performance IQ scores from the Wechsler Intelligence Scale for Children–Revised for children with spina bifida meningomyelocele (SBM) and aqueductal stenosis (AS). The children have lower Performance IQ than Verbal IQ scores.

served abilities on measures of facial recognition, simple visual discrimination, and the ability to match shapes. However, significant problems are apparent on complex visuospatial tasks involving form consistency, figure-ground relationships, memory for spatial location, and the location for stimuli and external space. These are certainly not the only deficiencies that children with early hydrocephalus display, but they are the most pronounced (Fletcher et al., 1995).

In a series of studies, we have shown that the motor and spatial deficits displayed by children with early hydrocephalus are strongly related to the integrity of the corpus callosum. In the initial study, Fletcher et al. (1992a) measured a variety of verbal and nonverbal skills in children with spina bifida meningomyelocele, aqueductal stenosis, and controls. From a concurrently obtained MRI, quantitative assessments were made of several white matter structures, including the corpus callosum, internal capsules, and centrum semiovale. Lateral ventricular volumes in both hemispheres were also computed. When the cognitive measures were correlated with the MRI measures, we found significant correlations of the cross-sectional area of the corpus callosum with measures of both verbal and nonverbal skills. However, the relationship was much stronger for nonverbal skills and held up across different measures.

In a subsequent study, Fletcher et al. (1996a) replicated the findings involving the corpus callosum and cognitive skills on a much larger sample of children who varied in the etiology of early hydrocephalus. Children with ventricular expansion who were not shunted for hydrocephalus were also included. Again, the MRI was quantitated, including an area of measure of the corpus callosum. As before, the corpus callosum was significantly smaller in children with shunted hydrocephalus, with no etiology effects. The correlation of the corpus callosum measure was significant with both verbal and spatial measurements, but the relationship was much stronger for nonverbal cognitive skills. In this study, measures of motor skills and skills in other domains involving problem-solving skills were also included. There were no significant relationships with problem-solving measures, but the corpus callosum measure also correlated robustly with the measure of fine motor dexterity. In general, these two studies showed a robust relationship between the area (measurement) of the corpus callosum and nonverbal cognitive and motor skills. This relationship is depicted in Figure 7-4, which plots the Performance IQ score from the Wechsler Intelligence Scale for Children–Revised (WISC-R; Wechsler, 1974) and the area of measurement of the corpus callosum. Figure 7-4 shows a strong relationship *within* children with shunted hydrocephalus, who have significantly smaller area measurements of the corpus callosum. Figure 7-4 also shows that there is little relationship between the size of the corpus callosum and the Performance IQ in children with arrested hydrocephalus and normal controls.

Experimental studies

On the basis of the correlational findings, we subsequently adopted an experimental approach based on the paradigms used to study acallosal subjects (Klaas et al., 1997). We specifically hoped to evaluate relationships of different task re-

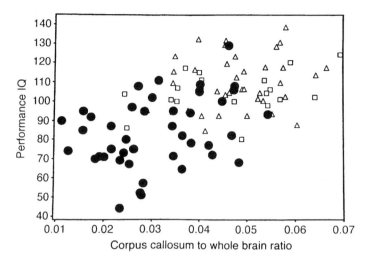

Figure 7-4. Correlation ($r = 0.55$) of the area measurement of the corpus callosum (mid-sagital slice) and Performance IQ for children with shunted, arrested, and no hydrocephalus. Children with hydrocephalus tend to have both lower Performance IQ scores and smaller corpus callosum measurements. ●, Shunted hydrocephalus; △, arrested hydrocephalus; □, no hydrocephalus. (From Fletcher et al., 1996a).

quirements to partial agenesis of the corpus callosum. Interhemispheric transfer of information was investigated in hydrocephalic children with spina bifida mening-omyelocele ($n = 8$) or aqueductal stenosis ($n = 5$). All of the children had partial agenesis of the corpus callosum, having no splenium and partial agenesis/hypoplasia of the body. There were also 13 normal controls of similar age, race, gender, and socioeconomic status. All subjects were right handed, with seven males and six females in each group. The age range was 10–17 years for the hydrocephalics and 9–15 years for the normal controls. Children with prior histories of head injury, neurological disorders not associated with shunting, or severe psychiatric disorders were excluded from the study. All children were required to have a WISC-R Verbal or Performance IQ ≥70 to avoid the effects of mental deficiency.

The children were administered a variety of sensory and perceptual tasks as well as interhemispheric transfer tasks. The sensory and perceptual tasks were used to determine if the ability to receive and interpret stimuli that did not have to cross the corpus callosum to be processed was in any way responsible for atypical performance on interhemispheric transfer tasks. A tachistoscopic laterality task (Fontenot, 1973; Dee and Hannay, 1981) was used to examine callosal transfer of high complexity–low association forms. A dichotic listening tasks (Hawles, 1991) was used to examine callosal transfer of auditory information. Tactile matching of objects in each hand was used as a control tasks for determining if the children could make appropriate tactile discrimination with each hand because it does not involve the callosal transfer of information. A tactile naming task requiring naming of objects felt out of sight with the right or left hand served as the tactile interhemispheric transfer test. Finally, an ITT task, developed based on studies reported by Bashore (1981), was used to assess visuomotor performance.

Visual tasks. The hypothesis that some neural reorganization takes place in hydrocephalic children with a missing splenium and hypoplasia of the body was tested. Specifically, it was hypothesized that the transfer of visual information by other pathways such as the anterior commissure should result in slower and more degraded transfer of the information. In comparison to normal children, the hydrocephalic children were predicted to show a larger left visual field superiority for recognition of high complexity–low association value forms because they correctly identified fewer of the forms presented in the right visual field, which presumably had to be transferred from the left to the right hemisphere to be processed effectively. In contrast to controls, the hydrocephalic children demonstrated a significant left visual field superiority for the forms, primarily because they made more errors when the forms were presented in the right visual field. This pattern of performance relative to the controls can be viewed as an exaggeration of normal performance related to poorer transfer of right visual field information from the left hemisphere to the right hemisphere for processing.

Auditory tasks. Because the body of the corpus callosum was primarily hypoplastic rather than missing in the hydrocephalic children, it was hypothesized that the anterior commissure would not be involved in neural reorganization in audition the same way as in vision. Instead, greater use of ipsilateral and/or subcortical pathways was expected because the callosal auditory fibers would not be fully capable of transferring auditory information. This would result in either a reduction in the normal right ear advantage for fused dichotic words or even a left ear advantage. Neither the normal nor the hydrocephalic group showed a significant ear advantage, and no significant differences were found between the hydrocephalic and control children in their ear effects. However, there was a significant relation between ear effect and group because more normal children showed right ear advantage than a left ear advantage and more hydrocephalic children showed a left ear advantage rather than a right ear advantage. This provides some support for the idea that the hydrocephalic children have stronger ipsilateral projections. We are replacing the dichotic listening procedure with one that is likely to produce clearer ear effects in normals in our future research.

Tactile tasks. Neural reorganization in somatosensory perception and visuomotor performance was predicted to involve greater use of ipsilateral and/or subcortical pathways. Because tactile naming is not lateralized in normals, greater use of ipsilateral and/or subcortical pathways might result in equally good naming in both hands like normals or only somewhat reduced left-hand naming. The hydrocephalic children should take longer to make their responses. Tactile naming performance was similar for both groups, who showed no difference in their ability to name objects presented to the left and right hands. The hydrocephalic children took significantly longer to name felt objects, regardless of hand. These findings support greater use of ipsilateral and or subcortical pathways by the hydrocephalic children. The hydrocephalic children also matched significantly fewer objects with each hand, which indicates poorer tactile perception.

Visuomotor task. We hypothesized that children with hydrocephalus would have a longer ITT because greater use would have to be made of ipsilateral and/or subcortical pathways. The ITT task involved the measurement of reaction time to a simple visual stimulus (a small white square) lateralized in the right visual field or the left visual field and responded to as quickly as possible by either the left or right hand. This procedure permits determination of reaction time when the response demands transmission of information across the corpus callosum (crossed reaction time) and when it does not (uncrossed reaction time). The crossed–uncrossed difference in reaction time provides an estimate of ITT. The crossed–uncrossed difference did not differ significantly between the hydrocephalic and normal children. This was, in part, because of the very large standard deviations for reaction time for all subjects. Indeed, the crossed–uncrossed difference was longer for the hydrocephalic children, as predicted. We used short practice and test sessions in an attempt to avoid fatiguing the subjects. Longer practice and test sessions, more like those used with adults, might stabilize the reaction times of individual subjects and result in smaller intrasubject variation. The reaction time was, in general, significantly longer for the hydrocephalic children on the ITT task, reflecting their motor slowness.

The results of this initial investigation were very promising. The findings suggested that there is functional reorganization of the nervous system to compensate for the loss or thinning of sections of the corpus callosum and that different mechanisms were probably involved. These mechanisms possibly include the enlargement of the anterior commissure to carry information between visual association areas when the splenium is missing. A significant correlation between the size of the anterior commissure and performance on the visual, but not the auditory, tactile, and visuomotor interhemispheric transfer tasks would provide further evidence for this interpretation of the data. The strengthening of ipsilateral and/or subcortical pathways for visuomotor information would be indicated by less lateralized or reversed ear, tactile, and motor performances and a relationship between these effects and the size of callosal regions transferring this information.

In the future, we plan much larger experimental investigations of children with early hydrocephalus who have congenital absence of the corpus callosum. Because spina bifida meningomyelocele is relatively common, we plan to focus on children with partial agenesis and hypoplasia of the corpus callosum in this population. Using a sagittal MRI, we will identify subgroups based on patterns of the corpus callosum defects. Although our initial investigation focused primarily on children who were missing the splenium, the rostrum is also commonly missing. Because the rostrum connects prefrontal areas, absence of the rostrum could be a potential mechanism that accounts for some of the difficulties with language organization and pragmatics commonly observed in children with spina bifida meningomyelocele (Dennis et al., 1994). In addition, using MRI, we will attempt to assess the integrity of the anterior commissure and evaluate hypotheses about the anterior commissure and other potential compensatory mechanisms. Anomalies of the corpus callosum will be assessed by performance on a revised battery of callosal transfer tasks. The key is a sufficiently large sample to permit identification of subgroups and to have enough statistical power to evaluate these potential relationships.

Conclusions

Children with congenital brain malformations commonly have abnormalities of the corpus callosum. Although the significance of these abnormalities may be obscured by the primary brain malformation, the corpus callosum is a significant factor in the long-term outcomes of these children. In most instances, the corpus callosum defects reflect part of the process that results in the defining cerebral malformation. For example, spina bifida meningomyelocele is a neural tube defect that is the product of abnormalities during the first month of gestation. However, the defect in neuroembryogenesis actually extends beyond the first trimester, not only resulting in the Arnold-Chiari II malformation but also reflecting the characteristic abnormalities of the corpus callosum. As Barkovich (1995) has suggested, the nature of these congenital defects may provide important clues as to the nature and timing of the neural migration defect characterizing any particular child.

Equally important is the role of the corpus callosum in the development of cognitive functions. Despite significant brain insults during the gestational period and shortly after birth, children with early hydrocephalus are infrequently mentally deficient. However, their characteristic motor and spatial deficits correlate robustly with measures of spatial cognition obtained many years after the primary brain malformation and subsequent insult. Hence, these children show substantial reorganization of function, but are hardly normal children. Future investigations of children with early hydrocephalus and congenital brain malformations may provide important insight as to the neural and environmental mechanisms responsible for reorganization of function.

Although a focus on structures such as the corpus callosum is important, the role of environmental factors should not be neglected. To use spina bifida meningomyelocele as an example, these children are born with characteristic oculomotor and physical disabilities. The children are often paralyzed and may have no control over the lower extremities. Upper extremity coordination is also frequently impaired. Consequently, these children may be less able to initiate motor-based activities or to attend consistently to features in their environment. They also may be less inclined to respond to motor and attentional contingencies introduced between the parent and the child. For example, one of the few studies of infants with spina bifida meningomyelocele found that those with spina bifida meningomyelocele displayed a higher rate of verbal imitation earlier in their development than normal children (Morrow and Wachs, 1992). This may reflect an attempt to compensate for their early motor-based deficits and the impact of these deficits on attention and motor functions.

Future investigations of children with spina bifida meningomyelocele and other congenital malformations should examine not only potential neural factors reflecting reorganization of function, but carefully evaluate the environment, particularly when these children are very young. This may lead to interventions that are effective in ameliorating the long-term deficiencies in motor and spatial skills characteristic of these children.

References

This work was supported in part by NINDS grant R01 NS25368, Neurobehavioral Development of Hydrocephalic Children, and NICHD grant P01 HD35946, Spina Bifida: Cognitive and Neurobiological Variability. The assistance of Patricia Klaas with data collection and Rita Taylor with manuscript preparation is gratefully acknowledged.

Barkovich, A. J. (1995). *Pediatric neuroimaging,* 2nd ed. New York: Raven Press.

Barkovich, A. J., and Norman, D. (1988). Anomalies of the corpus callosum: Correlation with further anomalies of the brain. *Am. J. Neuroradiol., 15,* 171–179.

Bashore, T. R. (1981). Vocal and manual reaction time estimates of interhemispheric transmission time. *Psychol. Bull., 89,* 352–368.

Bryden, M. P., and Zurif, E. B. (1970). Dichotic listening performance in a case of agenesis of the corpus callosum. *Neuropsychologia, 8,* 371–377.

Chiarello, C. (1980). A house divided? Cognitive functioning with callosal agenesis. *Brain Language, 11,* 128–158.

Chuang, S. (1986). Perinatal and neonatal hydrocephalus. Part 1: Incidence and etiology. *Perinatal Neonatol., 10,* 8–19.

Clarke, J. M., Lufkin, R. B., and Zaidel, E. (1993). Corpus callosum morphometry and dichotic listening performance: Individual differences in functional interhemispheric inhibition. *Neuropsychologia, 31,* 547–557.

Clarke, J. M., and Zaidel, E. (1989). Simple reaction times to lateralized light flashes. *Brain, 112,* 849–870.

Corbalis, M. C., and Morgan, M. J. (1978). On the biological basis of human laterality. *Behav. Brain Sci., 1,* 261–269.

Dee, H., and Hannay, H. J. (1981). Reversal of asymmetry in human perceptual performance as a function of labeling, mode of response, and familiarity. *Percept. Motor Skills, 52,* 183–193.

Del Bigio, M. R. (1993). Neuropathological changes caused by hydrocephalus. *Acta Neuropthol., 85,* 573–585.

Dennis, M. (1976). Impaired sensory and motor differentiation with corpus callosum: A lack of callosal inhibition during ontogeny? *Neuropsychologia, 14,* 455–469.

Dennis, M., Fitz, C. R., Netley, C. T., Sugar, J., Derek, C. F., Harwood-Nash, M. B., Hendrick, H. B., Hoffman, H. J., and Humphreys, R. P. (1981). The intelligence of hydrocephalic children. *Arch. Neurol., 38,* 607–715.

Dennis, M., Jacennik, B., and Barnes, M. (1994). The content of narrative discourse in children and adolescents after early-onset hydrocephalus in normally-developing age peers, *Brain and Language, 46,* 129–165.

Di Stephano, M., Sauerwein, H. C., and Lassonde, M. (1992). Influence of anatomical factors and spatial compatability on the stimulus–response relationship in the absence of the corpus callosum. *Neuropsychologia, 30,* 177–185.

Ettlinger, G., Blakemore, C. B., Milner, A. D., and Wilson, J. (1974). Agenesis of the corpus callosum: A further behavioral investigation. *Brain, 97,* 225–234.

Fischer, M., Ryan, S. B., and Dobyns, W. B. (1992). Mechanisms of interhemispheric transfer and patterns of cognitive function in acallosal patients of normal intelligence. *Arch. Neurol., 49,* 271–277.

Fletcher, J. M., Bohan, T. P., Brandt, M. E., Brookshire, B. L., Beaver, S. R., Francis, D. J., Davidson, K. C., Thompson, N. M., and Miner, M. E. (1992a). Cerebral white matter and cognition in hydrocephalic children. *Arch. Neurol., 49,* 818–824.

Fletcher, J. M., Bohan, T. P., Brandt, M. E., Kramer, L. A., Brookshire, B. L., Thorstad, K., Davidson, K. C., Francis, D. J., McCauley, S., and Baumgartner, J. E. (1996a). Morphometric evaluation of the hydrocephalic brain: Relationships with cognitive development. *Child's Nerv. Syst., 12,* 192–199.

Fletcher, J. M., Brookshire, B. L., Bohan, T. P., Brandt, M. E., and Davidson, K. C. (1995). Early hydrocephalus. In B. P. Rourke (ed.): *Syndrome of Nonverbal Learning Disabilities: Neurodevelopmental Manifestations.* New York: Guilford Publications, Inc., pp. 206–238.

Fletcher, J. M., Francis, D. J., Thompson, N. M., Brookshire, B. L., Bohan, T. P., Landry, S. H., Davidson, K. C., and Miner, M. E. (1992b). Verbal and nonverbal skill discrepancies in hydrocephalic children. *J. Clin. Exp. Neuropsychol., 14,* 593–609.

Fletcher, J. M., McCauley, S. R., Brandt, M. E., Bohan, T. P., Kramer, L. A., Francis, D. J., Thorstad, K., and Brookshire, B. L. (1996b). Regional brain tissue composition in children with hydrocephalus: Relationships with cognitive development. *Arch. Neurol., 49,* 818–824.

Fontenot, D. J. (1973). Visual field differences in the recognition of verbal and non-verbal stimuli in man. *J. Comp. Physiol. Psychol., 85,* 564–569.

Fox, C. A., and Schmitz, J. T. (1943). A Marchi study of the distribution of the anterior commissure in the cat. *J. Comp. Neurol., 89,* 297–304.

Geffen, G. M., Nelson, J., Simpson, D. A., and Jeeves, M. A. (1994). The development of interhemispheric transfer of tactile information in cases of callosal agenesis. In M. Lassonde and M. A. Jeeves (eds.): *Callosal Agenesis: A Natural Split Brain?* New York: Plenum Press, pp. 185–197.

Hawles, T. (1991). *User's Manual for the Fused Dichotic Words Test.* New Haven, CT: Precision Neurometrics.

Hines, M., Chiu, L., McAdams, L. A., Bentler, P. M., and Lipcamon, J. (1992). Cognition and the corpus callosum: Verbal fluency, visuospatial ability, and language lateralization related to midsagittal surface areas of callosal subregions. *Behav. Neurosci., 106,* 3–14.

Jeeves, M. A. (1965). Psychological studies of three cases of congenital agenesis of the corpus callosum. In E. G. Ettlinger (ed.): *Functions of the Corpus Callosum.* CIBA Foundation Study Groups, vol. 20. London: Churchill, pp. 79–94.

Jeeves, M. A. (1979). Some limits to interhemispheric integration in cases of callosal agenesis and partial commissurotomy. In I. S. Russell, M. W. Van Hof, and G. Berlucchi (eds.): *Structure and Function of the Cerebral Commissures.* London: MacMillan, pp. 449–474.

Jeeves, M. A. (1986). Callosal agenesis: Neuronal and developmental adaptations. In F. Lepore, M. Ptito, and H. H. Jasper (eds.): *Two Hemispheres—One Brain: Functions of the Corpus Callosum.* New York: Alan R. Liss, pp. 403–421.

Jeeves, M. A. (1994). Callosal agenesis—A natural split brain: Overview. In M. Lassonde and M. A. Jeeves (eds.): *Callosal Agenesis: A Natural Split Brain?* New York: Plenum Press, pp. 285–299.

Jeeves, M. A., and Milner, A. D. (1987). Specificity and plasticity in interhemispheric integration: Evidence from callosal agenesis. In D. Ottoson (ed.): *Duality and Unity of the Brain—Unified Functioning and Specialization of the Hemispheres.* London: MacMillan.

Jeeves, M. A., and Rajalakshmi, R. (1964). Psychological studies of a case of congenital agenesis of the corpus callosum. *Neuropsychologia, 26,* 153–159.

Jeeves, M. A., Silver, P. H., and Jacobson, I. (1988). Bi-manual coordination in callosal agenesis and partial commissurotomy. *Neuropsychologia, 26,* 833–850.

Karnath, H. O., Schumacher, M., and Wallesch, C. W. (1991). Limitations of interhemispheric extracallosal transfer of visual information in callosal agenesis. *Cortex, 27,* 345–350.

Klaas, P., Hannay, H. J., Caroselli, J., and Fletcher, J. M. (1997). Interhemispheric transfer of visual, auditory, tactile, and visuomotor information in hydrocephalic children with partial agenesis of the corpus callosum. Paper presented at the Twentieth Annual Mid-Year Meeting of the International Neuropsychological Society, Bergen, Norway, June 27.

Klinger, J., and Gloor, P. (1960). The connections of the amygdala and of the anterior temporal cortex in the human brain. *J. Comp. Neurol., 115,* 333–369.

Lassonde, M. (1986). The facilitatory influence of the corpus callosum on interhemispheric processing. In F. Lepore, M. Ptito, and H. H. Jasper (eds.): *Two Hemispheres—One Brain: Functions of the Corpus Callosum.* New York: Alan R. Liss, pp. 385–401.

Lassonde, M. (1994). Disconnection syndrome in callosal agenesis. In M. Lassonde and M. A. Jeeves (eds.): *Callosal Agenesis: A Natural Split Brain?* New York: Plenum Press, pp. 275–284.

Lassonde, M., Bryden, M. P., and Demers, P. (1990). The corpus callosum and cerebral speech lateralization. *Brain Language, 38,* 195–206.

Lassonde, M. C., Lortie, J., Ptito, M., and Geoffroy, G. (1981). Hemispheric asymmetry in callosal agenesis as revealed by dichotic listening performance. *Neuropsychologia, 19,* 455–458.

Lassonde, M., Sauerwein, H., Chicoine, A., and Geoffroy, G. (1991). Absence of disconnexion syndrome in callosal agenesis and early callosotomy: Brain reorganization or lack of structural specificity during ontogeny. *Neuropsychologia, 29,* 481–495.

Lassonde, M., Sauerwein, H., McCabe, N., Laurencelle, L., and Geoffroy, G. (1988). Extent and limits of cerebral adjustment to early section or congenital absence of the corpus callosum. *Behav. Brain Res., 30,* 165–181.

Lehmann, H. J., and Lampe, H. (1970). Observations on the interhemispheric transmission of information in 9 patients with corpus callosum defect. *Eur. Neurol., 4,* 129–147.

Loeser, J. D., and Alvord, E. C. (1968). Clinicopathological correlations in agenesis of the corpus callosum. *Neurology, 18,* 745–756.

Milner, A. D. (1994). Visual integration in callosal agenesis. In M. Lassonde and M. A. Jeeves (eds.): *Callosal Agenesis: A Natural Split Brain?* New York: Plenum Press, pp. 171–183.

Milner, A. D., and Jeeves, M. A. (1979). A review of behavioural studies of agenesis of the corpus callosum. In I. S. Russell, M. W. Van Hof, and G. Berlucchi (eds.): *Structure and Function of the Cerebral Commissures.* London: MacMillan, pp. 428–448.

Milner, A. D., Jeeves, M. A., Silver, P. H., Lines, C. R., and Wilson, J. (1985). Reaction time to lateralized visual stimuli in callosal agenesis: Stimulus and response factors. *Neuropsychologia, 23,* 323–331.

Morrow, J. D., and Wachs, T. D. (1992). Infant with meningomyelocele: Visual recognition memory and sensorimotor abilities. *Dev. Med. Child Neurol., 34,* 488–498.

Moscovich, M. (1977). Development of lateralization of language functions and its relations to cognitive and linguistic development: A review and some theoretical speculations. In S. J. Segalowitz and F. A. Gruber (eds.): *Language Development and Neurological Theory.* New York: Academic Press, pp. 193–211.

Norman, M. G., McGilliuray, B. C., Kalousek, D. K., Hill, A., and Poskitt, K. J. (1995). *Congenital Malformations of the Brain.* New York: Oxford University Press.

Pandya, D. N., Karol, E. A., and Heilronn, D. (1971). The topographical distribution of interhemispheric projections in the corpus callosum of the rhesus monkey. *Brain Res., 32,* 31–43.

Payne, B. R. (1986). Role of callosal cells in the functional organization of cat striate cortex. In F. Lepore, M. Ptito, and H. H. Jasper (eds.): *Two Hemispheres—One Brain: Functions of the Corpus Callosum.* New York: Alan R. Liss, pp. 385–401.

Preilowski, B. F. B. (1972). Possible contributions of the anterior forebrain commissures to bilateral motor coordination. *Neuropsychologia, 10,* 267–277.

Rauch, R. A., and Jinkins, J. R. (1994). Magnetic resonance imaging of corpus callosum dysgenesis. In M. Lassonde and M. A. Jeeves (eds.): *Callosal Agenesis: A Natural Split Brain?* New York: Plenum Press, pp. 83–95.

Reigel, D. H., and Rotenstein, D. (1994). Spina bifida. In W. R. Cheek (ed.): *Pediatric Neurosurgery* (3rd ed.). Philadelphia: W. B. Saunders, pp. 51–76.

Reynolds, D. M., and Jeeves, M. A. (1977). Further studies of tactile perception and motor coordination in agenesis of the corpus callosum. *Cortex, 13,* 257–272.

Risse, G. L., LeDoux, J., Springer, S. P., Wilson, D. H., and Gazzaniga, M. S. (1978). The anterior commissure in man: Functional variation in a multisensory system. *Neuropsychologia, 16,* 23–31.

Robertson, I. J. A., Leggate, J. R. S., Miller, J. D., and Steers, A. J. W. (1990). Aqueduct stenosis—presentation and prognosis. *Br. J. Neurosurg., 4,* 101–106.

Sauerwein, H. C., Nolin, P., and Lassonde, M. (1994). Cognitive functioning in callosal agenesis. In M. Lassonde and M. A. Jeeves (eds.): *Callosal Agenesis: A Natural Split Brain?* New York: Plenum Press, pp. 221–233.

Schmidt, S. L. (1994). Three different animal models of early callosal defects: Morphological and behavioral studies. In M. Lassonde and M. A. Jeeves (eds.): *Callosal Agenesis: A Natural Split Brain?* New York: Plenum Press, pp. 147–154.

Wahlsten, D., and Ozaki, H. S. (1994). Defects of the fetal forebrain in acallosal mice. In M. Lassonde and M. A. Jeeves (eds.): *Callosal Agenesis: A Natural Split Brain?* New York: Plenum Press, pp. 125–133.

Wechsler, D. (1974). *Wechsler Intelligence Scale for Children–Revised.* New York: Psychological Corporation.

Whitlock, D. G., and Nauta, W. J. H. (1956). Subcortical projections from temporal neocortex in *Macaca mulatta. J. Comp. Neurol., 106,* 183–212.

Wills, K. E. (1993). Neuropsychological functioning in children with spina bifida and/or hydrocephalus. *J. Clin. Child Psychol., 22,* 247–265.

Witelson, S. F. (1989). Hand and sex differences in the isthmus and genu of the human corpus callosum. *Brain, 112,* 799–835.

Yazgan, M. Y., Wexler, B. E., Kinsbourne, M., Peterson, B., and Leckman, J. F. (1995).

Functional significance of individual variations in callosal area. *Neuropsychologia, 33,* 769–779.

Zeki, S. M. (1973). Comparison of cortical degeneration in the visual regions of the temporal lobe of the monkey following section of the anterior commissure and the splenium. *J. Comp. Neurol., 43,* 167–175.

8

Functional Consequences of Congenital Cerebellar Dysmorphologies and Acquired Cerebellar Lesions of Childhood

MAUREEN DENNIS, C. ROSS HETHERINGTON,
BRENDA J. SPIEGLER AND MARCIA A. BARNES

Plasticity is a general property of the central nervous system. It is the brain's response to solving functional problems as they arise in both damaged and undamaged neural substrates. In the normally and abnormally developing brain, plasticity is the neurodevelopmental manifestation of the interaction between maturational and environmental forces. Plasticity may be analyzed at the level of brain microstructure (axonal regrowth, axonal rerouting) or brain macrostructure in immature or mature organisms and at the level of brain function or behavior. At the level of brain microstructure, synaptic plasticity within a neural network is responsible for the alterations in brain function responsible for learning and memory (Teyler et al., 1995). At a behavioral level, plasticity is the putative mechanism for emerging competencies and skill acquisition (Greenough et al., 1993).

Plasticity is an operative mechanism of change at any age (Stiles, 1995), but the functional challenges for brain-injured individuals are different depending on when in development the brain damage was sustained. Functional challenges for the mature organism with brain injury occur in a context in which many skills are developed to an adult level. The immature organism, in contrast, must master the maturational challenges involved in moving from one developmental level to the next, a task facilitated by the emergence of age-dependent structural changes such as myelination. After adult brain insult, the mature brain engages in recovery of lost functions, at whatever level; after congenital dysmorphologies and childhood lesions, the immature brain must attempt to master the problems of development, as well as recovering any functions that were lost in consequence of the lesion.

Children with brain damage are of interest in the context of functional plasticity. In children, both normal brain development and lesion-induced aberrant brain events affect the expression of previously acquired functions and the acquisition of new functions. Brain lesions during development disrupt the process of skill acquisition, offering unique challenges to the mechanisms of plasticity and unique opportunities to study not only functional recovery that can be compared with lesions in the mature brain but also deviations from anticipated developmental trajectories. Outcomes after early brain damage concern the skill itself, its course of development, and its long-term maintenance (Dennis, 1988).

At a single time point, outcome may be considered with reference to *skill level* and *skill automaticity.* Syntax provides an example. Massive early lateralized brain damage may result in impaired identification of syntactic form (Dennis and Whitaker, 1976), but it is also associated with compensatory mechanisms that are less efficient, exacting a price in terms of automaticity such that a skill or behavior breaks down under conditions of challenge. When children and adolescents with left hemispherectomy correctly understand grammar, they take longer to do so than do individuals with right hemispherectomy (Dennis and Kohn, 1975). They are also less able than individuals with right hemispherectomy to read the case assignment (who did what to whom) from the case markers, like the passive marker *by,* instead relying on a strategic recoding of complex grammar to a simpler, canonical form (Dennis, 1980a).

Because children grow and develop, outcome may also be viewed in terms of multiple measures over the course of development. Here, the variable of interest is the slope of the curve relating function and age, and the question is whether the slope differs in brain-damaged and normally developing individuals. Outcomes here are *the rate of skill acquisition,* the *stability of skill maintenance over the course of mature, optimal performance,* and the *rate of loss with aging.*

For a child with any form of brain injury, congenital or acquired, it is important to identify different types of outcome in relation to age expectations. Each type of brain injury also addresses a distinctive set of questions about age-based functional plasticity. The child with congenital brain injury provides an opportunity to study the effects of increasing age on a neural substrate that was dysmorphic from the time it was formed. Of special interest are rate of skill acquisition and level of adult mastery. The child with acquired brain injury provides a model for studying both age at injury and time since injury, the latter including both recovery of previously acquired skills lost as a result of the lesion and developmental advances in skill. *Age-based functional plasticity* concerns the study of these outcomes.

Two Views of Age-Based Functional Plasticity

Plasticity is inversely correlated with chronological age

Historically, *plasticity* was taken to mean that the adaptive functional response of an immature central nervous system was greater than that of the mature nervous system. Plasticity was thought to be a property of the brain at birth, something lost in linear quanta as the brain matured. The argument adduced in support of plasticity involved several propositions: that brain lesions in children produce fewer deficits, less severe deficits, and more rapid recovery of function than brain lesions in adults; that children with early lesions develop normal skills; that the milder lesion response in children is due to their younger age because brain immaturity conveys a functional advantage to an individual with a brain lesion; and that the degree of immaturity is related to the degree of functional lesion-induced deficit. Thus, Lenneberg (1967) proposed a positive linear relation between age and functional deficit, and he also sought to identify the "critical periods" within which the young brain could be damaged with no functional consequences.

Plasticity is inversely correlated with stability of regional neuronal connections.

Functional plasticity is not a universal response of the immature brain to a lesion. Regional rather than global brain maturation predicts the degree of age-based plasticity, and plasticity is correlated with regional stability of neuronal connections for which chronological age is a marker. Within the immature cortex, there appears to be a pattern of regional development that has consequences for the nature and the type of age-based functional plasticity.

More than half a century ago, Kennard and Fulton (1942, p. 601) proposed that adjacent, as-yet-uncommitted cortical areas contribute to functional reorganization in the infant more than in the adult:

> If, for instance, the frontal association areas are removed unilaterally or bilaterally from an adult before, after or simultaneously with areas 4, 6 and 8, no added motor deficit can be detected. . . . However, if, following bilateral removal of areas 4 and 6 in infancy, a young animal is allowed to grow until improvement in motor performance has ceased and then a frontal association area or postcentral gyrus is removed, a markedly increased deficit in motor performance appears. . . . The indication therefore is that, when the motor areas are removed in infancy, there is a reorganization of the remaining non-motor cortex.

The idea that a reorganization of neighboring brain regions may provide a mechanism for sustaining function has been supported by later studies. Early lesions may stabilize normally transient connections in neighboring brain regions, and these stabilized connections provide a substrate for function (Webster et al., 1991). Recruitment of brain regions with transient rather than stable connections, then, might be one viable mechanism of functional reorganization for parts of the immature cortex.

Within the cortex, some cortical regions exhibit an adult-type lesion response before others. Removal of area 8 in the infant monkey produces marked deviation of the head and eyes at a time in development when other motor skills are only slightly affected by cortical ablations elsewhere in the motor cortex (Kennard and Fulton, 1942). Anterior projections from temporal areas to some regions of cortex are adult-like within the first days of life (Webster et al., 1995). In keeping with this idea, medial temporal lesions in infancy produce pronounced and permanent memory deficits (Bachevalier and Mishkin, 1994). Early functional development presumably stabilizes transient connections in a brain region, which then are less available for recruitment after brain lesions.

Evaluation of Evidence for Age-Based Functional Plasticity

The evidence for age-based functional plasticity is not clear, even granted that it is regional rather than global. In fact, the evidence that adults and children show different adaptive responses to central nervous system lesions has proven ambiguous, incomplete, and difficult to interpret. One central problem has been that inferences about the age component of age-based functional plasticity have been confounded by factors other than age, making equivocal the comparison between child and adult lesions.

Children and adults exhibit different forms of neuropathology

For example, strokes from arteritis are common in adults but rare in children, which makes difficult any comparisons of the functional effects of the same pathology. Early evidence for age-based plasticity compared aphasia in adults with strokes and children with diffuse, infectious, or traumatic brain injury (e.g., Basser, 1962). It is now known that aphasic symptoms abate more quickly in individuals with traumatic pathology and less quickly, if at all, in those with vascular disorders, regardless of age (Dennis, 1996b). To accurately assess age-based plasticity, the mechanism of brain insult should remain constant across the age range studied.

The base rate of certain behavioral symptoms is different in children and adults even after similar pathology

This obviates any clear consideration of functional plasticity for these behaviors. For example, aphasic neologisms, which provide evidence about the functional plasticity of the phonological system, occur less frequently in children than in adults (Dennis, 1996b), so a comparison of neologisms in children and adults after brain injury would encounter problems in accruing comparable samples. Minimally, the groups would likely differ in dimensions other than age at injury.

The description of deficits after adult lesions is rarely investigated in the context of functional plasticity, so there is a dearth of adult plasticity studies with which to compare functional plasticity in children

Understanding functional plasticity requires separation of age at lesion and time since lesion variables, each of which may be associated with different effects on cognitive function (Dennis and Barnes, 1994). In classical studies of functional plasticity, time since lesion is often not considered. Typically, acute phase adults are compared with chronic phase children (for discussion, see Dennis, 1980b). Acute stage symptoms in the adult have been informative for theories of localization of function and cognitive architecture, but they are not pertinent to hypotheses about age-based functional plasticity. As it happens, time since lesion predicts outcome in adults. For example, recovery of some cognitive functions in adults with traumatic brain injury continues through the first decade after injury (Hetherington et al., 1996). What is lacking are direct comparisons of the rate and extent of recovery in children and adults in which time since lesion is explicitly considered.

Some functional deficits show inconsistent structure–function correlations

For example, visual neglect has been observed in both children and adults, but in neither group is there a fully consistent connection between high parietal lesions and neglect. For functions where the lesion effects are not fully predictable, questions about age-based plasticity become quite ambiguous.

Little is known about age-based functional plasticity after subcortical and subtentorial lesions

Subcortical lesions have been associated with non-verbal intellectual deficits (Dennis, 1985), and with adult-like aphasic syndromes (Aram et al., 1983). Compared with the data on cortical lesions, however, there is little evidence about the functional capacities of children after lesions in subcortical or subtentorial (below the tentorium cerebelli or tent) brain regions. These brain regions may differ from cortical regions in the nature and extent to which they exhibit age-based functional plasticity.

Acquisition of new functions and recovery of old functions may be separate processes

Age-based functional plasticity involves both recovery of old skills and acquisition of new skills. This complicates the comparison of child and adult lesions not only because the proportions of old and new skills is likely different in children and adults but also because recovery and new learning may depend on partially separate brain mechanisms.

Only at maturity can the effects of developmental brain perturbations on skill acquisition be fully assessed

Infant monkeys with lesions to the motor cortex appear functionally normal during early development, but begin to show paresis and spasticity as they reach maturity (Kennard, 1940). Ablation of the frontal association areas in infant monkeys causes no immediate visible motor change, but with age, a compulsive motor hyperactivity appears similar to that in monkeys with the same areas removed in adolescence or adulthood (Kennard et al., 1941). These delayed or latent (Taylor and Alden, 1997) effects, which are identified from longitudinal study of function into adulthood, are critical for understanding age-based functional plasticity.

Age-based Functional Plasticity: The Case of the Cerebellum

Although plasticity was once conceptualized as an all-or-none phenomenon, the studies on regional cortical plasticity show that this is far from the case, and adequate data for a clear view of plasticity are not available. One task is to define age based functional plasticity in terms of *the type of skill* and *how and when it develops* in particular brain regions. In this chapter, we evaluate age-based plasticity with assays that present testable hypotheses that require evidence-based verification about skill, rate, and parameters of brain injury in a brain region with well-defined functions in the adult nervous system.

The functional capacities of individuals who have sustained structural damage to the cerebellum early in development, either while the brain was being formed or later during childhood, represent important evidence with which to consider issues of functional plasticity:

- Various forms of cerebellar dysmorphologies affect children, and cerebellar lesions affect children as well as adults.
- Symptoms of cerebellar dysfunction occur in both children and adults. For example, cerebellar lesions produce truncal ataxia, limb ataxia, and eye movement deficits that include saccadic dysmetria, pursuit disturbances, and optokinetic nystagmus, and these are observed in infants, children, and adults following cerebellar lesions.
- Cerebellar perturbations in children provide a basis for studying the age basis of functional plasticity. Dysmorphologies of the cerebellum can occur during gestation, and children with these dysmorphisms who are of different chronological ages at test provide a model for studying time since lesion effects because age at lesion is constant. Lesions of the cerebellum acquired during childhood, in contrast, can be used to test functional recovery in relation to both age at lesion and time since lesion.
- Many cerebellar functions show a highly predictable association with the locus of cerebellar lesion in the developing and mature brains. For example, adult vermian cerebellar lesions reliably produce ataxia, and congenital agenesis and malformation of the cerebellar vermis are associated with slow motor development in infancy and ataxia in childhood (Fischer, 1973; Tal et al., 1980). Therefore, hypotheses about plasticity of function in relation to specific structural insult of the cerebellum ought to be readily testable.

In using the cerebellum as a model of functional plasticity, we discuss briefly the structure and function of the cerebellum and outline some common childhood conditions involving congenital and acquired lesions that produce significant structural and functional cerebellar compromise. We then apply assays for age-based functional plasticity to data from children and young adults with developmental lesions of the cerebellum in order to consider whether there exists age-based functional plasticity following early perturbations of the cerebellum.

Structure and functions of the cerebellum

The cerebellum consists of a large cortex that processes input, and deep nuclei, that process output. The lateral cerebellar cortex and the lateral deep nucleus, or dentate, became markedly expanded in the course of evolution and are phylogenetically newer (Passingham, 1975).

The cerebellum is one of the earliest discrete structures of the brain to differentiate and one of the last to achieve its mature configuration (Moore, 1982; Koop et al., 1986). The maturation of the cerebellum generally precedes that of the cortex, as measured by completion of myelination and adult number of cells (Martin et al., 1988). As with the cortex, however, there are regional cycles of maturation in the brain stem and cerebellum. Systems mediating vestibular response myelinate early and rapidly, before birth; the fiber systems mediating proprioceptive and exteroceptive somatic experience myelinate later and at a slower rate; and the fibers mediating the integrative activities of the cerebral hemispheres with the cerebellum myelinate only after birth and show a protracted cycle of maturation (Yakovlev and Lecours, 1967).

Because substantial changes occur in the cerebellar cellular organization for months after birth, disruption of the cerebellar formation can occur at times from early in embryonic development to well after birth. The prenatal course of cerebellar development is sensitive to disturbances in skull formation (Lechtenberg, 1993), which occur in some congenital brain malformations.

The cerebellum has a high degree of structural homogeneity, but mediates a heterogeneous array of functions through widespread interconnections (Bloedel, 1992). The cerebellum is important in the regulation of balance, posture and gait, dynamic motor programming, fine motor control, and motor timing (Ghez, 1991; Ito, 1993). It has long been observed that the cerebellum is essential for the *quality of limb and eye movements.* Lesions to the cerebellum impair the quality of movement but do not abolish it (Holmes, 1922); they are associated with failure at motor tasks such as touching a finger to the tip of the nose, the maintenance of posture, and walking a straight line. Defective motor coordination is a principal feature of diseases of the cerebellum, and disturbances of coordinated movements are manifest by lack of fluidity during movement execution (Gilman, 1994). Patients with cerebellar disorders show multiple peaks in the velocity profiles of movements, and movements are oscillatory as a limb approaches a target (Gilman et al., 1976).

The cerebellum may be responsible for patterning the sequences of contraction of agonist and antagonist muscles and may contribute to the temporal aspect of motor and pattern generation in neurons within the motor cortex (Hore and Flament, 1988). One explanation proposed for disturbances of coordinated movement involves disruption in the timing of the normal patterning of agonist and antagonist muscle activity in the course of a movement (Gilman, 1994); in support of this idea, individuals with cerebellar disease have delayed onset of antagonist activity and a time delay in tracking movements because of increased reaction time for movement initiation (Diener and Dichgans, 1992).

Timing is a part of movement, and timing deficits have been proposed as an explanation of clinical cerebellar symptoms; for example, dysmetria and dysdiadochokinesia after cerebellar lesions have been attributed to inability to time onset and offset of movements (Dichgans and Deiner, 1984). More broadly, the cerebellum has also been viewed as a component of a *cognitive timing system* that contributes to the control of movement but that is also involved in nonmotor tasks that require precise timing, for example, estimating duration of tones (Ivry and Keele, 1989). Timed periodic or rhythmic movement is central to any theory attempting to account for coordinated behavior (Turvey, 1990).

The contemporary view has supported the idea that the extensive connections between the cerebellum and higher brain structures are related to a role that involves more than coordinate movement. For example, it has been argued that the increase in size of the cortical areas influenced by cerebellar output is related to an expansion of cerebellar function to include *language and cognition* (Leiner et al., 1986, 1991). Evidence for this view is that the dentate nucleus of the cerebellum is activated during problem solving but not during simple movements (Kim et al., 1994), which suggests involvement of the cerebellum in motor learning and *the adaptive modification of motor output.*

The cerebellum also appears to be important for *the automatization of skills.* Automaticity, conceptualized as the noncognitive regulation of a movement or as the ability to perform more than one task without excessive performance decrement, is essential for the development of motor expertise (Lee and Swinnen, 1993). Functional neuroimaging has implicated the cerebellum in motor skill acquisition. Activation of the cerebellar hemispheres diminishes after a motor task has been practiced and becomes automatized (Friston et al., 1992); furthermore, individuals with cerebellar lesions perform visual selective attention tasks at a rate that is fivefold slower than controls (Courchesne et al., 1994).

Several issues are currently under active debate. One is whether the cerebellar involvement in higher brain function can be explained in terms of its motor control function. Specifically, the issue is whether the cerebellar role in cognition and timing is an expression of the well-documented cerebellar role in the *planning of movements,* especially those that require high-quality sensory information.

In summary, historical evidence gave rise to the traditional view of the cerebellum as a real-time mediator of fine motor control and coordination, capable of adjusting motor responses to varying environmental demands. An emerging contemporary view, based on functional neuroimaging studies in humans and lesion studies in humans and animals, supports a role for the cerebellum in motor learning (Thach, 1997). Although recent evidence implicates the cerebellum in higher cognitive functions such as language, attention, and spatial processing, the most robust support is for the role of the cerebellum as a component in a cognitive timing network. General roles for the cerebellum may be in learning or automatization of response sequences and participating in the linkage of experiential context with response sequences. In the absence of the cerebellum, prefrontal and premotor areas can still plan and effect movement, but the movement is not automatic, rapid, error free, or precisely linked to context (Thach, 1997).

Developmental anomalies of the cerebellum

A variety of conditions have long been observed to directly affect the structural development of the cerebellum (Sutton, 1887). Some involve genetic syndromes or congenital malformations that affect cerebellar development, while others involve acquired structural lesions. Congenital cerebellar dysmorphologies produce classic cerebellar signs and symptoms whether or not mental retardation exists. Conditions not associated with mental retardation or global developmental delay, however, provide particularly important evidence about plasticity of function because they allow the effects of cerebellar functional disorders to be measured independent of global cognitive impairment.

Genetic anomalies associated with mental retardation. Several genetic syndromes are characterized by structural anomalies of the cerebellum, and the functional disorders observed are those typically associated with acquired adult cerebellar lesions. Marinesco-Sjogren syndrome (Williams et al., 1996) is an autosomal recessive condition characterized by bilateral cataracts and mental retardation. Neuroimaging shows hypoplasia of the cerebellum, and ataxia is a prominent part of the clinical presentation. Machado-Joseph disease (Sudarsky and Coutinho, 1995) is a dominantly inherited condition involving a single mutant gene with an unstable CAG repeat on chromosome 14q32.1, and neuropathology has been found to involve both afferent and efferent cerebellar systems. The clinical spectrum of this single mutant gene involves nystagmus, dysarthria, postural instability, and ataxia, all classic signs of cerebellar dysfunction.

Congenital anomalies of the cerebellum congruent with broadly normal cognitive development. Two developmental anomalies that affect the cerebellum are of particular interest, the common Arnold Chiari-II malformation associated with spina bifida, and the rare disorder of the Dandy-Walker syndrome or Dandy-Walker variant, both of which have major cerebellar dysmorphologies as a diagnostic feature. These conditions have different patterns of neuropathology; they have different embryological timing and so occur at different points in gestation; they have separable regional neurotransmitters and neuromodulators; they are discordant for associated birth defects; and, if syndromal, they are part of different clinical genetic syndromes.

The Arnold-Chiari II malformation is frequently associated with spina bifida, which involves a defect in closure of the neural tube and occurs in 7 of 10,000 live births and which begins around gestational week 10. Within the spina bifida complex, there may be defects of both neuralization and canalization, marked by the vertebral level of the defect and associated with different malformations (Toriello and Higgins, 1985). Neuropathology involves a primary hindbrain deformity (Gilbert et al., 1986), a small posterior fossa, agenesis and/or hypoplasia of the lateral cerebellar hemispheres, and herniation of the cerebellum through the exits of the fourth ventricle (Barkovich, 1994). The Dandy-Walker syndrome occurs in 1 of 50,000 live births and originates in gestational weeks 6–7. It is a congenital midline field malformation involving the triad of complete or partial agenesis of the vermis, dysplastic cerebellar hemispheres, cystic dilation of the fourth ventricle, and an enlarged posterior fossa (Barkovich, 1994; Paidas and Cohen, 1994; Pellock and Johnson, 1993).

Both conditions are associated with hydrocephalus, but with different base frequencies (0.95 in Arnold-Chiari II, 0.77–0.91 in Dandy Walker syndrome). When hydrocephalus occurs during gestation or shortly after birth, it has a variety of neuropathological effects (reviewed by Del Bigio, 1993; Dennis, 1996a) that alter the development and function of the brain both directly and indirectly from ventricular enlargement (Harwood-Nash and Fitz, 1976; Hoffman, 1989).

Primary dysmorphologies are part of the basic formation of the brain and define these conditions. For example, agenesis of the cerebellar vermis is part of the triad that defines the Dandy-Walker syndrome (Pascual-Castroviejo et al., 1991). There are also *secondary dysmorphologies,* some related to increased intracranial pressure. For example, partial agenesis of the corpus callosum occurs as a primary dysmorphology in most cases of Arnold-Chiari II, but hydrocephalus can destroy an already-formed corpus callosum, causing a secondary hypoplasia (Fletcher et al., 1992).

The Arnold-Chiari II malformation and the Dandy-Walker syndrome are of considerable interest with respect to issues of plasticity. Both have defining dysmorphologies of the cerebellum that occur in the formation of the brain, even though other dysmorphologies (e.g., hypoplasia of the corpus callosum) are shared. They are consistent with normal intelligence and an extended life span, which means that important issues about rate of acquisition of function and adult stability of function may be addressed.

Acquired childhood lesions of the cerebellum

The posterior fossa is the site of half of all childhood brain tumors (Heideman et al., 1993). Posterior fossa tumors, of which medulloblastomas and astrocytomas are the most common types, are relatively frequent causes of childhood cerebellar lesions. Two tumors, medulloblastoma and astrocytoma, commonly occur in the posterior fossa and displace (but typically do not infiltrate) the cerebellum.

Medulloblastomas are malignant, primitive neuroectodermal tumors of childhood (Rorke et al., 1985) that account for about 25% of primary central nervous system tumors in the first two decades of life. Medulloblastomas have a typically midline locus, and most are located within the cerebellar vermis. With recent improvements in treatment (typically surgery, radiation, with or without chemotherapy), survival after childhood medulloblastoma has increased so that some 60% of children with medulloblastoma can expect to live 5 years or more (Packer et al., 1989). Cognitive morbidity is common, however, and survivors of medulloblastoma often have problems in both motor and cognitive domains (Dennis et al., 1996).

Cerebellar astrocytomas are benign glial tumors that constitute 13%–28% of posterior fossa tumors. Astrocytomas typically arise laterally, from the cerebellar hemispheres. Treatment involves surgery alone, and for children with low-grade astrocytomas the 5-year survival rate approaches 100% after gross total excision (Hoffman et al., 1990; see also Cohen and Duffner, 1994).

Medulloblastomas and cerebellar astrocytomas, acquired cerebellar lesions of childhood, provide a useful perspective on age-based functional plasticity by virtue of variations in the age of the child at onset of tumor symptoms. Comparison of the two tumor types is also of interest because malignant medulloblastomas typically require radiation treatment while astrocytomas rarely require radiation. Finally, the tendency for one type of tumor to arise medially and the other laterally allows a perspective on localization of function within the cerebellum.

Assays for functional plasticity: Conditions under which age-based plasticity may be inferred

How might we know if skill represents age-based plasticity in response to a brain lesion? To answer this question, we propose five assays, which we apply here to study age-based functional plasticity in the cerebellum but which might also be applied to the outcome of cortical lesions. In defining assays for functional plasticity, we outline hypotheses that can be confirmed or disconfirmed.

Functional competence assay. If a function is maintained at an age-appropriate level following a lesion to a brain region that would normally support it, then evidence exists that the function shows some degree of age-based plasticity. To apply this assay, however, the structure–function relations in the mature brain must be known, and both age-appropriate performance and the relevant structure–function relations must be defined in the immature organism. An hypothesis of age-based plasticity under this assay would require that age-appropriate skill be demonstrated at a given time point after a lesion to the immature brain; a null hypothesis is that deficits follow brain lesions in younger and older children as well as in adults.

Developmental rate assay. A skill exhibiting age-based functional plasticity would develop over time in an immature lesioned organism at a rate similar to that in nonlesioned individuals. That is to say, children with and without brain lesions should show similar slopes for the curve plotting functional skill acquisition against chronological age, if not in the time period immediately following the lesion then at least during further post-injury development of that skill. Under an age-based plasticity hypothesis, any difference between lesioned children and age peers is a developmental lag that will disappear or attenuate with time; a null hypothesis is that the difference is a deficit that is stable over the time and evident throughout the age of acquisition.

Full adult mastery assay. A skill exhibiting age-based functional plasticity would attain adult levels of mastery and be maintained throughout maturity. That is to say, children with brain lesions should eventually reach the same level of competence as adults without childhood brain lesions and maintain that level of competence. This assay requires longitudinal study from childhood to adulthood, so data from adults with a history of childhood lesions are a particularly important category of evidence for this assay.

Equivalence of developmental stability and decline assay. Many functions decline with aging. For this assay, the issue is whether the slope of cognitive decline with aging is similar in individuals with and without early brain insult. Under an age-based plasticity hypothesis, individuals with lesions would show the same negative slope as nonlesioned individuals, while a null hypothesis would propose that deterioration in skill with aging is more rapid in individuals with childhood brain lesions. There is almost no information pertinent to this important assay.

Functionality under challenge assay. A skill is instantiated in the real world in the presence of other behaviors and distraction; for example, it is common to walk and talk at the same time. A plastic function should be fully operational under a routine challenge. The idea of challenge is important because it is related to skill automaticity, and, as discussed earlier, the cerebellum has been implicated in the automatization of motor and cognitive skills. Evidence for an age-based plasticity hypothesis would require not only that skills in brain-injured individuals be as accurate and fluent as those in noninjured individuals but also that skill execution and fluency be equally resistant to cognitive and motor interference.

The following section describes data on motor and cognitive timing functions from groups with congenital and acquired cerebellar pathology. The data are used to confirm or disconfirm hypotheses from the assays, discussed above, for age-based functional plasticity of the cerebellum.

Application of Assays for Functional Plasticity in Children and Young Adults with Congential Dysmorphologies or Acquired Lesions of the Cerebellum

Functional competence: Motor function in congenital cerebellar dysmorphology

Cerebellar lesions produce problems with upper and lower limb coordination. One aspect of functional competence is whether congenital malformations of the cerebellum are associated with deficits similar to those in adult cerebellar lesions. To the extent that functional plasticity is present, performance on motor tasks will be age appropriate; an absence of functional plasticity would be inferred from significant skill impairments. Compromised skill would suggest that other neural structures involved in the motor system, for example, basal ganglia or motor cortex, may not be recruited as alternative substrates to support age-appropriate skill development.

Another aspect of functional competence concerns structure–function congruence. To the degree that skill is related to dysmorphism in functional regions of the cerebellum, structure–function congruence may be inferred, and this would support the involvement of specific mediating substrates for these tasks.

Do children with congenital cerebellar malformations show deficits on tests of limb ataxia and rapid finger movements? Is functional deficit on these tasks associated with the degree and type of cerebellar dysmorphology? As part of a larger study of motor skills in children with hydrocephalus (Hetherington and Dennis, 1999), we tested 17 children with spina bifida and hydrocephalus. Of these 11 were ambulatory, and 6 had ambulation difficulties requiring the use of a wheelchair, parapodium, or braces plus crutches. Two motor tasks were selected from an individually administered test of motor development with quantified scoring and scaled scores based on a sample of 2,000 normally developing children, as well as another adult sample (McCarron, 1976). The tasks were Limb Ataxia (the Finger-to-Nose test of a standard neurological examination) and Finger Tapping (rapid oscillation of the index finger against a restraining rubber band). Figure 8.1 shows obtained and age-expected scores.

The classic lateral cerebellar task of limb ataxia is performed poorly in children with spina bifida, showing that upper limb functions are impaired. The highest score is Finger Tapping, which, although better developed than Limb Ataxia in comparison with age expectations, is still at a borderline level.

Structure–function congruence was studied by comparing volumetric analyses of MRI scans and cerebellar function tests in two 13-year-old girls, one with spina bifida and one with Dandy-Walker syndrome (Hetherington et al., 1998). Im-

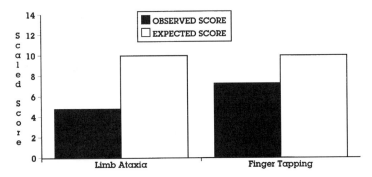

Figure 8-1. Functional competence. Limb Ataxia and Finger Tapping in individuals with Arnold-Chari II syndrome.

ages were acquired with a 1.5 tesla Siemens Magnetom 6300. Using a three-dimensional gradient echo sequence (3D MP RAGE: T_1 weighted, TE = 5, TR = 11.5, flip angle 10°), 128 contiguous 1.8-mm slices were acquired in the coronal plane. Image segmentation and analysis were performed on a SUN SPARCstation using Cardviews (Caviness et al., 1995). In the spina bifida brain, the ratio of cerebellar to cerebral volume was 28% less than that of a comparison group of children (Caviness et al., 1995). The spina bifida cerebellum was 19% smaller than the Dandy-Walker cerebellum; conversely, the Dandy-Walker medial cerebellum was 26% smaller than the spina bifida medial cerebellum. The smaller lateral cerebellar volume in the spina bifida brain was associated with a significantly greater impairment of Limb Ataxia (Z score, 3.0) compared with the Dandy-Walker syndrome subject (Z score, 0.33).

Taken together, the data on function and structure–function congruence suggest that many years after a developmental dysmorphology of the cerebellum, children with spina bifida have not attained age-appropriate levels of skill in motor skills that at maturity rely on the integrity of the lateral cerebellum. Morphometric analysis of the brains demonstrate some degree of structure–function congruence in 13 year olds with cerebellar dysmorphologies in that motor skills relying on the lateral cerebellum were impaired in the child with reduced volume in the lateral cerebellum despite cerebellar anomalies of various types in both children. Thus, the data on motor functions as assays of functional competence suggest limited age-based functional plasticity.

Developmental rate: Rapid automatized naming in spina bifida

Hydrocephalus in spina bifida develops from brain dysmorphologies with a known age at onset. Absent severe medical complications, the condition is nonprogressive and stable; therefore, time since onset is the same as age at cognitive testing, and this may be used as an index of how experience affects cognitive development in a dysmorphic brain substrate. This feature may be used to explore the question of developmental rate for skill acquisition.

Rapid automatized naming (Denckla and Rudel, 1974), which requires naming of visual items on a chart as rapidly as possible, was studied in 95 children, five age groups with spina bifida and five age-matched control groups. Damage to the cerebellum in adulthood is associated with difficulty in attaching morphemes to words in running speech (Silveri et al., 1994), so this task is of some interest with respect to the known cerebellar abnormalities of spina bifida.

The results, shown in Figure 8-2, indicate a significant effect of condition (F [1, 85] = 19.9, $p < 0.0001$) such that the spina bifida group was slower at automatized naming than controls and a significant effect of age group (F [4, 85] = 24.7, $p < 0.0001$) such that the youngest children were slower than all other ages and the 8- and 10-year-olds were slower than the 14-year-olds, but there was no interaction between condition and age group.

The slower performance of the spina bifida group was not due to poorer naming ability. Errors were coded (details in Dennis et al., 1987) into linguistic errors

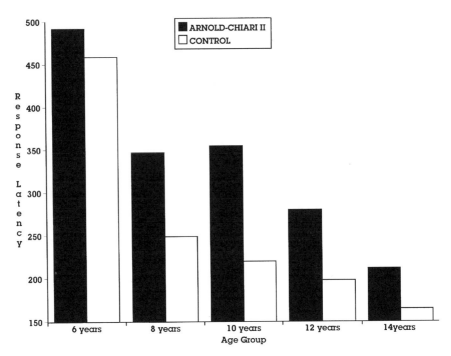

Figure 8-2. Developmental rate. Rapid automatized naming tested cross-sectionally from 6 to 14 years of age in normally developing children and in children with Arnold-Chari II syndrome.

(semantic paraphasias, phonemic paraphasia, distortions, and the like) and pacing errors (errors involving extraneous elements: sound cues, stammering, fillers like *Um* or addition of definite/indefinite articles). There was a significant effect of condition (F [1, 71] = 7.9, p = 0.0065), such that the spina bifida group made more errors than controls, a significant effect of error type, (F [1, 71] = 45.2, p < 0.0001), such that pacing errors were more common than linguistic errors, and a significant interaction between condition and error type (F [1, 71] = 5.6, p < 0.0210). The spina bifida and control groups had a similarly low linguistic error rate (2.6 vs. 1.1), but the spina bifida group made many more pacing errors (19.7 vs. 9.7).

The view that emerges from these data is that of a stable cognitive deficit rather than a developmental lag. The slope of the curve plotting functional skill against chronological age is similar in spina bifida and age-matched controls; however, with advancing age, the difference between them is maintained, not attenuated. The spina bifida groups do not catch up over the years tested. While it remains to be seen how this task is performed in adulthood, the present cross-sectional evidence suggests that the brain dysmorphism associated with spina bifida, of which cerebellar dysmorphologies are prominent, disrupts speeded and automatized naming. The spina bifida groups had difficulty not with naming, but with the rapid recruitment of linguistic elements in ongoing speech, which is consistent with the putative cerebellar role in the automatization of cognitive operations. Age appropriate function in these timing skills was not observed by adolescence, despite developmental increments.

Performance on a duration discrimination task by long-term survivors of posterior fossa tumors provides further evidence for the compromise of a cognitive timing mechanism, in this case in the presence of acquired cerebellar lesions (Hetherington et al., 1999). Twenty-nine long-term medulloblastoma survivors, 29 long-term astrocytoma survivors, and 58 controls were compared on a task requiring the discrimination of intervals in the range of 400 msec. The medulloblastoma group, but not the astrocytoma group, was impaired relative to controls (F [2, 113] = 5.5, $p < 0.006$). The timing deficit in the medulloblastoma group may have been more pronounced than that of the astrocytoma group because of the greater severity of the cerebellar lesion produced by the additive effects of the tumor, surgery, and focal radiation. The three groups did not differ on a control task of frequency discrimination, so the cognitive timing deficit does not represent a global perceptual impairment.

Taken together, the data from the congenital and acquired cerebellar lesions demonstrate that childhood disorders of the cerebellum produce not only chronic motor deficits, but cognitive timing deficits as well. The apparent absence of age-based functional plasticity in these tasks is further evidence that functions associated with the cerebellum are not readily compensated, even in the long term.

Full adult mastery: Tandem walk tested longitudinally in a long-term medulloblastoma survivor

Longitudinal studies of recovery into adulthood provides valuable evidence about age-based functional plasticity. Such data allow the observation of *plasticity for recovery of lost functions,* of which the raw score at the time of the lesion is an index, and *plasticity for recovery-plus-development,* which can only be established at maturity and which requires long-term longitudinal observations.

The heel-to-toe tandem walk of a standard neurological examination, using a method of McCarron (1976), was used in a longitudinal study of an individual treated for medulloblastoma, beginning at the time of tumor diagnosis and treatment, age 4 years, through to adulthood, age 24. The tandem walk task is performed on a calibrated 3-m floor mat, and factors evaluated in the test score include arm movement, foot placement, heel–toe orientation and distance, smoothness of gait progression, trajectory, and time required to walk the tape. The same task was given at all ages, using the child and adult norms, as appropriate. The data are shown in Figure 8-3.

Before the onset of tumor symptoms (Time 1), motor function was reported as normal, so we have assumed in Figure 8-3 that observed and expected skills were congruent and age appropriate. Functional effects of the lesion are evident at initial tumor presentation and surgery and radiation treatment (Time 2), at which time there was an *absolute loss of function* involving profound impairment in perfor-

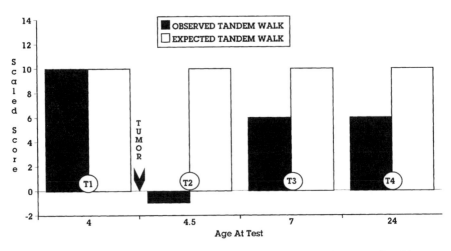

Figure 8-3. Full adult mastery. Tandem Walk tested longitudinally from ages 6 to 24 years in an individual who is a long-term (>5 years post-treatment) survivor of childhood posterior fossa medulloblastoma. T1 = Time 1; T2 = Time 2; T3 = Time 3; T4 = Time 4.

mance of the tandem walk, in keeping with a clinically florid ataxia. The difference between observed and expected tandem walk at tumor onset is a measure of the acute effects of the cerebellar tumor.

The *recovery phase* was measured here at age 7 years (Time 3), some 2.5 years after tumor treatment. Although skill improvement is evident, her scaled score of 6 was well below age expectations. The slope of the curve during the recovery phase provides some index of rate of recovery. Consideration of raw rather than age-scaled scores shows that the slope of the curve is steeper than that of normally developing peers from ages 4 to 7 years. It may be inferred that this slope represents additive effects of recovery and development processes because later, postrecovery, the slope of the development curve is similar to that of normally developing peers. When a skill is abolished in an adult after a lesion, recovery involves returning to pre-lesion skill mastery; in a 4-year-old it means returning to the level of mastery of a 4-year-old; thus, requirements for recovery are much more stringent in the adult than in the child. *Skill mastery* is impaired in the long term. The difference between observed and expected tandem walk remains significant at Time 4, nearly 20 years after tumor diagnosis and treatment.

The issues relevant to age-based functional plasticity are recovery of what was lost, new learning, and final mastery. If recovery is defined as restoration of previously lost skill, then, by age 7 years, this girl has recovered the same level of skill in terms of raw scores that she had lost at the time of the lesion. During the recovery from 4 to 7 years, the slope of the performance on the age curve is steeper for the child with the tumor than for normally developing children (i.e., there are more rapid increases in raw scores during this time). Between ages 7 and 24 years, the slope of the curve showing raw score increases is less steep and remains parallel with that of age peers, which suggests perhaps that there is ongoing development in the tumor individual but more limited or negligible recovery. At age 24, her raw score would be normal for 9–11-year-olds, and the fact of a chronic adult deficit means that this survivor of childhood medulloblastoma has not reached the same level of skill mastery at maturity as adults without childhood lesions.

Developmental stability or decline of function: Tandem walk in younger (16–19 years) and older (32–36 years) adult survivors of childhood medulloblastoma

Some genetically based neurodevelopmental disorders show accelerated cognitive aging (e.g., Down syndrome; Devenny et al., 1996). The question arises whether individuals with other neurodevelopmental and childhood acquired lesions also exhibit aging profiles that differ from normally developing peers. In this section, we consider this issue with reference to late adolescent and early middle-aged survivors of medulloblastomas. Investigations of function in adult survivors of acquired childhood lesions are important for testing the limits and nature of plasticity. Possible outcomes include full recovery of function maintained across the life span, impaired skill relative to nonlesioned age peers maintained across the life span, or a greater rate of skill decline than age peers with increasing age. Although the following data do not address performance in elderly survivors of medulloblastoma (of whom, as yet, there are few because survival rates have increased only recently), they do show the form that such data would take into middle adulthood.

Scores from the tandem walk test described earlier (McCarron, 1976) were converted to age-adjusted scaled scores for four groups, each comprising five individuals: 18-year-old younger controls, 18-year-old younger medulloblastoma survivors, 34-year-old older controls, and 34-year-old older medulloblastoma survivors. The tumor groups were long-term survivors who were five years or more post-treatment. The issue of interest is whether the ability to perform a tandem walk is constant with time since tumor (i.e., whether it changes at the same rate as controls) or whether skill is lost more rapidly in the tumor group than in the control groups. The data are shown in Figure 8-4.

The older groups, both tumor and control, perform slightly better than the younger groups. It remains to be seen whether other cerebellar functions are similar with aging in the two groups and also whether the performance by age curve in the tumor group will continue to have a similar slope to that of controls as its members move into middle age and beyond. Meanwhile, the present preliminary data suggest that the rate of change in tandem walk from 16 to 36 years in young adult survivors of childhood medulloblastoma appears similar to nonlesioned age peers.

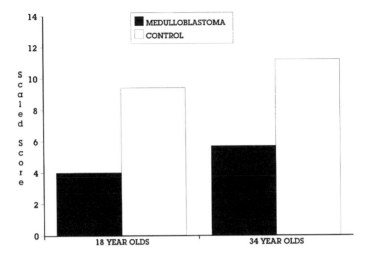

Figure 8-4. Equivalence of developmental stability and decline. Tandem Walk in younger (16–19) and older (32–34) adults, normally developing or survivors of childhood posterior fossa medulloblastoma.

Functionality under challenge: Motor function in long-term survivors of childhood posterior fossa tumors

To test the limits of plasticity in individuals with childhood onset of cerebellar pathology, relevant motor skills should be robust to the extent that performance is not more significantly disrupted than that of control children under conditions that place a load on, or challenge to, the function in question. In assaying whether individuals with compromised cerebellums can perform to the same levels as controls under conditions of routine challenge, we test whether the function in question is similarly robust in both groups.

As part of our analysis of motor function, we have examined cerebellar function under routine conditions and also under conditions of challenge (Dennis et al., 1996). The tandem walk task (McCarron, 1976) was presented under four conditions: routine (walking forward), physical challenge (walking backward), cognitive challenge (walking forward while counting backward from 50), and physical–cognitive challenge (walking backward while counting backward from 50). Two groups of individuals 5 or more years since diagnosis of posterior fossa tumors, 29 treated for astrocytoma and 33 treated for medulloblastoma or ependymoma, were compared to a group of 59 young adult controls. The results, shown in Figure 8-5, indicate a significant effect of group (F [2, 118] = 31.2, $p < 0.0001$) such that astrocytomas and medulloblastomas were each different from controls but not from each other, and a significant effect of tandem walk condition (F [3, 118] = 24.8, $p < 0.0001$), such that the challenge conditions were more difficult than the routine task. There was no interaction between group and condition.

The results are not due to radiation treatment because the radiated (medul-

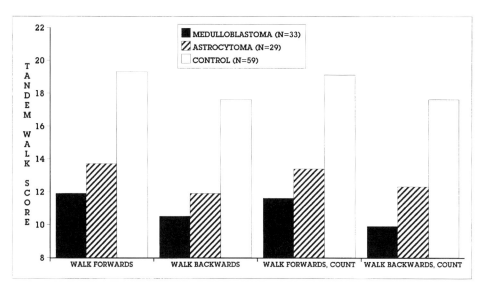

Figure 8-5. Functionality under challenge. Tandem Walk under conditions of challenge in children and young adults who are long-term survivors (>5 years post-treatment) of posterior fossa tumors of childhood.

loblastoma) and nonradiated (astrocytoma) groups do not differ. With respect to the assay of functionality under challenge, these data suggest that acquired cerebellar tumors are associated with significant and long-lasting deficits in gait. Some support for one aspect of the age-based plasticity hypothesis is provided here in that adding a challenge to the task does not increase its difficulty disproportionately for the tumor groups. However, the support is limited because the challenges reduce the performance of the medulloblastoma group to clinical impairment.

Discussion

This paper has described the use of behavioral assays for exploring the issue of age-based functional plasticity in response to developmental dysmorphologies and childhood lesions of the cerebellum. The methodologies used here have some heuristic value for understanding age-based functional plasticity. The importance of specifying hypotheses was stressed, as was the need to adduce long-term observations in support or disconfirmation of these hypotheses. The data considered were from the chronic phase of brain lesions: By middle childhood, lesions sustained during gestation are by definition chronic and all the tumor cases were long-term survivors.

The implications of the data are fivefold:

1. Cerebellar lesions in the immature brain are associated with stable functional deficits into middle adulthood rather than with developmental lags.

2. Functional deficits after childhood lesions are related to the type of brain damage in that they are similar to what has been observed after cerebellar damage in adulthood. These deficits appear related to the location and extent of cerebellar dysmorphology.

3. Cerebellar function was not related to age at lesion onset. Congenital cerebellar dysmorphologies are not associated with better development of cerebellar functions than are cerebellar lesions acquired later in development.

4. Recovery of lost function and development of new function may both continue after cerebellar dysmorphology or injury, but full age-appropriate functional level may not be attained. Developmental advances in function after childhood cerebellar lesions may be somewhat independent of processes relevant to recovery of function.

5. Age-based plasticity in the cerebellum may be overall less evident than in the cortex, although there are regional patterns of maturation in both that are relevant to the level of recovery.

Cerebellar lesions in the immature brain produce deficits rather than lags. Generally, the data support the view of stable, long-lasting deficits rather than developmental lags following congenital or childhood-acquired cerebellar lesions. Compensation for cerebellar lesions was incomplete, at best, by the time of maturity, despite many years of recovery. Longitudinal studies over childhood suggest that the difference between spina bifida and control subjects with respect to cognitive–motor timing tasks is constant over the main ages of skill mastery (6–14 years). Long-term follow-up studies into adulthood suggest further that the difference between acquired lesion groups and controls is maintained at a fairly constant rate into middle adulthood. To suggest that skills compromised by congenital malformations and acquired lesions of the cerebellum produce deficits from which the individual will "catch up" represents a strong hypothesis about age-based functional plasticity that receives no support from the present data.

The data from children with cerebellar lesions suggest a pattern of *predictable functional deficit* after cerebellar lesions that is similar to that in the adult brain. Childhood lesions of the cerebellum produce similar symptoms to cerebellar lesions in adulthood, and these symptoms persist, producing compromised functions associated with the cerebellum.

From the evidence available, there is also *structure–function congruence,* suggesting that the type of deficit and the type of lesion are predictable from knowledge of the same structure–function relations in the adult. In the two congenital dysmorphology cases with morphometric analyses of magnetic resonance scans, there was a *quantitative relation* between the degree of cerebellar dysmorphology and the magnitude of cerebellar functional deficit, as well as specificity between location of cerebellar dysmorphology and the type of functional cerebellar deficit, whereby medial tumors of the cerebellum in childhood were associated with problems in gait.

Functional plasticity was not age related in that cerebellar dysfunction was demonstrated after lesions with onset times ranging from 6 weeks of gestation to adolescence. Therefore, the data are relevant to hypotheses about *the age-based component* of plasticity. The skills studied here provide no evidence for a progressive reduction in functional plasticity with increased age at lesion. In this connection, cerebellar agenesis is *always* associated with profound motor deficits (Glickstein, 1994).

Neither congenital nor acquired cerebellar lesions precluded some continuing development of pertinent functions. Individuals with cerebellar compromise, although consistently performing below normative age expectations, were able to maintain their standing relative to age peers, and, for this to have occurred, there had to have been continued functional increments. The effects of development and recovery-plus-development may be differentiated on the basis of skill acquisition (or re-acquisition) gradients. The degree of developmental acceleration produced post-lesion by the combined processes of recovery and development and the duration of this acceleration establishes the extent to which age-appropriate function may be attained.

Long-term, longitudinal studies are essential for understanding the relation of recovery to development and the role of age at lesion in determining outcome. The 10-year follow up of tandem walk in a survivor of childhood medulloblastoma is a case in point. She recovered pre-lesion skill levels by the age of 7 years, 3 years after treatment for the cerebellar tumor. During this period, her skill acquisition gradient was greater than that of normally developing peers. The gradient decreased after this time, but was equal to that of normally developing peers. Although she did not obtain full adult mastery of this skill, continued development after recovery was possible. Post-lesion skill acquisition gradients provide a direct metric for comparison of functional plasticity. After comparable lesions, skill acquisition gradients may be compared longitudinally among individuals of different ages. Greater functional plasticity may be inferred from steeper slopes of longer duration.

Cerebellar lesions in children are associated with measurable recovery of lost functions and with new learning. Following cerebellar insult, skills are learned, sometimes at a normal developmental rate. However, the *base rate* of skill development and its *mature functional level* are attenuated relative to age peers. These findings are likely not unique to children. Even in adults, there is partial recovery from severe cerebellar symptoms and generally full recovery from more limited lesions (Glickstein, 1994).

More generally, the outcome of cerebellar lesions may depend not on age, per se, but on both the *type of cerebellar function* and the *location of the cerebellar lesion.* The functions of some structures may be structure specific, as in the case of the mediation of vegetative functions by nuclei in the medulla or mediation of body equilibrium during stance and gait by the vestibulocerebellum. These functions may not be compensated for by other neural structures. Other functions, such as oculomotor responses mediated by the cerebellar cortex, may be compensated for by structures in the cerebrum or by intact cerebellar nuclei. Mutism occurs commonly in acute stage posterior fossa lesions of childhood (Dennis, 1996) and occurs especially with posterior fossa tumors located in the midline and vermis of the cerebellum that include both cerebellar hemispheres or the deep nuclei (Humphreys, 1989; Rekate et al., 1985). In animals with cerebellar ablation that includes the intracerebellar nuclei, functional compensation is never complete, even years later (Eckmiller and Westheimer, 1983). The dysmorphologies and lesions reported here were generally extensive and likely involved in many cases significant compromise of deep cerebellar nuclei, which may have contributed to the limited functional outcome.

To be sure, the data presented here provide only a preliminary sketch of age-based plasticity in the cerebellum. Additional data are required to amplify and confirm these observations. For example, the role of motor and cognitive timing should be further explored, as should the processes of skill automatization; long-term follow-up studies that continue into the period of aging are now possible with increased survival rates of children with cerebellar injury and tumors; and quantitative neuroimaging studies are important in pursuing issues of structure–function congruence in the cerebellum. Of particular value will be studies that compare earlier and later established cerebellar skills with respect to the type and extent of cerebellar dysmorphology and lesion.

Even with the limits of the observations and studies presented here, one may infer that the degree and type of age-based functional plasticity following congenital malformations or childhood acquired lesions of the cerebellum are likely to differ in measurable and significant ways from those governing the response to childhood focal cortical lesions. Global age-based functional plasticity—whatever its status in the immature cortex—does not appear to be the rule with congenital dysmorphologies and childhood lesions below the tent, and cerebellar dysmorphologies and lesions do not confer any reorganizational advantage to the young brain.

References

This research was supported by project grants from the Ontario Mental Health Foundation and the National Cancer Institute of Canada.

Aram, D. M., Rose, D. F., Rekate, H. L., and Whitaker, H. A. (1983). Acquired capsular/striatal aphasia in childhood. *Arch. Neurol., 40,* 614–617.

Bachevalier, J., and Mishkin, M. (1994). Effects of selective neonatal temporal lobe lesions on visual recognition memory in rhesus monkeys. *J. Neurosci., 14,* 2128–2139.

Barkovich, A. J. (1994). Congenital malformations of the brain and skull. In A. J. Barkovich (ed.): *Pediatric Neuroimaging* (2nd ed.). New York: Raven Press, pp. 177–275.

Basser, L. S. (1962). Hemiplegia of early onset with special reference to the effects of hemispherectomy. *Brain, 85,* 427–460.

Bloedel, J. R. (1992). Functional heterogeneity with structural homogeneity: How does the cerebellum operate? *Behav. Brain Sci., 15,* 666–678.

Caviness, V. S., Kennedy, D. N., Bates, J., and Makris, N. (1995). The developing human brain: A morphometric profile. In R. W. Thatcher, G. R. Lyon, J. Rumsey and N. Krasnegor (eds.): *Developmental Neuroimaging: Mapping the Development of Brain and Behavior.* New York: Academic Press, pp. 3–14.

Cohen, M. E., & Duffner, P. K. (1994). *Brain Tumors in Children. Principles of Diagnosis and Treatment* (2nd ed.). New York: Raven Press.

Courchesne, E., Townsend, J., and Akshoomoff, N. A. (1994). Impairment in shifting attention in autistic and cerebellar patients. *Behav. Neurosci., 108,* 848–865.

Del Bigio, M. R. (1993). Neuropathological changes caused by hydrocephalus. *Acta Neuropathol., 85,* 573–585.

Denckla, M. B., and Rudel, R. (1974). Rapid "automatized" naming of pictured objects, colors, letters, and numbers by normal children. *Cortex, 10,* 186–202.

Dennis, M. (1980a). Capacity and strategy for syntactic comprehension after left or right hemidecortication. *Brain Lang., 10,* 287–317.

Dennis, M. (1980b). Strokes in childhood: I. Communicative intent, expression, and comprehension after left hemisphere arteriopathy in a right-handed nine-year-old. In R. Rieber (ed.): *Language Development and Aphasia in Children.* New York: Academic Press, pp. 45–67.

Dennis, M. (1985). Intelligence after early brain injury: I. Predicting IQ scores from medical history variables. *J. Clin. Exp. Neuropsychol., 7,* 526–554.

Dennis, M. (1988). Language and the young damaged brain. In T. Boll and B. K. Bryant (eds.): *Clinical Neuropsychology and Brain Function: Research, Measurement, and Practice.* Master Lecture Series, vol. 7. Washington, DC: American Psychological Association, pp. 85–123.

Dennis, M. (1996a). Hydrocephalus. In J. G. Beaumont, P. Kenealy, and M. Rogers (eds.): *Blackwell Dictionary of Neuropsychology.* Oxford: Blackwell, pp. 406–411.

Dennis, M. (1996b). Acquired disorders of language in children. In T. E. Feinberg and M. J. Farah (eds.): *Behavioral Neurology and Neuropsychology.* New York: McGraw-Hill, pp. 737–754.

Dennis, M., and Barnes, M. A. (1994). Developmental aspects of neuropsychology: Childhood. In D. Zaidel (ed.): *Handbook of Perception and Cognition, vol. 15.* New York: Academic Press, pp. 219–246.

Dennis, M., Hendrick, E. B., Hoffman, H. J., and Humphreys, R. P. (1987). The language of hydrocephalic children and adolescents. *J. Clin. Exp. Neuropsychol., 9,* 593–621.

Dennis, M., and Kohn, B. (1975). Comprehension of syntax in infantile hemiplegics after cerebral hemidecortication: Left hemisphere superiority. *Brain Lang., 2,* 472–482{**EP**}.

Dennis, M., Spiegler, B. J., Hetherington, C. R., and Greenberg, M. L. (1996). Neuropsychological sequelae of the treatment of children with medulloblastoma. *J. Neuro-Oncol., 29,* 91–101.

Dennis, M., and Whitaker, H. A. (1976). Language acquisition following hemidecortication: Linguistic superiority of the left over the right hemisphere. *Brain Lang, 3,* 404–433.

Devenny, D. A., Silverman, W. P., Hill, A. L., Jenkins, E., Sersen, E. A., and Wisniewski, K. E. (1996). Normal ageing in adults with Down's syndrome: A longitudinal study. *J. Intell. Disabil. Res., 40,* 208–221.

Dichgans, J., and Deiner, H. (1984). Clinical evidence for functional compartmentalization of the cerebellum. In J. Bloedel, J. Dichgans, and W. Precht (eds.): *Cerebellar Functions.* Berlin: Springer, pp. 126–147.

Diener, H. C., and Dichgans, J. (1992). Pathophysiology of cerebellar ataxia. *Mov. Disord., 7,* 95–109.

Eckmiller, R., and Westheimer, G. (1983). Compensation of oculomotor deficits in monkeys with neonatal cerebellar ablations. *Exp. Brain Res., 49,* 315–326.

Fischer, E. G. (1973). Dandy Walker syndrome: An evaluation of surgical treatment. *J. Neurosurg., 39,* 615–621.

Fletcher, J. M., Bohan, T. P., Brandt, M. E., Brookshire, B. L., Beaver, S. R., Francis, D. J., Thompson, N. M., and Miner, M. E. (1992). Cerebral white matter and cognition in hydrocephalic children. *Arch. Neurol., 49,* 818–824.

Friston, K. J., Frith, C. D., Passingham, R. E., Liddle, P. F., and Frackowiak, R. S. J. (1992). Motor practice and neurophysiological adaptation in the cerebellum: A positron tomography study. *Proc. R. Soc. Lond. B., 248,* 223–228.

Ghez, C. (1991). The cerebellum. In E. R. Kandel, J. H. Schwartz, and T. M. Jessell (eds.): *Principles of Neural Science* (3rd ed.). New York: Elsevier Science, pp. 626–646.

Gilbert, J. N., Jones, K. L., Rorke, L. B., Chernoff, G. F., and James, H. E. (1986). Central nervous system anomalies associated with meningomyelocele, hydrocephalus, and the Arnold-Chiari malformation: Reappraisal of theories regarding the pathogenesis of posterior neural tube closure defects. *Neurosurgery, 18,* 559–564.

Gilman, S. (1994). Cerebellar control of movement. *Ann. Neurol., 35,* 3–4.

Gilman, S., Carr, D., and Hollenberg, J. (1976). Kinematic effects of deafferentiation and cerebellar ablation. *Brain, 99,* 311–330.

Glickstein, M. (1994). Cerebellar agenesis. *Brain, 117,* 1209–1212.

Greenough, W. T., Wallace, C. S., Alcantara, A. A., Anderson, B. J., Hawrylak, N., Sirevaag, A. M., Weiler, I. J., and Withers, G. S. (1993). Development of the brain: Experience affects the structure of neurons, glia, and blood vessels. In N. J. Anastasiow and S. Harel (eds.): *At-risk Infants. Interventions, Families and Research.* New York: Paul H. Brookes, pp. 173–185.

Harwood-Nash, D. C. F., and Fitz, C. R. (1976). *Neuroradiology in Infants and Children,* vol. 2. St. Louis, MO: C. V. Mosby Co.

Heideman, R. L., Packer, R. J. Albright, L. A., Freeman, C. R., and Rorke, L. B. (1993). Tumors of the central nervous system. In P. A. Pizzo and D. G. Poplack (eds.): *Principles and Practice of Pediatric Oncology* (2nd ed.). Philadelphia: J. B. Lippincott Company, pp. 633–681.{EP}

Hetherington, R., and Dennis, M. (1999). Motor function profile in children with early onset hydrocephalus. *Dev. Neuropsychol., 15,* 25–51.

Hetherington, C. R., Dennis, M., Kennedy, D., Barnes, M., and Drake, J. (1998). Congenital cerebellar dysmorphology: Motor function and MRI-based morphometric analyses. *Brain Cog., 37,* 34–40.

Hetherington, C. R., Dennis, M., and Spiegler, B. (1999). Temporal discrimination is impaired in survivors of childhood cerebellar tumors. *Journal of the International Neuropsychological Society 5,* 101.

Hetherington, C. R., Stuss, D. T., and Finlayson, M. A. J. (1996). Reaction time and variability 5 and 10 years after traumatic brain injury. *Brain Injury, 10,* 473–486.

Hoffman, H. J. (1989). Diagnosis and management of posthemorrhagic hydrocephalus in the premature infant. In K. E. Pape and J. S. Wiggleworth (eds.): *Perinatal Brain Lesions.* Oxford: Basil Blackwell, pp. 219–229.

Hoffman, H. J., Berger, M. S., and Becker, L. E. (1990). Cerebellar astrocytomas. In M. Deutsch (ed.): *Management of Childhood Brain Tumors.* Boston: Kluwer Academic Publishers, pp. 441–456.

Holmes, G. (1922). The clinical symptoms of cerebellar disease and their interpretation. *Lancet, 1,* 1177–1182.

Hore, J., and Flament, D. (1988). Changes in motor cortex neural discharge associated with the development of cerebellar limb ataxia. *J. Neurophysiol., 60,* 1285–1302.

Humphreys, R. P. (1989). Mutism after posterior fossa tumour surgery. *Con. Pediatr. Neurosurg., 9,* 57–69.

Ito, M. (1993). Movement and thought: Identical control mechanisms by the cerebellum. *Trends Neurosci., 16,* 448–450.

Ivry, R., and Keele, S. (1989). Timing functions of the cerebellum. *J. Cog. Neurosci., 1,* 136–151.

Kennard, M. A. (1940). Relation of age to motor impairment in man and in subhuman primates. *Arch. Neurol. Psychiatry, 44,* 377–397.

Kennard, M. A., and Fulton, J. F. (1942). Age and reorganization of central nervous system. *Mt. Sinai Hosp. J., 9,* 594–606.

Kennard, M. A., Spencer, S., and Fountain, G. (1941). Hyperactivity in monkeys following lesions of the frontal lobes. *J. Neurophysiol. 4,* 512–524.

Kim, S.-G., Ugurbil, K., and Strick, P. L. (1994). Activation of a cerebellar output nucleus during cognitive processing. *Science, 265,* 949–951.

Koop, M., Rilling, G., Herrmann, A., and Kretschmann, H. J. (1986). Volumetric development of the fetal telencephalon, cerebral cortex, diencephalon, and rhombencephalon including the cerebellum in man. *Bibl. Anat., 28,* 53–78.

Lechtenberg, R. (1993). Embryogenesis of the cerebellum. In R. Lechtenberg (ed.): *Handbook of Cerebellar Diseases.* New York: Marcel Dekker, pp. 1–16.

Lee, T. D., and Swinnen, S. P. (1993). Three legacies of Bryan and Harter: Automaticity, variability and change in skilled performance. In J. L. Starkes and S. Allard (eds.): *Cognitive Issues in Motor Expertise.* New York: Elsevier Science Publishers, pp. 295–315.

Leiner, H. C., Leiner, A. L., and Dow, R. S. (1986). Does the cerebellum contribute to mental skill? *Behav. Neurosci., 100,* 443–453.

Leiner, H. C., Leiner, A. L., and Dow, R. S. (1991). The human cerebrocerebellar system: Its computing, cognitive, and language skills. *Behav. Brain Res., 44,* 113–128.

Lenneberg, E. (1967). *Biological Foundations of Language.* New York: Wiley.

Martin, E., Kikinis, R., Zuerrer, M., et al. (1988). Developmental stages of human brain: An MR study. *J. Comput. Assist. Tomogr., 12,* 917–922.

McCarron, L. T. (1976). McCarron assessment of neuromuscular development. Dallas, TX: McCarron-Dial Systems.

Moore, K. L. (1982). *The Developing Human: Clinically Oriented Embryology* (3rd ed.). Philadelphia: W. B. Saunders.

Paidas, M. J., and Cohen, A. (1994). Disorders of the central nervous system. *Semin. Perinatol., 18,* 463–482.

Packer, J. R., Sutton, L. N., Atkins, T. E., Radcliffe, J., Bunin, G. R., D'Angio, G., Siegel, K. R., and Schut, L. (1989). A prospective study of cognitive function in children receiving whole-brain radiotherapy and chemotherapy: 2-year results. *J. Neurosurg., 70,* 707–713.

Pascual-Castroviejo, I., Velez, A., Pascual-Pascual, S. I., Roche, M. C., and Villarejo, F. (1991). Dandy-Walker malformation: Analysis of 38 cases. *Childs Nerv. Syst., 7,* 88–97.

Passingham, R. E. (1975). Changes in the size and organization of the brain in man and his ancestors. *Brain Behav. Evol., 11,* 73–90.

Pellock, J. M., and Johnson, M. H. (1993). Dandy-Walker malformation. In R. Lechtenberg (ed.): *Handbook of Cerebellar Diseases.* New York: Marcel Decker, pp. 147–162.

Rekate, H. L., Grubb, R. L., Aram, D. L., Hahn, J. F., and Ratcheson, R. A. (1985). Muteness of cerebellar origin. *Arch. Neurol., 42,* 697–698.

Rorke, L. B., Gilles, F. H., Davis, R. L., and Becker, L. E. (1985). Revision of the World Health Organization classification of brain tumors for childhood brain tumors. *Cancer, 56,* 1969–1986.

Silveri, M. C., Leggio, M. G., and Molinari, M. (1994). The cerebellum contributes to linguistic production: A case of agrammatic speech following a right cerebellar lesion. *Neurology, 44,* 2047–2050.

Stiles, J. (1995). Plasticity and development: Evidence from children with early occurring focal brain injury. In M. H. Johnson (ed.): *Brain Development and Cognition,* vol. 23. Cambridge: Blackwell Publishers, pp. 217–237.

Sudarsky, L., and Coutinho, P. (1995). Machado-Joseph disease. *Clin. Neurosci., 3,* 17–22.

Sutton, J. B. (1887). The lateral recesses of the fourth ventricle; their relation to certain cysts and tumors of the cerebellum, and to occipital meningocele. *Brain, 9,* 352–361.

Tal, Y., Freigang, B., Dunn, H. G., Durity, F. A., and Moyes, P. D. (1980). Dandy-Walker syndrome: Analysis of 21 cases. *Dev. Med. Child Neurol., 22,* 189–201.

Taylor, H. G., and Alden, J. (1997). Age-related differences in outcomes following childhood brain insults: An introduction and overview. *J. Int. Neuropsychol. Soc., 3,* 555–567.

Teyler, T. J., Cavus, I., Coussens, C., DiScenna, P., Grover, L., Lee, Y.-P., and Little, Z. (1995). Advances in understanding the mechanisms underlying synaptic plasticity. In A. Schurr and B. M. Rigor (eds.): *Brain Slices in Basic and Clinical Research.* Boca Raton, FL: CRC Press, pp. 1–25.

Thach, W. T. (1997). On the specific role of the cerebellum in motor learning and cognition: Clues from PET activation and lesion studies in man. In P. J. Cordo, C. C. Bell, and S. Harnad (eds.): *Motor Learning and Synaptic Plasticity in the Cerebellum.* New York: Cambridge University Press, pp. 73–93.

Toriello, H. V., and Higgins, J. V. (1985). Possible causal heterogeneity in spina bifida cystica. *Am. J. Med. Genet., 21,* 13–20.

Turvey, M. T. (1990). Coordination. *Am. Psychol., 45,* 938–953.

Webster, M. J., Bachevalier, J., and Ungerleider, L. G. (1995). Transient subcortical connections of interior temporal areas TE and TEO in infant macaque monkeys. *J. Comp. Neurol., 352,* 213–226.

Webster, M. J., Ungerleider, L. G., and Bachevalier, J. (1991). Connections of inferior temporal areas TE and TEO with medial temporal-lobe structures in infant and adult monkeys. *J. Neurosci., 11,* 1095–1116.

Williams, T. E., Buchhalter, J. R., and Sussman, M. D. (1996). Cerebellar dysplasia and unilateral cataract in Marinesco-Sjogren syndrome. *Pediatr. Neurol., 14,* 158–161.

Yakovlev, P. I., and Lecours, A.-R. (1967). The myelogenetic cycles of regional maturation of the brain. In A. Minkowski (ed.): *Regional Development of the Brain in Early Life.* Oxford: Blackwell Scientific, pp. 3–65.

9

Recovery from Acquired Reading and Naming Deficits Following Focal Cerebral Lesions

BARRY GORDON, DANA BOATMAN,
RONALD P. LESSER, AND JOHN HART, JR.

Trying to improve function in children with developmental deficits—particularly the higher level, symbolic functions that allow humans to reason and to communicate—requires attempting to establish abilities that these children may never have developed. In addressing this problem of training abilities *de novo,* it is reasonable to consider the data and insights that can be derived from studies of recovery of functions that were once present but that have been extirpated due to brain injury or disease. Recovery of cognitive functions after brain injury is a common occurrence, particularly in children. Yet it has been difficult to establish the precise functional and neuroanatomical bases for such recoveries.

One major problem is that human cognitive abilities are uniquely human, precluding any strictly analogous animal models. Another problem is that cognitive abilities are complex, the product of many underlying mental operations. The exact nature, sequence, and properties of the many mental operations underlying most abilities are not well understood. This situation is further complicated by the likelihood that putatively similar mental abilities in different individuals may be subserved by different combinations or weighings of the more basic mental abilities, making cross-subject comparisons difficult. Moreover, acquired impairments are usually due to conditions such as infarction, trauma, hemorrhage, and encephalitis. Because they occur without warning, determination of pre-lesion cognitive status is often indirect and speculative. In addition, cognitive function is often not the most important issue in the immediate post-lesion period, and evaluation of recovery at that time is often scanty and relatively superficial. The full course of recovery may therefore not be well documented. Functionally, such lesions tend to be large and affect many different cognitive, sensory, and motor functions, making it difficult to determine with accuracy the nature of the disruption in any particular one. Their boundaries are often poorly defined, making it hard to specify the extent to which various structures are actually involved. Because such accidental lesions tend to be quite traumatic to the brain and associated structures, processes such as inflammation and edema may confound attempts to determine responsibility for decline or for improvement.

The principal study discussed in this chapter avoids some of these difficulties by studying the recovery of reading impairments in patients undergoing planned focal surgical cerebral resections. The surgeries were planned in advance so that data on reading level were collected before any resection occurred. Because these were surgical patients, the resected area was relatively small, and the resection was done as atraumatically as possible. The patients were under hospital care, and their immediate post-lesion status was closely monitored. It was possible to get later measures of their status because they needed to return for continuing care.

The task used with these surgical patients, reading of single words, and the task used with another case to be described, naming of objects, have several advantages for studying recovery. These tasks are representative of higher cognitive functions. They require learning of complex visual stimuli (words or objects), complex phonological forms (words), and, most importantly, learning of a noninnate linkage between these inputs and outputs. There is general agreement about the broad outlines of the stages and processes responsible for reading and for naming. There are, of course, debates about the exact mental functions that are yoked to generate either of these abilities. These details are not of central importance for the issues discussed here. What is critical is that it is self-evident that the arbitrariness of the mapping from vision to speech means that accurate reading aloud or naming requires *knowing* the association between a visual representation and sound. Accurate reading and naming cannot be innate abilities; some information must be learned to perform them accurately. For naming, it is likely that the association between vision and speech is mediated by semantic representations, for most items, at least in adults (for review, see Gordon, 1997a). In reading single words out loud, semantic mediation is generally not thought to be either necessary or typically used. Instead, reading aloud depends on either recognition of the whole word and matching to phonology or recognition of parts of the word (letters and letter combinations), retrieving the phonological representations of these parts, and then blending these parts into the whole word for pronunciation. Because many words share parts (e.g., *lint* and *mint*) and because some letters or letter combinations are pronounced identically or with lawful regularity in many words, these latter, sublexical mechanisms may be fairly general. How much the whole-word or sublexical routes contribute to reading in general, and the nature of sublexical-to-phonological processing, are matters of considerable debate. There is general agreement, however, that words can be roughly ranked along a dimension of orthographical-to-phonological regularity (Coltheart et al., 1993; Plaut et al., 1996). *Regular* words have pronunciations that are predictable from the pronunciation of other words. In contrast, the pronunciation of less regular words requires more specific knowledge. For example, while *lint, mint,* and *tint* all have the same pronunciation of the body of the words, *pint,* with the same letter combinations, does not. The extreme examples of irregular pronunciation are the *unique* words, such as *yacht,* which can only be pronounced by knowing their specific pronunciation.

The theoretical debates about the details of these processes should not obscure the major points of relevance for the data to be presented. The processes involved in naming and reading are examples of just those kinds of higher order, complex symbolic processes that are desirable for humans to learn. Successful performance on naming or reading tasks requires acquired knowledge. Acquisition of that knowledge is generally a relatively slow process. Acquisition of object names happens very early in development, and the processes involved in name acquisition itself are strongly conflated with maturation of the sensory systems, the speech apparatus, and perhaps general cognitive abilities. Acquisition of reading typically occurs later, when the capabilities of the child's nervous system more closely approach those of the adult. It is still difficult to be sure of how much training is required to learn specific orthographic-to-sound associations apart from the learning of new orthographical representations and new phonological representations themselves; these are all normally interactive, bootstrapping processes. But it does seem to be the case that learning the information required for successful reading out loud can be a relatively slow and effortful process for both children and illiterate adults (Adams, 1990).

What also makes naming and reading useful for investigating the mechanisms involved in recovery is that the processes that produce them are relatively straightforward. Under normal circumstances for adults, the internal steps involved in reading or naming out loud are generally rapid, automatic, and processed only in a forward direction. There are no conscious strategies, searches, or feedback. Input stimuli are sharply defined in time and space (in essence, step functions), which also makes subsequent processing easier to track. Responses are also relatively discreet. The precise definitions of inputs and outputs also make these tasks more experimentally tractable.

In addition to a reasonable understanding of the functional processes involved, there is also now a general understanding of the neuroanatomical structures involved in these tasks and functions. In particular, the areas involved in accessing visual representations and in linking them to phonological representations appear to be in the posterior temporal region and in the inferior frontal region, perhaps bilaterally but particularly on the dominant (left) side. (It should be noted, however, that investigations based on imaging [Fiez and Petersen, 1998; Shaywitz et al., 1998] have perhaps come to different anatomical conclusions than those based on lesion data [Gordon, 1997a; Henderson et al., 1985].)

This outline is the context within which we have tried to understand the following examples of recovery of function of reading and naming. The data and analyses we report are preliminary, and some of the specific details and results may require revision because of complexities in the data and in the analyses. However, these data- and theory-specific issues should not affect the broad characterizations we present here. Portions of these studies have been previously presented and published in abstract form (Boatman et al., 1988, 1991a,b, 1994; Hart et al., 1990).

A complete description of these studies is being prepared (Gordon et al., manuscript in preparation).

Prospective Study of Recovery of Single-Word Reading

Subjects were a subset of those Johns Hopkins Medical Institution patients being considered for focal cerebral resections for treatment of intractable epilepsy, tumors, or arteriovenous malformations. Before any surgery, all patients had thorough medical, educational, and work histories; neurological examinations; neuropsychological testing; brain MRI scans; continuous video-EEG monitoring; and intracarotid amobarbital injections to test for language dominance and memory functions. Before any resections were done, all the patients considered here also had surgical implantation of subdural electrodes for prolonged surface EEG recording and for clinical mapping of language and related functions. Of specific relevance to the current report, all patients, prior to any resection, also had clinical and experimental testing of single-word reading.

The materials used to test reading were 118 words (together with 118 pseudowords, which will not be further discussed). Sixty-eight of the words were specifically selected to test knowledge of various orthographical-to-phonological mappings and were drawn from a published experimental study of such mappings (Brown, 1987). They were four to six letters in length. Words were presented one at a time either on cards or on a computer screen. The patient's task was to pronounce the words as rapidly and as accurately as possible. If testing was on the computer, response latencies were recorded by voice key. Responses were transcribed as they were uttered by an experienced speech–language therapist who watched the patient's mouth and also recorded by a high-quality tape recorder. Only first responses were counted (although others were noted). Later, a second technician trained in speech–language pathology, who was blinded to the stimuli, also transcribed the responses from the tapes. Transcriptions used a broad International Phonetic Alphabetic coding scheme. The inter-rater reliability of the two transcribers was high ($r = 0.92$; $p < 0.005$).

Focal resections were done for clinical purposes 1–2 weeks after initial implantation of the subdural arrays. The resections consisted of tailored resections or corticectomies. Thirty-three had resections in the dominant (left) temporal, temporo-occipital, or occipital areas. Of these, seven developed specific impairments. Four had impairments principally of reading and are the focus of this section; two had impairments primarily involving naming, and one had both reading and naming deficits. Of the four with reading impairments, three had resections of the inferior temporal region, while one had a left lateral occipital corticectomy.

In one of the patients with a reading deficit, the deficit occurred in the course of the resection, which was being done stepwise, under local anesthesia, to minimize the chances of causing a persistent focal deficit (Gordon et al., 1991b).

Patients were tested as soon as possible after surgery, sometimes 1–2 days later, and at periodic intervals after that (often at 1 week, 6 months, and 1 year).

All patients were informed about any deficits that were found. They were also informed that any deficits were expected to resolve spontaneously. For the first patient, this prediction was on the basis of clinical experience (see below); for the others, it was based on the empirical data from the prior cases. Other than the testing itself, subjects were not explicitly shown the stimuli again. Whether a subject read independently was neither encouraged nor discouraged. Whether they read in the hospital or at home was assessed informally on return interviews. No one reported reading out loud, and none reported any training in reading aloud.

None of these subjects had impairments of basic visual functions, word meaning, or word production. Three of the four had intact visual lexical decision ability (for discriminating words from nonwords). Instead, they had a relatively specific deficit in reading aloud. Performance on the reading aloud task in the subset of patients with reading deficits is schematized in Figure 9-1, which shows the proportions correct and mean correct reaction times for pre- and postoperative testings.*

As Figure 9-1 shows, all subjects recovered to nearly their baseline levels. This was true not only for the formal test data (allowing for the fact that not all subjects had pre-resection testing on the computer) but also from subjects' reports and the reports from their families that the reading abilities recovered to premorbid levels.

The deficits and recoveries affected words of all the different orthographical-to-phonological classes equally, at least in our preliminary analyses. An example from one subject is shown in Figure 9-2. Reading of words with irregular orthographical-to-phonological mappings was no more susceptible to disruption than was reading of words with regular orthographical-to-phonological mappings, and the recoveries of these classes of word were also of comparable rates.

Before discussing the significance of all these data, another relevant patient study is presented.

Patient 5

Patient 5 was a 31-year-old right-handed female with 16 years of education, working in journalism. A small, left posterior inferior temporal oligodendroglioma was diagnosed by needle biopsy. The biopsy was followed by a small hemorrhage, as shown by MRI scan. With the hemorrhage, she developed more marked subjective difficulties with word-finding in spontaneous speech. These difficulties were not apparent even to close family members, but Patient 5 was certain that she was expending far more effort on generating words than she had before the hemorrhage occurred. As part of her evaluation, we administered the Boston Naming Test,

---

*Analysis and representation of these data are complex issues, partly because of theoretical concerns over the justifications for pooling data across subjects and items. The detailed results from these and other subjects are being written up for publication (Gordon et al., manuscript in preparation). The raw data (for each subject, for each item, and for each testing session) will be made available to reviewers and to other researchers as needed.

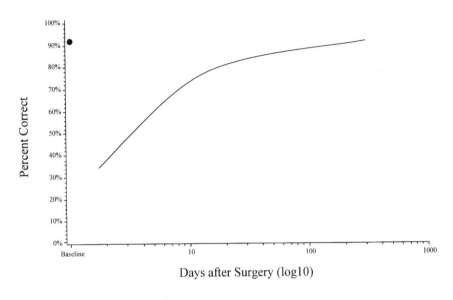

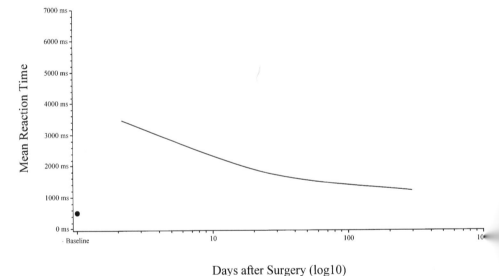

Days after Surgery (log10)

Figure 9-1. Performance on reading out loud for cases 1–4 (schematic summary of data). (*Top*) Proportions correct. (*Bottom*) Mean correct voice onset time (from onset of word presentation).

which elicits single-word names of objects represented by line drawings. The 85-item research edition (Goodglass et al., 1976) was used. Her initial performance was 48% correct, which is quite poor (Fig. 9-3). She was quite surprised at this performance. Other testing showed intact visual perceptual abilities, intact speech production abilities, and intact semantic comprehension (through other routes).

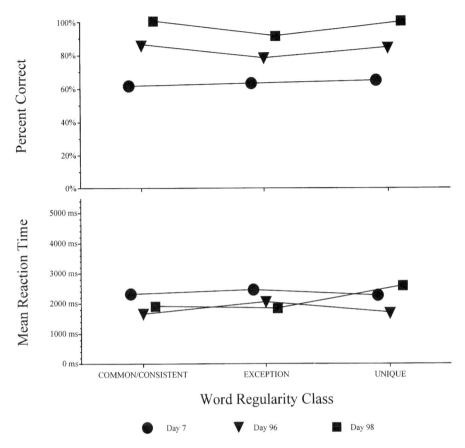

Figure 9-2. Reading out loud of words of different classes of orthographical-to-phonological regularity, by one subject, over time.

Without warning, she was retested the next day on the same naming task. This time, she was 88% correct, a highly significant improvement (using Liddell's exact test for matched pairs, $p < 0.001$).

Discussion

Recovery of function after central nervous system damage is widely assumed to be due mostly to the recruitment of other regions, either adjacent cortical tissue, subcortical structures, or more widely removed ipsilateral and contralateral cortex (Nudo et al., 1996; Yamaski and Wurtz, 1991). However, this mechanism can only account for why *capabilities* can be restored; it cannot account for how prior *knowledge* can be restored. Knowledge of orthographical-to-phonological associations, or of picture-to-phonological associations, is not innate; the specifics of

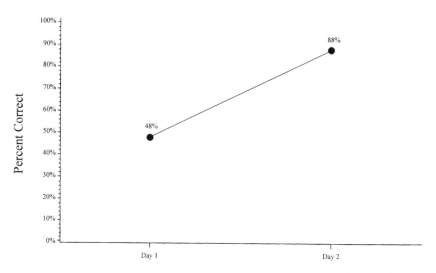

Figure 9-3. Boston Naming Test (Experimental Edition) performance of Patient 5 on two successive days of testing.

such knowledge must be learned. The cases we have presented all were able to recover this specific knowledge in some fashion. How?

It is seemingly easy to account for their initial deficits. Use of item- and stage-specific information is an on-line, implicit process. Storage of the specific knowledge is thought to be within the regions in which it is actually used (Gordon, 1997b). It is widely assumed that the specific knowledge is in the form of patterns of synaptic connectivity and latent changes in synaptic conductance (see Gordon, 1997a). With appropriate inputs, these latent changes become expressed as different patterns of neuronal electrical activity. It is also generally assumed that the types of information needed for reading words out loud or for naming objects out loud is dependent on the activity of thousands if not tens of thousands of neurons and neuronal elements. Nonetheless, even though the information is distributed across many neurons and neuronal connections, these cells still only represent a small subset of cortical cells and probably a geographically delimited subset.

Given these assumptions about the mechanisms and elements involved, there is a ready explanation for why these patients developed impairments. The resection or lesion, respectively, damaged some critical part of the sequence of processes required. More specifically, the damage affected the neuronal elements or connections involved in image-to-sound translation (or, in the case of one of the postsurgical patients, more likely damaged her initial orthographical access mechanism (Gordon et al., 1991a). The other component processes necessary for reading and for naming were intact. Damage to portions of the neural network responsible for a function, or to the connections between component networks, is thought to be capable of causing the types of degraded performance observed in these patients.

But if damage to the neuronal networks that held the implicit knowledge necessary for performance of a task was the cause of the deficits in these subjects, how can the deficit improve? How can the knowledge that was acquired with such effort and so slowly appear so quickly again in Patient 5 and more slowly but still remarkably in the patients with focal resections?

The most direct explanation for the partial loss and nearly complete recovery of information is that the network corresponding to the relevant stage of naming or reading, or its connecting pathways, was not completely destroyed by the surgical resection (in the patients undergoing focal resections) or by the tumor/hematoma (in Patient 5's case). The partial damage allowed some words through, at slower speeds. Recovery would then come about when adjacent cerebral regions were recruited and trained. However, because some of the original neural net and its latent knowledge were intact, there would be substantial savings, and relearning could be far more rapid. This might appear to be spontaneous recovery, but it is really just accelerated learning off of a partial knowledge base. Neural network simulations of learning can readily show the acceleration of learning after some weights (knowledge) have become established in the network (McClelland, 1989).

One important corollary of this explanation of the recovery is that it does require that the original damage is relatively restricted to a single stage of processing and incomplete even at the stage. The reason relearning can be relatively rapid is because it is not necessary to relearn all the steps in the process, and all of the knowledge in each of those steps. Instead, only one step has to be relearned, and only part of the information in that step. Teaching focused in this manner can be vastly more efficient and rapid than teaching of a whole, multistep process from scratch. This is both intuitively obvious and also buttressed by neural simulation studies (Cohen et al., 1990; McClelland, 1989).

As straightforward as this explanation of recovery of knowledge may be, there are other possible explanations that need to be considered. One possibility is that the recovery was not restoration of prior knowledge, or partial relearning, but instead complete relearning. This was possible in the patients with focal cerebral resections. They were not prevented from having exposure to printed words. However, relearning from a zero knowledge baseline (for those words that could not be produced) seems unlikely. Normal learning of naming (Bloom and Markson, 1998) and reading (Adams, 1990) is relatively slow. It does not seem possible for the population of items from which our materials were sampled to have been relearned in the time period under study. More convincingly, Patient 5 made a marked improvement in naming after only one presentation. She had been given no explicit feedback. This strongly suggests that such recovery is drawing on a latent store of pre-existing knowledge; it does not represent complete relearning. Why, then, would this store of prior knowledge be hidden at first and then become accessible?

Inflammation and other structural changes might be part of the answer, at least in the postsurgical patients. In this hypothesis, critical neurons and neuronal connections are disturbed and irritated by these outside influences; as inflammation and edema resolve, the neurons function normally again, their latent knowledge (and their ability to express that knowledge) intact. This mechanism may be an important factor in recovery from the usual accidental brain injury. However, it would have been expected that tissue trauma, inflammation, and edema would have been appreciably less in these postsurgical cases, cases 1–4. In addition, other visual and language functions in these patients were also closely monitored after surgery and did not show any changes. Moreover, such a mechanism is totally unable to explain the rapid, 24-hour recovery of a function in Patient 5, which occurred some time after her second insult (a hemorrhage).

A comparable, but more direct possibility is that localized neural damage causes dysfunction or inhibition, or both, in adjacent cortical tissue. (This hypothesis is of course related to the broader idea of diaschesis [Gazzaniga, 1975].) Electrolytic lesions of the visual cortex have been shown to produce increased excitability and reduced inhibition in the surrounding cortex that was otherwise spared from the direct lesion (Eysel, 1997). Resolution of these more or less direct disruptions would allow apparent recovery of the functions that the adjacent tissue previously was able to perform. This might appear as an apparent restoration of previously stored information.

Yet another possible explanation for the recovery that we observed is that the lesion(s) did not directly affect the neuronal elements and connections that were directly responsible for the on-line retrieval of information. Instead, the lesions affected mechanisms that controlled or regulated this on-line access or retrieval. Such a mechanism has not been invoked in the literature on reading or naming themselves, but does appear in a computational model of reading and naming in the Stroop task proposed by Cohen et al. (1990). They postulated a mechanism that gates processing channels and response options. If such gating and channeling mechanisms were damaged, the prior knowledge could appear to be lost, but still appear to recover with recovery of the switch. There must exist mechanisms for gating or switching information flow to allow underlying processing modules to participate in many different overt tasks and functions. To endow such a switching or channeling mechanism with the single-item specificity needed to account for the processing of some items but not others, a way must be found to differentiate items along dimensions that are different than the ones usually thought to influence processing (e.g., frequency; see Gordon, 1997a). But given that some of the dimensions that are known to influence higher order processing are far from intuitive (Hart and Gordon, 1992), this latter requirement may not be completely inplausible. It will certainly bear examining stimuli and responses in detail to determine if there are any commonalities in their possible central processing components that might determine success or failure of processing at any given stage of recovery.

It is also possible that the mechanisms involved in reading and naming are more complicated than we have presupposed. Instead of single-pass, purely unidirectional processing, full activation of the accurate phonological output might depend on constant feedback between, for example, output phonology and the just-prior orthographical stage. This feedback would normally allow the pattern of superimposed neural activity to locate and to settle into the appropriate basin of attraction (see Gordon, 1997a). Any interference with this rapid feedback and feed-forward—for example, by a partial lesion of the connections between the two stages (Gordon, 1982)—would slow down the settling process and perhaps prevent it completely. The net result would be slow, erroneous naming or reading, yet the knowledge of those functions would still be latent in the neurons and their connections, more clearly visible as feedback is restored to normal.

It is clear that a large number of possible explanations may need to be considered to explain the phenomenon of restoration of information that we describe; the discussion of possibilities given above is not necessarily complete. It is also clear that discriminating among these various possibilities will require experimental designs that have not been part of most experiments, let alone the ones we describe. However, drawing on both these observations and prior studies, we can make some tentative conclusions about the possibilities for recovery or restoration of item-specific information after central nervous system lesions:

1. Damage to the central nervous system that seemingly abolishes a behavioral ability (e.g., reading a word aloud, naming a picture) may nonetheless still leave a residual of neural tissue that retains in some fashion some of the specific knowledge necessary to perform that function. Therefore, loss of a function behaviorally does not necessarily imply loss of a function neurally.

2. This latent neural knowledge may recover quickly, as in the case of Patient 5. Such rapid recovery may require "prompting" by specific stimuli. It may also only be possible if there is relative preservation of the stages leading into and out of the affected stage so that the effects of the stimulus–response attempt are focused in some fashion on the rate-limiting stage. This rapid, prompted recovery may actually be a widespread phenomenon, but one that has generally not been recognized, as repeat testing for deficits is generally not done in close succession.

3. It has frequently been noted that far less neural tissue is required to support a function than the nervous system devotes to the function. A general rule seems to be that only about 10%–20% of neural tissue is necessary for fairly adequate functioning to occur and perhaps even slightly less for recovery of function (Sabel, 1997). Whether the "extra" tissue is necessary for peak performance (to push performance along a sigmoidal curve of declining yield), part of a common pool whose allocation gets shifted with different needs, or truly superfluous (which seems unlikely) is not known. What is important about these data, in considering children with developmental impairments and children and adults with brain injuries, is that they suggest that even 10%–20% of the tissue that would otherwise normally be present may be capable of achieving up to 90% of the normal function, in some fashion.

4. These data and speculations provide additional hope for attempts at trying to teach or restore learned, symbolic behavior. Human symbolic behavior is typically the product of multiple underlying processing stages. For each of these stages, enough item-specific information must be learned to ade-

quately support processing by the entire chain of stages. However, to the extent such systems are taught only by relatively external stimuli and errors, it is not surprising that they will learn relatively slowly and erratically in the early phases of teaching. The stages in the middle of the processing sequence are simply not getting clear inputs or clear indications of their desired outputs. But the fact that learning is not rapid in the system as a whole (before each component has reached a sufficient threshold for rapid learning) may not mean that each individual stage cannot learn rapidly. Learning at the level of isolated stages may be as efficient as it can be. In this scenario, it may then also be the case that even a damaged network or network connections can still be capable of extremely rapid learning if the stimulus is delivered directly to the responsible stage (as may have been the case with Patient 5). Therefore, training of a complex cognitive function *de novo* may proceed best by focusing training first on each component stage to get each up to the level of functioning necessary for the most efficient learning of the multistage function as a whole. Achieving this threshold of ability for efficient learning may not require full training of each and every stage; very partial training may be adequate for learning of the overall behavior to start on a more accelerated schedule. Of course, the training may have to be quite precise to enhance the specific neural circuits involved.

The same general principles may be even more applicable to attempts to teach each complex symbolic function to networks and to chains of networks that are impoverished due to developmental disorders. It may be, in some of these cases, that the developmental impairment has resulted in the existing neural tissue having diminished capacities, but not absent ones. If so, then the developmental disorder may seriously handicap initial learning, but not be as much of an impediment to nearly normal learning and functioning once learning passes a threshold. If this is the case, then it suggests a specific teaching strategy for the initial phases of learning. The first step would be to bring each stage up to a sufficient level of functioning by focusing learning on that particular subcomponent of information. Learning these initial steps would be expected to be slow and laborious. Tasks would have to be subdivided much more than is normally the case, and the initial learning for each stage would be expected to take far longer than normal. But the net result might be to create a chain of stages that can support complex symbolic functions, with more normal rates of learning and more normal levels of performance than might have otherwise been the case with less specific training. This program is admittedly very speculative. Yet several lines of research on enhancing functions by specific training can be viewed as examples of such training strategies (e.g., Tallal et al., 1996; Merzenich et al., 1996; see also Merzenich, Chapter 15).

The evidence we have touched on here, both from our own data and from other investigators' experiments and hypotheses, suggest a number of points that build toward a suggestion for how functions may be improved in children with developmental deficits. It is widely assumed that complex symbolic abilities are the products of separable underlying stages. We and others have data suggesting that damage can affect such stages more or less specifically. There are presumably developmental disorders in which the necessary stages are present, but not operating at normal capacity. Simulation studies on how complex, multistage processes learn and can be taught suggest that normal teaching strategies may simply not be capable of pushing developmentally impaired systems to their fullest capacities. There may be strategies for teaching such multistage processes that may ultimately result in greater yields. The work of Merzenich and colleagues (Chapter 15) suggests one such focus and method for these efforts; there are likely to be others.

References

The work presented and the preparation of this chapter were supported in part by NIH grants R01-NS26553, R01-29973, and K08-DC00099; the Seaver Foundation; the Whittier Foundation; the McDonnell-Pew Program in Cognitive Neuroscience; the Benjamin A. Miller Family Fund; and the Hodgson Fund of the New York Community Trust. Sumio Uematsu, M.D. (deceased) was the neurosurgeon for all of the Johns Hopkins cases; we deeply appreciated his medical wisdom, his surgical skills, and his permission to study his patients. We thank Drs. Robert Fisher, John Freeman, Greg Krauss, and Eileen Vining for permission to study their patients and Dr. Guy McKhann for referring Patient 5. We thank Barbara Cysyk, Coleman Hill, Mark Pettis, Dr. Sarah Reusing, Dr. Pamela Schwerdt, and Mark Tesoro for data collection; Jeffrey Sieracki for programming; Dr. Karen Bandeen-Roche, Dr. Charles B. Hall, and Diana Miglioretti, Sc.M., for advice and statistical analyses; Robert Glatzer for preparing the illustrations; and Drs. Jack Fletcher and Sarah Broman for organizing the meeting, for encouraging the preparation of this chapter, and for their scientific and editorial acumen. Portions of this work were presented at the annual meetings of the Academy of Aphasia (1988, 1994), the American Academy of Neurology (1990), the American Neurological Association (1991), and the American Epilepsy Society (1991).

Adams, M. J. (1990). *Beginning To Read.* Cambridge: The MIT Press.

Bloom, P., and Markson, L. (1998). Capacities underlying word learning. *Trends Cog. Sci., 2,* 67–73.

Boatman, D., Pettis, M., Hart, J., Lesser, R., and Gordon, B. (1991). Reading deficits revealed by interruption of external auditory feedback [Abstract]. *Neurology, 41(suppl. 1),* 408.

Brown, G. D. A. (1987). Resolving inconsistency: A computational model of word naming. *J. Memory Lang., 26,* 1–23.

Cohen, J. D., Dunbar, K., and McClelland, J. L. (1990). On the control of automatic processes: A parallel distributed processing account of the stroop effect. *Psychol. Rev. 97,* 332–361.

Coltheart, M., Curtis, B., Atkins, P., and Haller, M. (1993). Models of reading aloud: Dual-route and parallel-distributed-processing approaches. *Psychol. Rev., 100,* 589–608.

Eysel, U. T. (1997). Perilesional cortical dysfunction and reorganization. *Adv. Neurol., 73,* 195–206.

Fiez, J., and Petersen, D. (1998). Neuroimaging studies of word reading. *Proc. Natl. Acad. Sci. U.S.A., 95,* 914–921.

Gazzaniga, M. S. (1975). The concept of diaschisis. In O. C. K. J. Zulch and G. C. Galbraith (eds.): *Cerebral Localization: An Otfrid Foerster Symposium.* New York: Springer-Verlag.

Goodglass, H., Kaplan, E., and Weintraub, S. (1976). *Boston Naming Test (Experimental Edition)*. Boston: Boston University.

Gordon, B. (1982). Confrontation naming: Computational model and disconnection simulation. In D. C. M. A. Arbib and J. C. Marshall (eds.): *Neural Models of Language Processes*. New York: Academic Press, pp. 511–530.

Gordon, B. (1997a). Models of naming. In H. Goodglass and A. Wingfield (eds.): *Anomia*. San Diego: Academic Press, pp. 31–64.

Gordon, B. (1997b). Neuropsychology and advances in memory function. *Curr. Opin. Neurol., 10*, 306–312.

Gordon, B., Hart, J., Jr., Lesser, R. P., Boatman, D., Uematsu, S., Fisher, R. S., and Masdeu, J. (1991a). Loss of visual word recognition in pure alexia from left lateral occipital lesion: A prospective, longitudinal study [Abstract]. *Ann. Neurol., 30*, 240.

Gordon, B., Hart, J., Lesser, R. P., and Selnes, O. A. (1994). Recovery and its implications for cognitive neuroscience. *Brain Lang., 47*, 521–524.

Gordon, B., Hart, J., Lesser, R. P., Uematsu, S., and Resor, S. (1988). *Pure Alexia and Models of Orthographic to Phonologic Mapping*. Paper presented at the Academy of Aphasia Annual Meeting, Montreal.

Gordon, B., Uematsu, S., Lesser, R., Schwerdt, P., Fisher, R., Vining, E. P. G., and Hart, J. (1991b). Utility of intraoperative neuropsychological testing with stepwise resection [Abstract]. *Epilepsia, 32(Suppl. 3)*, 87.

Hart, J., Jr., and Gordon, B. (1992). Neural subsystems of object knowledge. *Nature, 359*, 60–64.

Hart, J., Gordon, B., Lesser, S., Uematsu, S., Schwerdt, P., Pettis, M., and Zinreich, S. J. (1990). Alexia without agraphia from restricted inferotemporal lesions [Abstract]. *Neurology, 40(Suppl. 1)*, 171.

Henderson, V. W., Friedman, R. B., Teng, E. L., and Weiner, J. M. (1985). Left hemisphere pathways in reading: Inferences from pure alexia without hemianopia. *Neurology, 35*, 962–968.

McClelland, J. L. (1989). Parallel distributed processing: Implications for cognition and development. In R. G. M. Morris (ed.): *Parallel Distributed Processing: Implications for Psychology and Neurobiology*. Oxford: Clarendon Press, pp. 8–45.

Merzenich, M. M., Jenkins, W. M., Johnston, P., Schreiner, C., Miller, S. L., and Tallal, P. (1996). Temporal processing deficits of language-learning impaired children ameliorated by training. *Science, 271*, 77–81.

Nudo, R. J., Wise, B. M., SiFuentes, F., and Milliken, G. W. (1996). Neural substrates for the effects of rehabilitative training on motor recovery after ischemic infarct. *Science, 272*, 1791–1794.

Plaut, D. C., McClelland, J. L., Seidenberg, M. S., and Patterson, K. (1996). Understanding normal and impaired word reading: Computational principles in quasi-regular domains. *Psychol. Rev., 103*, 56–115.

Sabel, B. A. (1997). Unrecognized potential of surviving neurons: Within-systems plasticity, recovery of function, and the hypothesis of minimal residual structure. *Neuroscientist, 3*, 366–370.

Shaywitz, S. E., Shaywitz, B. A., Pugh, K. R., Fulbright, R. K., Constable, R. T., Mencl, W. E., Shankweiler, D. P., Liberman, A. M., Skudlarski, P., Fletcher, J. M., Katz, L., Marchione, K. E., Lacadie, C., Gatenby, C., and Gore, J. C. (1998). Functional disruption in the organization of the brain for reading in dyslexia. *Proc. Natl. Acad. Sci. U.S.A., 95*, 2636–2641.

Tallal, P., Miller, S. L., Bedi, G., Byma, G., Wang, X., Nagarajan, S. S., Schreiner, C., Jenkins, W. M., and Merzenich, M. M. (1996). Language comprehension in language-learning impaired children improved with acoustically modified speech. *Science, 271,* 81–84.

Yamaski, D. S., and Wurtz, R. H. (1991). Recovery of function after lesions of the superior temporal sulcus in the monkey. *J. Neurophysiol. 66,* 651–673.

10

Plasticity, Localization, and Language Development

ELIZABETH BATES

The term *aphasia* refers to acute or chronic impairment of language, an acquired condition that is most often associated with damage to the left side of the brain, usually due to trauma or stroke. We have known about the link between left hemisphere damage (LHD) and language loss for more than a century (Goodglass, 1993). For almost as long, we have also known that the lesion–symptom correlations observed in adults do not appear to hold for very young children (Basser, 1962; Lenneberg, 1967). In fact, in the absence of other complications, infants with congenital damage to one side of the brain (left or right) usually go on to acquire language abilities that are well within the normal range (Eisele and Aram, 1995; Feldman et al., 1992; Vargha-Khadem et al., 1994). To be sure, children with a history of early brain injury typically perform below neurologically intact age-matched controls on a host of language and nonlanguage measures, including an average full-scale IQ difference somewhere between 4 and 8 points from one study to another (especially in children with persistent seizures; Vargha-Khadem et al., 1994). Brain damage is not a good thing to have, and some price must be paid for wholesale reorganization of the brain to compensate for early injuries. But the critical point for present purposes is that these children are not aphasic, despite early damage of a sort that often leads to irreversible aphasia when it occurs in an adult.

In addition to the reviews by other authors cited above, my colleagues and I have also published several detailed reviews, from various points of view, of language, cognition, and communicative development in children with focal brain injury (e.g., Bates et al., 1997, 1998; Elman et al., 1996; Reilly et al., 1998; Stiles, 1995; Stiles et al., 1998; Stiles and Thal, 1993; Thal et al., 1991). As these reviews attest, a consensus has emerged that stands midway between the historical extremes of *equipotentiality* (Lenneberg, 1967) and *innate predetermination* of the adult pattern of brain organization for language (e.g., Curtiss, 1988; Stromswold, 1995). The two hemispheres are certainly not equipotential for language at birth;

214

indeed, if they were it would be impossible to explain why left hemisphere dominance for language emerges 95%–98% of the time in neurologically intact individuals. However, the evidence for recovery from early LHD is now so strong that it is no longer possible to entertain the hypothesis that language *per se* is innately and irreversibly localized to perisylvian regions of the left hemisphere.

The compromise view is one in which brain organization for language emerges gradually over the course of development (Elman et al., 1996; Karmiloff-Smith, 1992) based on "soft constraints" that are only indirectly related to language itself. Hence the familiar pattern of language localization in adults is the product rather than the cause of development, an end product that emerges out of initial variations in the way that information is processed from one region to another. Crucially, these variations are not specific to language, although they do have important implications for how and where language is acquired and processed. In the absence of early brain injury, these soft constraints in the initial architecture and information-processing proclivities of the left hemisphere will ultimately lead to the familiar pattern of left hemisphere dominance. However, other "brain plans" for language are possible and will emerge when the default situation does not hold.

In the pages that follow, I do not intend to provide another detailed review of the outcomes associated with early brain injury; the reader is referred elsewhere for a more complete catalogue of such findings. What I do instead is to go beyond these findings to their implications for the nature and origins of language localization in the adult, providing an account of how this neural system might emerge across the course of development. With this goal in mind, the chapter is organized as follows: (*1*) a very brief review of findings from developmental neurobiology that serve as animal models for the kind of plasticity that we see in human children; (*2*) an equally brief illustration of results from retrospective studies of language development in the focal lesion population; (*3*) the distinction between prospective and retrospective studies, including a discussion of putative "critical periods" for language development; (*4*) an overview of prospective findings on language development in children with congenital lesions to one side of the brain; and (*5*) a new view of brain organization for language in the adult, an alternative to the static phrenological view that has dominated our thinking for two centuries, one that takes into account the role of experience in specifying the functional architecture of the brain.

Developmental Plasticity: Animal Models

Evidence for the plasticity of language in the human brain should not be surprising in light of all that has been learned in the last few decades about developmental plasticity of isocortex in other species (Bates et al., 1992; Deacon, 1997; Elman et al., 1996; Janowsky and Finlay, 1986; Johnson, 1997; Killackey, 1990; Mueller, 1996; Quartz and Sejnowski, 1998; Shatz, 1992). Without attempting an exhaustive or even a representative review, here are just a few of my favorite examples of research on developmental plasticity in other species, studies that provide animal models for the kind of plasticity that we have observed in the human case.

Isacson and Deacon (1996) have transplanted plugs of cortex from the fetal pig into the brain of the adult rat. These "foreigners" (called *xenotransplants*) develop appropriate connections, including functioning axonal links down the spinal column that stop in appropriate places. Although we know very little about the mental life of the resulting rat, no signs of pig-appropriate behaviors have been observed.

Stanfield and O'Leary (1985) have transplanted plugs of fetal cortex from one region to another (e.g., from visual to motor or somatosensory cortex). Although these cortical plugs are not entirely normal compared with "native" tissue, they set up functional connections with regions inside and outside the cortex. More importantly still, the transplants develop representations (i.e., cortical maps) that are appropriate for the region in which they now live and not for the region where they were born. ("When in Rome, do as the Romans do")

Sur and his colleagues (see Pallas and Sur, 1993; Sur et al., 1990) have rerouted visual information from visual cortex to auditory cortex in the infant ferret. Although (again) the representations that develop in auditory cortex are not entirely normal, these experiments show that auditory tissue can develop retinotopic maps. It seems that auditory cortex becomes auditory cortex under normal conditions primarily because (in unoperated animals) it receives information from the ear; but if it has to, it can also process visual information in roughly appropriate ways.

Killackey and colleagues (1994) have modified the body surface of an infant rat by removing whiskers that serve as critical perceptual organs in this species. Under normal conditions, the somatosensory cortex of the rat develops representations ("barrel cells") that are isomorphic with input from the whisker region. In contrast, the altered animals develop somatosensory maps reflecting changes in the periphery, with expanded representations for the remaining whiskers; regions that would normally subserve the missing whiskers are reduced or absent (Killackey, 1990). In other words, the rat ends up with the brain that it needs rather than the brain that Nature intended.

Finally, in an example that may be closer to the experience of children with early focal brain injury, a recent study by Webster et al. (1995) shows that the "where is it" system (mediated in dorsal regions, especially parietal cortex, including area MT) can take over the functions of the "what is it" system (mediated in ventral regions, especially inferior temporal cortex, including area TE). When area TE is bilaterally removed in an adult monkey, that animal displays severe and irreversible amnesia for new objects, suggesting that this area plays a crucial role in mediating object memory and detection (i.e., the so-called what is it system). However, as Webster et al. (1995) have shown, bilateral removal of area TE in infant monkeys leads to performance only slightly below age-matched unoperated controls (at both 10 months and 4 years of age). If area TE is no longer available, where has the "what is it" system gone? By lesioning additional areas of visual cortex, Webster et al. (1995) showed that the object detection function in TE-lesioned infant monkeys is mediated by dorsal regions of extrastriate cortex that usually respond to motion rather than form (i.e., the "where is it" system). In other words, a major higher cognitive function can develop far away from its intended site, in areas that would ordinarily play little or no role in the mediation of that function.

These examples and many others like them have led most developmental neurobiologists to conclude that cortical differentiation and functional specialization are largely the product of input to the cortex, albeit within certain broad architectural and computational constraints (Johnson, 1997). Such findings provide a serious challenge to the old idea that the brain is organized into largely predetermined, domain-specific faculties (i.e., the phrenological approach). An alternative proposal that is more compatible with these findings is offered later.

Language Outcomes in Children with Early Focal Brain Injury: Retrospective Findings

As noted earlier, retrospective studies of language outcomes in children with unilateral brain injury have repeatedly found that these children are not aphasic; they usually perform within the normal range, although they often do perform slightly below neurologically intact age-matched controls (cf. Webster et al., 1995). More importantly for our purposes here, there is no consistent evidence in these retrospective studies to suggest that language outcomes are worse in children with LHD than in children whose injuries are restricted to the right hemisphere. Without attempting an exhaustive review, three examples are given to illustrate these points.

Figure 10-1 presents idealized versus observed results for verbal versus nonverbal IQ scores in a cross-sectional sample of children with congenital injuries who were tested at various ages between 3 and 10 years. Figure 10-1A illustrates what we might expect if the left–right differences observed in adults were consistently observed in children: higher verbal than nonverbal IQ scores in children with right hemisphere damage (RHD), which means that these children should line up on the upper diagonal; higher nonverbal than verbal IQ scores in children with LHD, which means that these children ought to fall on the lower diagonal. These idealized scores were obtained by taking actual pairs of scores for individual children in our focal lesion sample and reversing any scores that were not in the predicted direction. In contrast with this idealized outcome, Figure 10-1B illustrates the actual verbal and performance IQ scores for 28 LHD and 15 RHD cases (note that there are no differences between these two groups in gender or chronological age and no mean differences in full-scale IQ). The actual data in Figure 10-1B illustrate several points. First, in line with other studies of this population, the mean full-scale IQ for the sample as a whole is 93.2, within the normal range but below the mean of 100 that we would expect if we were drawing randomly from the normal population. Second, the range of outcomes observed in the focal lesion population as a whole is extraordinarily broad, including some children who can be classified as mentally retarded (i.e., 16.3% of this sample have full-scale IQs at or below 80) and some with IQs over 120. Third, the correlation between the verbal

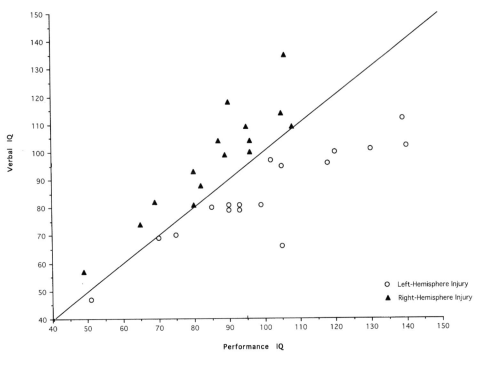

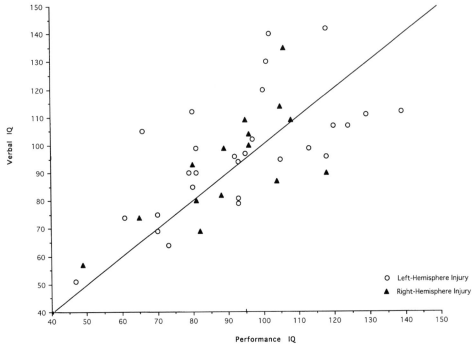

218

and nonverbal subscales is relatively strong (+ 0.65, $p < 0.0001$), which means that verbal and nonverbal IQs do not dissociate markedly in this group. In fact, as we can clearly see from the difference between Figure 10-1A (predicted outcomes) and 10-1B (the outcomes actually observed in these children), there is absolutely no evidence in these data for a double dissociation between verbal and nonverbal IQ as a function of LHD versus RHD.

Figure 10-2 presents results from a more focused study of grammatical development, illustrating the number of different complex syntactic forms produced in a narrative discourse tasks by LHD, RHD, and neurologically intact controls who were tested between 6 and 12 years of age. Figure 10-2 demonstrates (once again) that children with focal brain injury perform within the normal range in production of complex syntax, even though they do (as a group) score significantly below neurologically intact controls. In this respect, the Reilly et al. (1998) result for grammatical development in human children is remarkably similar to the findings reported by Webster et al. (1995) on the relative preservation of memory for novel objects in infant monkeys with bilateral TE lesions (i.e., performance roughly 10% below that of normal controls). In addition, Figure 10-2 shows that there is no evidence in this age range for a difference in syntactic production as a function of lesion side or site.

Finally, Figure 10-3 compares results for adults and 6–12-year-old children with LHD versus RHD on the same sentence comprehension task. All data are based on z-scores, with patients at each age level compared with the performance of age-matched normal controls (hence the difference in performance between normal adults and normal 6–12-year-old children is factored out of the results). In this particular procedure, subjects are asked to match each stimulus sentence to one of four pictured alternatives. Half the items are familiar phrases (well-known metaphors and figures of speech like "She took a turn for the worse"), and the other half are novel phrases matched to the familiar phrases in length and complexity. As Figure 10-3A shows, there is a powerful double dissociation between novel and familiar phrases in adult victims of unilateral brain injury: Adults with LHD score markedly better on the familiar phrases, while adults with RHD score better on the novel phrases. This is one example of a growing body of evidence challenging the old assumption that the left hemisphere is "the" language hemisphere, even in adults. The right hemisphere does make an important contribution to language processing, but its contribution is qualitatively different from that of the left hemisphere, involving a number of functions including emotionality, intonation contours, and (as this example illustrates) figurative, metaphorical, and/or formulaic speech (all forms of speech in which the meaning of the sentence as a whole goes beyond the meaning one would obtain by computing across the separate elements in the sentence). A comparison between Figure 10-3A and 10-3B helps to clarify three important points. First, children with focal injuries fare far better than

Figure 10-1. *(Top)* Idealized relation between verbal and performance IQ in children with left versus right hemisphere injury. *(Bottom)* Observed relation between verbal and performance IQ in children with left versus right hemisphere injury. (Adapted from Bates et al., 1998b).

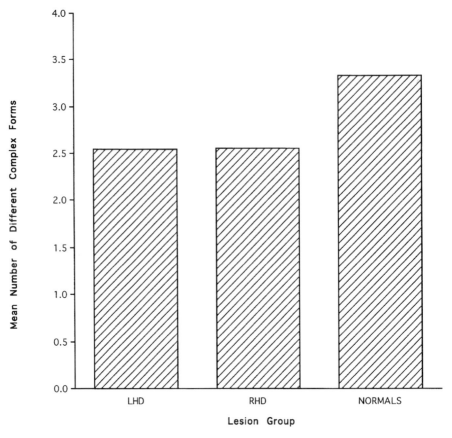

Figure 10-2. Number of different complex syntactic forms produced by children with left (LHD) versus right (RHD) hemisphere damage in a story-telling task (ages 6–12 years). (Adapted from Reilly et al., 1998).

adults with comparable damage when they are compared with age-matched controls. Second, the powerful double dissociation observed in adults is not observed in children. Third, novel sentences are more susceptible to the effects of brain injury than are familiar phrases in the child group, but RHD children actually perform below the LHD group in comprehension of novel sentences (significant by a one-tailed *t* test), the opposite of what we might expect if the adult pattern held for children with focal brain injury.

In short, whether we are talking about global measures like IQ or more subtle measures of sentence production and comprehension, children with LHD versus RHD do not display the profiles of impairment that we would expect based on the adult aphasia literature—at least not in these and other retrospective studies, with outcome measures at or above 6 years of age (i.e., beyond the point at which fundamental aspects of grammar and phonology are usually in place; Bates et al., 1995).

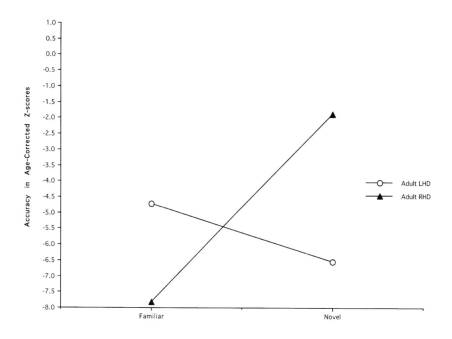

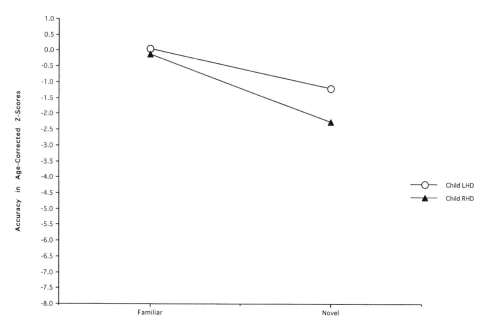

Figure 10-3. (*Top*) Performance on familiar versus novel sentences in adults with left (LHD) versus right (RHD) hemisphere injury. (*Bottom*) Performance on familiar versus novel sentences in children with left versus right hemisphere damage. (Adapted from Kempler et al., 1999).

221

Age of Lesion Onset and the Problem of Critical Periods

The distinction between retrospective and prospective studies is related to the controversial problem of "critical periods" for language, with special focus on the age at which a lesion is acquired. By definition, prospective studies focus on children whose lesions are acquired very early, preferably before the point at which language learning normally begins. In contrast, many retrospective studies collapse across children who acquired their lesions at different points across the course of language learning. Our own prospective studies are based exclusively on children with congenital injuries, defined to include pre- or perinatal injuries that are known to have occurred before 6 months of age, restricted to one side of the brain (left or right), confirmed through one or more forms of neural imaging (computed tomography or magnetic resonance imaging). Hence our results may differ from studies of children with injuries acquired at a later point in childhood.

What might those differences be? Unfortunately, there is very little empirical evidence regarding the effect of age of lesion onset on subsequent language outcomes. Only one fact is clear: that the outcomes associated with LHD are much better in infants than they are in adults. This means, of course, that plasticity for language must decrease markedly at some point between birth and adulthood (Lenneberg, 1967). But when does this occur, and how does it happen?

Many investigators have argued that this decrease in plasticity takes place at the end of a "critical period" for language, a window of opportunity that is also presumed to govern the child's ability to achieve native-speaker status in a second language (for discussions, see Bialystok and Hakuta, 1994; Curtiss, 1988; Elman et al., 1996; Johnson and Newport, 1989; Marchman, 1993; Oyama, 1993; Weber-Fox and Neville, 1996). So much has been said about this presumed critical period that a newcomer to the field (and many consumers within it) would be justified in assuming that we know a great deal about its borders (i.e., when it begins and when it comes to an end) and about the shape of the learning function in between these points. The very term *critical period* suggests that the ability to acquire a native language and/or the ability to recover from brain injury both come to a halt abruptly, perhaps at the same time, as the window of opportunity slams shut. The fact is, however, that we know almost nothing about the shape of this function. In fact, we are not even justified in assuming that the function is monotonic (i.e., that it gets progressively harder to learn a native language and progressively harder to recover from injuries to the left hemisphere).

With regard to the presumed critical period for recovery from brain injury, we are aware of only two large cross-sectional studies that have compared language and cognitive outcomes in children who acquired their lesions at different ages from congenital injuries (at or before birth) through early adolescence (Vargha-Khadem et al., unpublished results, cited with permission in Bates et al., 1999; Goodman and Yude, 1996). Figure 10-4 compares results from both these studies for verbal IQ. As Figure 10-4 indicates, the effect of age of injury is nonmonotonic in both studies: The worst outcomes are observed in children who suffered their injuries between approximately 1 and 4 years of age. In support of the critical pe-

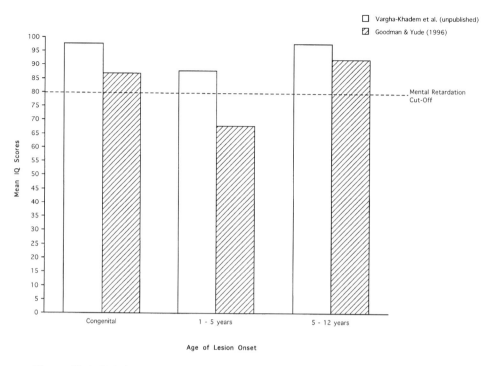

Figure 10-4. Relationship between age of lesion onset and IQ scores in two samples of children with focal brain injury.

riod hypothesis, better outcomes are observed following congenital injuries. However, in direct contradiction to the critical period hypothesis, better outcomes are also observed in children whose injuries occurred between approximately 5 and 12 years of age, which means that there is no monotonic drop in plasticity. To some extent, these unpleasant wrinkles in the expected function could be due to uncontrolled differences in etiology (e.g., the factors leading to injury may differ at birth, 1–5 years, and later childhood). At the very least, however, these results ought to make us skeptical of claims about a straightforward critical period for recovery from brain injury.

Similar nonmonotonic findings have been reported in at least one study of second-language acquisition and first-language loss (Liu et al., 1992). To illustrate, compare the results in Figure 10-5 (adapted from a famous study of second-language acquisition) and Figure 10-6. Figure 10-5 illustrates results from a grammaticality judgment task administered to first- and second-language learners of English, comparing performances of individuals who arrived in the United States at different points spanning the period from birth to early adulthood. This well-known figure suggests that there is no single point at which the window of opportunity for second-language learning slams shut. However, it does provide evidence for a monotonic drop in language learning ability from birth to adolescence.

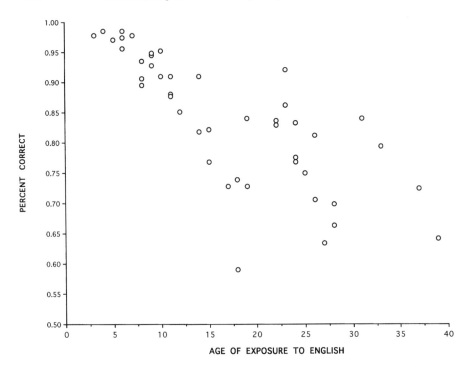

Figure 10-5. Performance on a grammaticality judgment task in non-native speakers of English as a function of age of exposure to English. (Adapted from Newport and Johnson, 1989.)

Consider, however, the results in Figure 10-6, based on a sentence interpretation task administered to Chinese–English bilinguals in both Chinese and English. In this task, subjects were able to use semantic or word order information to interpret "odd" sentences like "The rock chased the dog." Native speakers of English invariably choose the first noun, using word order to make their interpretation. Native speakers of Chinese invariably choose the second noun, ignoring word order in favor of semantic information. Both these strategies make perfect sense in terms of the information value of standard word order in these two languages (Chinese permits so much word order variation that a persistent word order strategy like the one used in English would not be very useful). Hence this little task serves as a useful litmus test for retention of the first language (L1) as well as acquisition of the second (L2). The interesting point for our purposes is that Chinese–English bilinguals often perform somewhere in between these two extremes, in one or both of their two languages, and these different "weightings" of word order and semantic information vary as a function of age of acquisition. Notice that results for English (L2) are generally in agreement with Johnson and Newport's results (1989) for a very different task: Although our results asymptote at an earlier point than those of Johnson and Newport (1989), they do provide evidence for a monotonic shift from "English-like" interpretations of English sentences in those who learned their Eng-

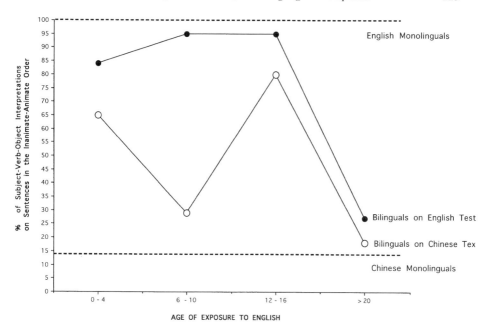

Figure 10-6. "English-like" versus "Chinese-like" grammatical comprehension as a function of age of exposure to English. (Adapted from Liu et al., 1992.)

lish very early to "Chinese-like" interpretation of English sentences in those who learned their English relatively late. However, results for Chinese (L1) show a very different function, a nonmonotonic curve in which the best results (movement toward the second language without loss of the first language) are observed in those who are exposed to a second language sometime between 4 and 7 years of age.

Although this is a complex result, the point of this comparison for our purposes here is a simple one: There is no single "critical period" for language learning; results depend on many different factors, and the probability of a positive outcome can rise or fall at different points in development, in L2 learning, and in recovery from brain injury. This is when prospective studies can be particularly illuminating: By studying children during their first encounters with language and other forms of higher cognition, we can learn more about effects associated with the initial state of the brain, together with the processes of development and (re)organization that lead these children to a normal or near-normal outcome.

Language Outcomes in Children With Early Focal Brain Injury: Prospective Findings

All theories that take some form of plasticity into account (including theories that assume a critical period) would lead us to expect relatively good outcomes in children with congenital injuries (i.e., the group that we have studied in our laboratory). Evidence for the developmental plasticity of language in this group has mounted in the last few years due in part to improved techniques for identifying children with early brain injury, including precise localization of the site and extent of damage through neuroradiology. In some cases, we have been able to identify such children in the first weeks of life, prior to the time when language acquisition would normally begin, permitting us to chart the course of language, cognition, and communicative development from the very beginning (Bates et al., 1997; Reilly et al., 1995; Stiles et al., 1998; Stiles and Thal, 1993), before the point at which alternative forms of brain organization have emerged.

In fact, the prospective studies that we have carried out so far provide compelling evidence for initial deficits and subsequent processes of recovery—phenomena that are not visible later on, when most retrospective studies take place. For example, prospective studies of nonverbal cognitive development by our colleague Joan Stiles have revealed subtle but consistent patterns of deficit in visuospatial cognition. For example, children with RHD appear to have difficulty perceiving and/or producing the global or configural aspects of a complex visual array; children with LHD are generally spared at the global level, but they have difficulty with the perception and/ or production of local details (Note: I will return to this example later on, relating it to our findings for language.) These visuospatial deficits are qualitatively similar to those observed in LHD versus RHD adults, although they are usually more subtle in children, and they resolve over time as the children acquire compensatory strategies to solve the same problems (Stiles et al., 1998; Stiles and Thal, 1993).

If a similar result could be found in the domain of language, then we might expect (by analogy to the literature on adult aphasia) to find the following results in the first stages of language development:

> **Left hemisphere advantage for language:** Children with LHD will perform below the levels observed in children with RHD on virtually all measures of phonological, lexical, and grammatical development, as well as measures of symbolic and communicative gesture.
> **The Broca pattern:** By analogy to Broca's aphasia in adults, children with damage to the frontal regions of the left hemisphere will be particularly delayed in expressive but not receptive language and may (on some accounts) be particularly delayed in the development of grammar and phonology.
> **The Wernicke pattern:** By analogy to Wernicke's aphasia in adults, children with damage to the posterior regions of the left temporal lobe will be particularly delayed in receptive language, perhaps (on some accounts) with sparing of grammar and phonology but selective delays in measures of semantic development.

Our group set out to test these three hypotheses in a series of prospective studies of early language development. In every case, we have uncovered evidence for early deficits, and these deficits do appear to be associated with specific lesion sites. However, in contrast with Stiles' findings for visuospatial cognition, results for language provide very little evidence for hypotheses based on the adult aphasia literature.

The first study (Marchman et al., 1991) focused on the emergence of babbling and first words in a small sample of five children with congenital brain injury, two with RHD and three with LHD, including one LHD case with injuries restricted to the left frontal region. All the children were markedly delayed in phonological development (babbling in consonant–vowel segments weeks or months behind a group of neurologically intact controls) and in the emergence of first words. However, three of the children moved up into the normal range across the course of the study. The two who remained behind had injuries to the posterior regions of the left hemisphere, results that fit with the first hypothesis (left hemisphere advantage for language) but stand in direct contradiction to both the Broca and the Wernicke hypotheses.

The second study (Thal et al., 1991) focused on comprehension and production of words from 12 to 35 months in a sample of 27 infants with focal brain injury based on a parental report instrument that was the predecessor of the MacArthur Communicative Development Inventories (MCDI) (Fenson et al., 1993, 1994). In complete contradiction to Hypothesis 1 (left hemisphere mediation of language) and Hypothesis 3 (the Wernicke hypothesis), delays in word comprehension were actually more likely in the RHD group. In line with Hypothesis 1, but against Hypothesis 2 (the Broca hypothesis), delays in word production were more likely in children with injuries involving the left posterior quadrant of the brain.

A more recent study built on the findings of Thal et al. (1991) with a larger sample of 53 children, 36 with LHD and 17 with RHD (Bates et al., 1997), and a combination of parent report (the MCDI) and analyses of free speech. This report is broken into three substudies, with partially overlapping samples. Study 1 used the MCDI to investigate aspects of word comprehension, word production, and gesture at the dawn of language development in 26 children between 10 and 17 months of age. Study 2 used the MCDI to look at production of both words and grammar in 29 children between 19 and 31 months. Study 3 used transcripts of spontaneous speech in 30 children from 20 to 44 months, focusing on mean length of utterance in morphemes (MLU). In all these studies, comparisons between the LHD and RHD groups were followed by comparisons looking at the effects associated with lesions involving the frontal lobe (comparing children with left frontal involvement to all RHD cases as well as LHD cases with left frontal sparing) and the temporal lobe (comparing children whose lesions include the left temporal lobe with all RHD cases and all LHD cases in which that region is spared). Results were compatible with those of Marchman et al. (1991) and Thal et al. (1991), but were quite surprising from the point of view of lesion/symptom mappings in adult aphasia, as follows.

First, in a further disconfirmation of Hypotheses 1 and 3, Bates et al. (1997) report that delays in word comprehension and gesture were both more likely in children with unilateral damage to the right hemisphere at least likely in the 10–17-month window examined here. Further studies of gestural development in our laboratory have confirmed that the gestural disadvantage for RHD children is still present between 20 and 24 months (Stiles et al., 1998).

Second, in a partial confirmation of Hypothesis 2 (the Broca hypothesis), frontal involvement was associated with greater delays in word production and the emergence of expressive grammar between 19 and 31 months. However, in a surprising partial disconfirmation of Hypothesis 2, this frontal disadvantage was equally severe with either left frontal or right frontal involvement. In other words, the frontal lobes are important during this crucial period of development (which includes the famous "vocabulary burst" and the flowering of grammar), but there is no evidence for a left–right asymmetry in the frontal regions and hence no evidence in support of the idea that Broca's area has a privileged status from the very beginning of language development.

Third, in line with Hypothesis 1 (left hemisphere mediation of language) but in direct contradiction to Hypotheses 2 and 3 (analogies to Broca's and Wernicke's aphasia), delays in word production and the emergence of grammar were both more pronounced in children with injuries involving the left temporal lobe. In contrast with the above two findings (which only reached significance within a restricted period of development), this left temporal disadvantage was reliable across all three substudies by Bates et al. (1997) from the very first words (between 10 and 17 months of age) through crucial developments in grammar (between 20 and 44 months of age). Hence we do have evidence for the asymmetrical importance of Wernicke's area, but that evidence pertains equally to grammar and vocabulary (with no evidence of any kind for a dissociation between the two) and seems to be restricted to expressive language.

Reilly et al. (1998) conducted similar comparisons by lesion side and lesion site in a cross-sectional sample of 30 children with focal brain injury (15 LHD and 15 RHD) between 3 and 12 years of age; these results were also compared with performances by a group of 30 age-matched controls with no history of neurological impairment. Analyses were based on lexical, grammatical, and discourse measures from a well-known story-telling task. For children between 3 and 6 years of age, Reilly et al. (1998) replicated the specific disadvantage in expressive language for children with lesions involving the temporal region of the left hemisphere. However, this effect was not detectable in children between 6 and 12 years of age—even though all children in this study had the same congenital etiology. In fact, data for the older children provided no evidence of any kind for an effect of lesion side (left versus right) or lesion site (specific lobes within either hemisphere). The only effect that reached significance in older children was a small but reliable disadvantage in the brain-injured children as a group compared with neurologically intact age-matched controls. Figure 10-7 compares results for younger versus older children on one grammatical index (mean number of errors in grammatical morphology per proposition), divided into children with left temporal involvement (+LTemp), focal lesion cases without left temporal involving (−Ltemp, combining all RHD cases and all LHD cases with temporal sparing), and neurologically intact normal controls. Although we must remember that these are cross-sectional findings, they suggest that a substantial degree of recovery takes place in the LHD group during the first few years of life. In subsequent longitudinal studies, Reilly and her colleagues have followed a smaller group of chil-

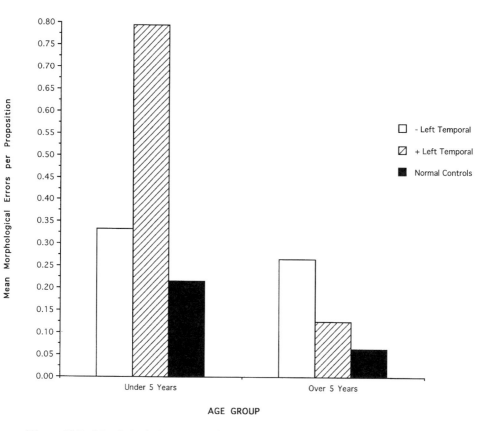

Figure 10-7. Morphological errors as a function of age and presence/absence of left temporal damage. (Adapted from Reilly et al., 1998.)

dren across this period of development. These longitudinal findings are compatible with the cross-sectional evidence in Figure 10-7, suggesting that the crucial period of recovery takes place before the age range covered by most of the retrospective studies in the literature on cognitive and linguistic outcomes in children with focal brain injury.

To summarize, our prospective studies of language development in children with early focal brain injury have provided evidence for specific delays, correlated with specific lesion sites. However, the nature of these lesion–symptom correlations differs markedly from those that we would expect based on the adult aphasia literature. Furthermore, these correlations are only observed within specific windows of development, followed by evidence for recovery and (by implication) reorganization. None of these results are evident in retrospective studies (including our own), where children are tested beyond the point at which this presumed reorganization has taken place.

We are occasionally asked why our results appear to be incompatible with an earlier literature on the effect of hemispherectomy (e.g., Dennis and Whitaker, 1976; but see Bishop, 1983) and/or effects of early stroke (e.g., Aram, 1988; Aram et al., 1985a,b; Woods and Teuber, 1978). Our first answer is that our results are *not* incompatible with the vast majority of studies. However, they do *appear* to be incompatible with a handful of studies that were cited (usually in secondary sources) as evidence in favor of an innate and irreversible role for the left hemisphere in some aspects of language processing. As we have noted elsewhere (Bates et al., 1999; see also Vargha-Khadem et al., 1994), apparent inconsistencies between the earlier studies and our more recent work disappear when one looks carefully at the fine print.

First, many of the earlier studies combined data for children whose injuries occurred at different points in development, and they also combined results (usually on rather global measures) for children at widely different ages at time of testing. As we saw in the previous section, there may not be a monotonic relation between age of injury and language outcomes, and the nature of the lesion–symptom mappings that we observe may be quite different depending on the age at which children are tested and the developmental events that are most prominent at that time.

Second, some of the earlier studies had methodological limitations that we have been able to overcome in the studies described above. In particular, a number of well-known studies could not perform direct comparisons of children with LHD versus RHD because of uncontrolled differences in age, education, and/or etiology. Instead, the RHD and LHD groups were each compared with a separate group of matched controls. For example, Dennis and Whitaker (1976) report that their left-hemispherectomized children performed below normal controls on subtle and specific aspects of grammatical processing; no such difference was observed between right-hemispherectomized children and their controls. These results were interpreted as though they constituted a significant difference between the LHD and RHD groups even though the latter two groups were never compared directly. As Bishop (1983) has pointed out in her well-known critique, a careful examination of results for the two lesion groups suggest that this interpretation is not warranted. The general problem that one encounters with the separate control group approach is illustrated in Figure 10-8, which compares hypothetical data for an LHD group, an RHD group, and their respective controls. As we can see, performance by the LHD group does fall reliably below performance by their controls (albeit just barely); performance by the RHD does not fall outside the confidence intervals for their control group. And yet, in this hypothetical example, performance is actually better in the LHD cases! The key to this conundrum lies in the standard deviations for each control group: The standard deviation is larger for the RHD controls, which means that a larger difference between RHD and controls is required to reach statistical significance. Clearly, it would be unwise to draw strong conclusions about left–right differences from a data set of this kind.

Finally, some of the better-known claims in favor of an early and irreversible effect of LHD have been based on single-case studies or very small samples (in-

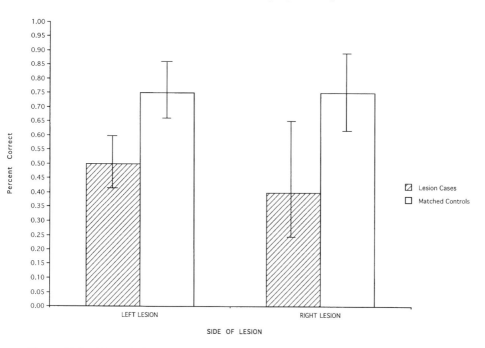

Figure 10-8. A hypothetical example of comparisons between left (LHD) and right (RHD) hemisphere groups with their respective controls (LHD, control difference is reliable; RHD, control difference is not).

cluding the hemispherectomy studies cited above). This fact limits the generalizability of results, and the same result is often contradicted by other individual-case or small-group studies.

For example, Stark and McGregor (1997) have recently described an interesting contrast between one child with a left hemispherectomy (seizure onset at 1;6, surgery at 4;0) and another with a right hemispherectomy (seizure onset at 2;0, surgery at 5;8). Both children were followed longitudinally with testing at 1– 2-year intervals through 9;0 and 9;6 years of age, respectively. Although both children did show substantial development in language and cognition across the course of the study, they fell behind age-matched normal controls at every point. At the end of the study, the LHD case had a full-scale IQ of 71 and the RHD case had a full-scale IQ of 81, well behind the norms for development in children who are neurologically intact. For Stark and McGregor (1997), the most interesting findings lie in the contrasting patterns observed for each child for performance IQ, verbal IQ, and a series of more specific language tests. For the LHD case, verbal and performance IQ were both quite low (separated by only four points). However, performance on the specific language tasks followed a profile typical of the pattern observed in children with Specific Language Impairment, i.e., greater impairment in language measures (especially morphosyntax) than we would expect for her mental age. In contrast, the RHD case displayed a sharp dissociation at the end of the study between Verbal IQ (95) and Performance IQ (70), with scores on most of the specific language measures that were appropriate for her mental age.

This is an interesting and provocative result, and it might indeed reflect evidence for the emergence of some kind of left hemisphere specialization for language prior to the age at which the surgery occurred. However, our own experience with a relatively large focal lesion sample has made us wary of basing strong results on case studies. Individual differences in language and cognitive ability are immense, even in perfectly normal children with no history of brain injury (Bates et al., 1995; Fenson et al., 1994). A similar degree of variation is observed even within the small cadre of cases that have undergone hemispherectomy.

Evidence for such variation comes from the case of Alex, recently reported by Vargha-Khadem et al. (1997). Alex was nearly mute prior to his surgery between 8 and 9 years of age and (to the extent that he could be tested at all) demonstrated levels of language comprehension similar to those of a normal 3-year-old. Soon after his surgery, he demonstrated remarkable recovery in both receptive and expressive language and continued to make progress into adolescence. Although Alex did suffer some degree of mental retardation (as an adolescent, he has the mental age of a 10–12-year-old on most measures), his language abilities are entirely commensurate with his mental age. In fact, his level of performance on language measures is superior to both of the cases reported by Stark and McGregor (1997), even though his surgery took place several years later. The contrast between this study and that of Stark and McGregor (1997) underscores two important points. First, it provides further evidence against the assumption that plasticity drops monotonically across a supposed critical period for language. Second, it reminds us that the effects of brain injury are superimposed on the vast landscape of individual variation observed in normally developing children (for an elaboration of this point, see Bates et al., 1995). Because there is so much variation in the normal population, it is difficult to know in a single-case or small-sample study whether the cognitive profiles we observe are statistically reliable. Indeed, they may be no different from the patterns that would be observed if brain damage were imposed randomly on cases selected from the population at large (Bates et al., 1991a; Bishop, 1997; see also Basser, 1962, for evidence that the vast majority of cases in a large sample of hemispherectomized children show no evidence at all of a speech–language impairment, regardless of side of surgery).

Despite these concerns, our results for older children are largely compatible with the retrospective literature on language development in the focal lesion population: Children with early injuries to one side of the brain usually acquire language abilities within the normal or low-normal range, with little evidence for effects of lesion side or lesion site (as reviewed by Bates et al., 1999; Eisele and Aram, 1995; Vargha-Khadem et al., 1994). Our prospective findings for children under 5 years of age are qualitatively different, but they are also so new that there is little or no comparable information in the literature, aside from a few single-case or small-sample studies with very different goals (e.g., Dall' Oglio et al., 1994; Feldman et al., 1992). Of course it will be important to replicate all these prospective findings with other samples of children, and in other laboratories. In the meantime, we can take some comfort in the fact that these results are based on the largest and most homogeneous sample of children with focal brain injury that has ever been studied in a prospective framework. Although in some cases the same children participate in more than one prospective study, the full sample across our two largest studies (Bates et al., 1997; Reilly et al., 1998) includes 72 cases of children with focal brain injury from three different laboratories. With sample sizes of 26 or more from one substudy to another, we have been able to use experimental designs and inferential statistics that would not be appropriate in a single-case or small-sample study, revealing new information about the changing nature of lesion–symptom correlations. In short, the findings are solid enough to justify some speculation about the development of brain organization for language under normal and pathological conditions.

How Brain Organization for Language Emerges
Across the Course of Development

The literature on language outcomes in human children with early unilateral brain injury is quite compatible with the burgeoning literature on neural plasticity in other species. Many of the human results are new, but the information from developmental neurobiology is now well established. Although few neurobiologists would argue in favor of *equipotentiality,* that is, the idea that all areas of cortex are created equal (Lenneberg, 1967), there is now overwhelming evidence in favor of *pluripotentiality*—the idea that cortical tissue is capable of taking on a wide array of representations, with varying degrees of success, depending on the timing, nature, and extent of the input to which that tissue is exposed (Elman et al., 1996; Johnson, 1997).

This conclusion is well attested in the developmental neurobiology literature, but it has had surprisingly little impact in linguistics, cognitive science, and cognitive neuroscience. In fact, the old phrenological approach to brain organization has found new life in the last two decades in various proposals that language is an "instinct" (Pinker, 1994), a "mental organ" (Chomsky, 1980a,b, 1995), or an "innate module" (Fodor, 1983; Pinker, 1997a), with its own neural architecture and its own highly specific genetic base (see also Gopnik, 1990; Pinker, 1991; Rice, 1996; Van der Lely, 1994). Indeed, Fodor's 1983 monograph celebrates the contributions of Franz Gall, the original phrenologist, and proudly bears a classic drawing of Gall's subdivided and numbered brain on its cover. The only real surprise is how little the claims have changed across the last 200 years.

Phrenology in all its reincarnations can be characterized as the belief that the brain is organized into spatially and functionally distinct faculties, each dedicated to and defined by a different kind of intellectual, emotional, or moral content. In some of the proposals put forward by Gall, Spurzheim, and others in the eighteenth century, these included areas for hope, combativeness, conjugal love, veneration, cautiousness, calculation, tune, memory, and, of course, language. A modern vari-

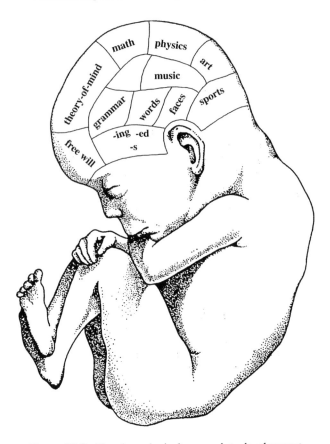

Figure 10-9. The phrenological approach to development.

ant of phrenology is represented in cartoon form in Figure 10-9, which differs from the old version in at least two respects. First, the content of the proposed modules has changed a great deal in the last two centuries: With some exceptions, most of the ethical content is gone (but see Ramachandran et al., 1997, for a proposed "religiosity module"), replaced by a smaller set of species-specific cognitive and linguistic domains (e.g., music, faces, mathematics, grammar, the lexicon). To be sure, the particular entries and placements in Figure 10-9 are of my own making, but each one represents explicit claims that have been made in the last 5–10 years in the *New York Times* and other public outlets. Second, and most important for our purposes here, the modern version of phrenology has a strong nativist component. In contrast with the nineteenth century phrenologists (some of whom underscored the role of experience in setting up the functional organization of the brain—see especially Wernicke, 1977), twentieth century champions like Fodor and Pinker have wedded their theory of modular localization to the doctrine of innateness. In this variant of phrenology, the adult brain is organized along modular lines because the brain came packaged that way, in its fetal form, with specific functions assigned to specific regions by a genetic program (see also Gopnik and Crago, 1991; Rice, 1996; Van der Lely, 1994).

In part, the phrenological approach may persist because alternative accounts are difficult to understand. The adult brain is a highly differentiated organ, and the infant brain (though underspecified in comparison to the adult brain) is certainly not a *tabula rasa.* And yet efforts to reintroduce experiential effects on this brain organization (e.g., Bates and Elman, 1996; Elman and Bates, 1997) have been met with great suspicion by those who fear a reintroduction of old behaviorist accounts (Clark et al., 1997; Jenkins and Maxam, 1997; Pesetsky et al., 1997; Pinker, 1997b). Some of the heat in this exchange comes from the fact that several logically and empirically distinct issues are conflated in the argument about mental organs for language. As a result, anyone who opposes the modern doctrine of phrenology in its full-blown form is accused of (gasp!) behaviorism. To clarify the difference between old-fashioned *tabula rasa* behaviorism and the emergentist perspective that I am espousing here, we need to break the mental organ doctrine down into a series of separate and separable assumptions about *(1) innate representations* (i.e., synaptic connections are determined by a genetic program), *(2) domain-specific processing* (each region of the brain is designed to handle a specific kind of content), and three corollaries about localization, *(3) compact location, (4) fixed location,* and *(5) universal location.* Table 10-1 summarizes the five claims of modern phrenology, together with a characterization of the emergentist alternative on each of these five counts.

Consider first the assumption of innate representations. As my colleagues and I have acknowledged repeatedly, throughout this chapter and elsewhere (Bates et al., in press; Elman et al., 1996), cortex is not equipotential. There are powerful endogenous constraints in the infant brain that bias the way that brain organization will proceed under normal circumstances. However, claims about the nature of these innate constraints can be made on several different levels: *innate representations* (where "representations" are operationally defined as the patterns of cortical connectivity that comprise knowledge), *innate architecture* (defined in terms of the global input–output architecture of the brain and local variations in density, speed, and style of information processing), and *innate timing* (including variations in length of neurogenesis and the onset and offset of neurotrophic factors). The mental organ doctrine is deeply committed to the existence of innate representations. The emergentist alternative is committed to the idea that knowledge

Table 10-1. Two views of brain organization for language

Phrenological View	Emergentist View
Innate representations	Emergent representations
Dedicated, domain-specific neural mechanisms for learning and processing	Domain-general neural mechanisms for learning and processing
Fixed localization	Plastic localization
Compact localization	Distributed localization
Universal localization	Variable localization

itself is not innate, but emerges across the course of development, through the interaction of innate architecture, innate timing, and input to the cortex.

In fact, the case for innate representations looks very bad right now. Thirty years ago, representational nativism was a perfectly plausible hypothesis. That is, it was reasonable to suppose that knowledge is built into the infant cortex in the form of detailed and well-specified synaptic connections, independent of and prior to the effects of input to the cortex (what Pinker [1997a] refers to as an innate "wiring diagram"). Indeed, such an assumption is critical for strong forms of linguistic nativism (i.e., the idea that children are born with Universal Grammar; Chomsky, 1980a,b; Pinker, 1994; Rice, 1996) because synaptic connectivity is the only level of brain organization with the necessary coding power for complex and domain-specific representations of the sort that would be required to support an innate grammar. However, this particular form of innateness is difficult to defend in the face of mounting information on the activity-dependent nature of synaptic connectivity at the cortical level. Of course the infant brain is certainly not a *tabula rasa*. At other levels of organization, we have ample evidence for endogenous effects that bias the learning game in significant ways. These include constraints on the global input–output architecture of the brain (e.g., the fact that information from the eye usually does end up in visual cortex, in the absence of wicked interventions by Sur and his colleagues [1990]), local variations in architecture and style of computation (e.g., primary visual cortex starts out with roughly twice as many neurons as any other area), and variations in timing (e.g., variations from one region to another in the length of neurogenesis) and in the availability of nerve growth factor. It now seems that the difference between the human brain and that of other primates must be determined primarily by nonrepresentational variations of this kind, controlled by a genetic program small enough to fit into the mere 1%–2% difference between the human genome and the genome of a chimpanzee (King and Wilson, 1975; Wilson, 1985).

The second assumption in Table 10-1, domain-specific processing, is a key component of the mental organ doctrine, i.e., that distinct regions of the brain have evolved to deal with particular kinds of content of compelling interest to our species (Barkow et al., 1992; Pinker, 1997a). In addition to language (and perhaps to distinct subcomponents of language, e.g., a distinction between grammar and the lexicon), proposed modules or mental organs include a face detector, a theory-of-mind module (that contains algorithms for detecting dishonest behavior by other members of the species), a mathematics module, a music module, and so forth. These systems have presumably evolved to deal optimally with their assigned content and only with that content. Indeed, Pinker (1997a) has proposed that diverse and specific forms of psychopathology may result if a module is applied to the wrong domain (although it is not entirely clear how this might occur, given the perceptual biases that define a mental organ).

The emergentist alternative to domain-specific processing is that domain-specific knowledge can be acquired and processed by domain-general mechanisms, that is, by mechanisms of attention, perception, memory, emotion and motor planning that are involved in many different aspects of learning, thought, and behavior. In other words, the cognitive machinery that makes us human can be viewed as a new machine constructed out of old parts (Bates et al., 1979). All of the component parts that participate in language are based on phylogenetically ancient mechanisms, with homologues up and down the vertebrate line. The specific functions that make humans different from other species are superimposed on this Basic Vertebrate Brain Plan. Of course it is likely that some and perhaps all of the neural components that participate in human activity have undergone quantitative changes that permit new behaviors like language to emerge, but these components still continue to carry out older and more general functions of object detection, shifting attention, formation of new memories, motor planning, and so forth (i.e., they have kept their day jobs.).

To help us think about the kind of adaptation that would permit the construction of a new machine from old parts, consider the metaphor of the giraffe's neck. Giraffes have the same number of neckbones that you and I have, but these bones are elongated to solve the peculiar problems that giraffes are specialized for (i.e., eating leaves high up in the tree). As a result of this particular adaptation, other adaptations were necessary as well, including cardiovascular changes (to pump blood all the way up to the giraffe's brain), shortening of the hindlegs relative to the forelegs (to ensure that the giraffe does not topple over), and so on. Should we conclude that the giraffe's neck is a "high-leaf-reaching organ"? Not exactly. The giraffe's neck is still a neck, built out of the same basic blueprint that is used over and over in vertebrates, but with some quantitative adjustments. It still does other kinds of "neck work," just like the work that necks do in less specialized species, but it has some extra potential for reaching up high in the tree that other necks do not provide. If we insist that the neck is a leaf-reaching organ, then we have to include the rest of the giraffe in that category, including the cardiovascular changes, adjustments in leg length, and so on.

In the same vein, our "language organ" can be viewed as the result of quantitative adjustments in neural mechanisms that exist in other mammals, permitting us to walk into a problem space that other animals cannot perceive much less solve. Of course, once language finally appeared on the planet, it is quite likely that it began to apply its own adaptive pressures to the organization of the human brain, just as the leaf-reaching adaptation of the giraffe's neck applied adaptive pressure to other parts of the giraffe. Hence the neural mechanisms that participate in language still do other kinds of work, but they have also grown to meet the language task. In fact, it seems increasingly unlikely that we will ever be in a position to explain human language in terms of clear and well-bounded differences between our brain and that of other primates. Consider, for example, the infamous case of the planum temporale (i.e., the superior gyrus of the temporal lobe reaching back to the temporal–parietal–occipital juncture). It was noted many years ago that the planum temporale is longer on the left side of the brain in the majority of normal, right-handed human adults. Because the temporal lobe clearly does play a special role in language processing, it was argued that the asymmetry of the planum may play a key role in brain organization for language. However, surprising new evidence has just emerged showing that the same asymmetry is also observed in chimpanzees (Hollaway et al., 1997). In fact, the asymmetry is actually larger and more consistent in chimpanzees that it is in humans! I do not doubt for a moment that humans use this stretch of tissue in a quantitatively and qualitatively different way, but simple differences in size and shape may not be sufficient or even relevant to the critical difference between us and our nearest relatives in the primate line. In response to findings of this sort, Pinker (1997a) has insisted that the answer lies in the cortical microcircuitry within relevant areas. And yet, as we have seen over and over, developmental neurobiologists have abandoned the idea that detailed aspects of synaptic connectivity are under direct genetic control, in favor of an activity-dependent account. There has to be something special about the human brain that makes language possible, but that "something" may involve highly distributed mechanisms that serve many other functions.

My own favorite candidates for this category of "language-facilitating mechanisms" are capacities that predate language phylogenetically and undoubtedly involve many different aspects of the brain. They include our rich social organization and capacity for social reasoning, our extraordinary ability to imitate the things that other people do, our excellence in the segmentation of rapid auditory and visual stimuli, and our fascination with joint attention (looking at the same events together, sharing new objects just for the fun of it; for an extended discussion, see Bates et al., 1991b). These abilities are all present in human infants within the first year, and they are all implicated in the process by which language is acquired. None of them is specific to language, but they make language possible, just as quantitative adjustments in th giraffe's neck make it possible for the giraffe to accomplish something that no other ungulate can do.

Is there any evidence in favor of this domain-general "borrowed system" view? I would put the matter somewhat differently: Despite myriad predictions that such evidence will be found, there is still no unambiguous evidence in favor of the idea that specific parts of the brain are dedicated to specific kinds of objects and *only* those objects. For example, there are cells in the brain of the adult primate that respond preferentially to a particular class of stimuli (e.g., faces). However, recent studies have shown that the same cells can also respond to other kinds of content, spontaneously and/or after an extended period of training (Das and Gilbert, 1995; De Weerd et al., 1995; Fregnac et al., 1996; Pettet and Gilbert, 1992; Ramachandran and Gregory, 1991; Tovee et al., 1996). Similarly, certain cortical regions around the sylvian fissure are invariably active in neural imaging studies of language processing, including some of the same areas that are implicated in fluent and nonfluent aphasia. However, each of these regions can also be activated by one or more forms of nonlinguistic processing. This point was made eloquently clear in a recent study by Erhard et al. (1996), who looked at all the proposed subcomponents of Broca's area while subjects were asked to carry out (covertly) a series of verbal and nonverbal actions, including complex movements of the mouth and fingers. Every single component of the Broca complex that is active during speech is also active in at least one form of covert nonverbal activity. In short, even though there is ample evidence for stretches of tissue that participate in language, there appears to be no candidate anywhere in perisylvian cortex for a pure language organ.

This brings us to three key assumptions about the nature of localization, the final three of the five contrasting issues listed in Table 10-1. On the phrenological account, precisely because of the assumptions about *(1)* innate representations and *(2)* dedicated architecture, it is further assumed that brain organization for language involves *(3)* a fixed architecture that cannot be replaced and cannot be modified significantly by experience, *(4)* a universal architecture that admits to very little individual variability, and *(5)* a compact and spatially contiguous architecture that operates as a coherent and autonomous unit in neural imaging studies and creates distinct deficits in or dissociations between cognitive functions when it is lesioned ("disconnection syndromes"; Caramazza, 1986; Caramazza and Berndt, 1985; Geschwind, 1965; Shallice, 1988). By contrast, the emergentist account is more compatible with forms of localization that are *(3)* plastic and modifiable by experience, *(4)* variable in form as a result of variations in experience as well as individual differences in the initial architecture, and *(5)* distributed across stretches of tissue that may participate in many different tasks (including spatially discontinuous systems that can perform separately or together depending on the task). Because of these properties, the emergentist view is much more compatible with all the mounting evidence from developmental neurobiology for the plasticity and activity dependence of cortical specialization, including plasticity for language in brain-injured children.

The emergentist view is also more compatible with the complex and variable findings that have emerged in recent neural imaging studies of normal adults (Courtney and Ungerleider, 1997; Poeppel, 1996). Indeed, new areas for language are multiplying at an alarming rate in language activation studies, including studies using positron emission tomography (PET), functional magnetic resonance imaging (fMRI), magnetoencephalography (MEG), and/or event-related brain potentials (ERP). Although activation is usually larger on the left than it is on the right in language activation studies, and the familiar perisylvian regions of the left hemisphere show up in study after study, there is increasing evidence for participation of homologous regions in the right hemisphere (e.g., Just et al., 1996), although there is substantial variation over individuals, tasks, and laboratories in the extent to which this occurs. Language activation studies that involve generation and maintenance of codes and/or a decision between behavioral options seem to result in reliable activation of several different prefrontal regions that were not implicated in older studies of language breakdown in aphasia (e.g., Raichle et al., 1994; Thompson-Schill et al., 1997). New regions that appear to be especially active during language activation have also appeared in basal temporal cortex (on the underside of the brain; Nobre et al., 1994), in some portions of the basal ganglia, and in the cerebellum (especially on the right side of the cerebellum). Many different aspects of both sensory and motor cortex seem to be activated in language tasks that involve imageable stimuli. More interesting still for our purposes here, these patterns of activation vary as a function of development itself, including variations with chronological age and language level in children (Hirsch et al., 1997; Mills et al., 1997; Mueller, 1996), and varying levels of expertise in adults (Hernandez et al., 1997; Kim et al., 1997; Perani et al., 1997; Raichle et al., 1994).

The picture that has emerged is one in which most of the brain participates in linguistic activity, in varying degrees, depending on the nature of the task and the individual's expertise in that task. In many respects, this is exactly what we should expect: Language is a system for encoding meaning, and there are now good reasons to believe that the activation of meaning involves activation of the same regions that participate in the original experiences on which meanings are based. Because most of the brain participates in meaning, we should expect widely distributed and dynamically shifting patterns of participation in most language-based tasks. The fact that these patterns of activation change over time is also not surprising, reflecting changes in experience as well as changes in the level of skill that individuals attain in activation and maintenance of both meaning and form.

Clearly, however, there are some important differences in the view of language organization that emerges from neural imaging studies and lesion studies. Neural imaging techniques can tell us about the areas of the brain that *participate* in language. From this point of view, we may conclude that the participation is very broad. Lesion studies can tells us about the areas of the brain that are *necessary* for normal language. The list of areas that are necessary for language (in children or adults) appears to be much smaller than the list of areas that participate freely in a language task. Even in this case, however, improved techniques for structural imaging and lesion reconstruction have yielded more and more evidence for individual variability in lesion–symptom mapping (Goodglass, 1993; Willmes and Poeck, 1993), and for compensatory organization in patients who display full or partial recovery from aphasia (Cappa et al., 1997; Cappa and Vallar, 1992).

There are of course some clear limits on this variability. Some areas of the brain simply cannot be replaced, in children or adults. For example, Bachevalier and Mishkin (1993) have shown that infant monkeys with bilateral lesions to the medial temporal regions (including the amygdala and the hippocampus) display a dense and apparently irreversible form of amnesia that persists for the rest of the animal's life, in marked contrast to the striking recovery that follows bilateral lesions to lateral temporal cortex (Webster et al., 1995). The key lies in the global input–output architecture of those medial temporal regions, a rich and broad form of connectivity that cannot be replaced because no other candidate has that kind of communication with the rest of the cortex. Other parts of the brain cannot be replaced because they are the crucial highways and offramps for information from the periphery (e.g., the insula, which receives crucial kinaesthetic feedback from the oral articulators, or the auditory nerve, which carries irreplaceable auditory input to the waiting cortex; Dronkers, 1996; Dronkers et al., 1994, 1999). These irreplaceable regions form the anchor points, the universal starting points for brain organization in normal children, and they are difficult if not impossible to replace once all the exuberant axons of the fetal brain have been eliminated.

Within this framework, learning itself also places limits on plasticity and reorganization in the developing brain. For example, Marchman (1993) has shown that artificial neural networks engaged in a language-learning task (i.e., acquiring the past tense of English verbs) can recover from "lesions" (i.e., random removal of connections) that are imposed early in the learning process. The same lesions result in a substantially greater "language deficit" when they are imposed later in the learning process. This simulation of so-called critical period effects takes place in the absence of any extraneous change in the learning potential of the network (i.e., there is no equivalent of withdrawal of neurotrophins or reduction in the learning rate). Marchman (1993) reminds us that critical period effects can be explained in at least two ways (and these are not mutually exclusive): exogenously imposed changes in learning capacity (the usual interpretation of critical periods) or the entrenchment that results from learning itself. In other words, learning changes the nature of the brain, eliminating some connections and tuning others to values that are difficult to change. Eventually the system may reach a point of no return, a reduction in plasticity that mimics critical period effects without any change in the architecture other than the changes that result from normal processes of learning and development. Marchman (1993) does not deny the possibility of exogenous effects on plasticity, but she argues convincingly that there are other ways to explain the same result, including gradual changes in the capacity to learn (and recover what was learned before) that are the product of learning itself—changes that are more compatible with the current developmental evidence than the idea of an abrupt and discontinuous critical period (see also Bates and Carnevale, 1993; Elman et al., 1996).

Finally, the emergentist view makes room for the possibility of systematic developmental changes in localization due to a shift in the processes and operations that are required to carry out a function at different points in the learning process. On the static phrenology view, a language area is a language area, always and forever. There may be developmental changes that are due to maturation (i.e., an area that was not "ready" before suddenly "comes on-line"), but the processes involved in that content domain are always carried out in the same dedicated regions. On the emergentist account, the areas responsible for learning may be totally different from the areas involved in maintenance and use of the same function in its mature form. In fact, there are at least three reasons why we should expect differences in the patterns of brain activity associated with language processing in children versus adults.

Early competition

We may assume (based on ample evidence from animal models) that the early stages of development involve a competition among areas for control over tasks. This competition is open to any region that can receive and process the relevant information, but that does not mean that every region has an even chance of winning. In fact, as the competition proceeds, those regions that are better equipped to deal with that task (because of differences in efficiency of access and type of processing) will gradually take more responsibility for the mediation of that function. In prospective studies of language development, we are looking at this process of competition as it unfolds. This leads to the prediction that the earlier stages of development will involve more diffuse forms of processing, a prediction that is borne out by ERP studies of changes in activation across the first 3 years of language development (from activation to known words that is bilateral but slightly larger in the right toward activation that is larger on the left and localized more focally to frontotemporal sites; Mills et al., 1997).

Expertise

We may also expect quantitative and qualitative change in the regions that participate in a given task as a function of level of expertise. These changes can take three different forms: expansion within regions, retraction within regions, and a wholesale shift in mediation from one region to another. An example of expansion comes from a recent fMRI study of skill acquisition in adults (Karni et al., 1995). In this study, the first stages of learning in a finger-movement task tend to involve smaller patches of somatosensory cortex; with increased skill in this task, the areas responsible for the motor pattern increase in size. Examples of retraction come from studies that show larger areas of activation in the early stages of second-language learning compared with activation in native speakers and in more experienced second-language learners (Hernandez et al., 1997; Perani et al., 1997). Presumably this is because the novice speaker has to recruit more neural resources to achieve a goal that was far easier for a more advanced speaker (equivalent to the amount of muscle a child versus an adult must use to lift a heavy box). The third possibility may be the most interesting, and the one with greatest significance for our focal injury results. In the earliest stages, areas involved in attention, perceptual analysis, and formation of new memories may be particularly important. As the task becomes better learned and more automatic, the baton may pass to regions that are responsible for the reactivation of over-learned patterns, with less attention and less perceptual analysis. A recent example of this kind of qualitative shift is reported by Raichle et al. (1994), who observed strong frontocerebellar activation in the early stages of learning, replaced by activation in perisylvian cortex after the task is mastered.

Maturation and "readiness"

Finally, the emergentist approach does not preclude the possibility of maturational change. Examples might include differential growth gradients for the right versus left hemisphere (Chiron et al., 1997), differential rates of synaptogenesis ("synaptic sprouting") from one region to another within the two hemispheres (Huttenlocher et al., 1982), changes from region to region in the overall amount of neural activity (as indexed by positron emission tomography; Chugani et al., 1987), variation in rates of myelination, and so forth. As a result of changes of this kind (together with the effects of learning itself in reshaping the brain; Marchman, 1993), we should expect to find marked shifts in the patterns of activity associated with language processing at different points in early childhood.

Based on these assumptions, let us return to our findings on the early stages of language development in children with early focal brain injury to see what these results suggest about the emergence of brain organization for language in normal children.

Right hemisphere advantage for word comprehension and gesture from 10 to 17 months

Contrary to expectations based on the adult aphasia literature, we found evidence for greater delays in word comprehension and gesture in children with RHD. This is exactly the opposite of the pattern observed in adults, where deficits in word comprehension and in production of symbolic gesture are both associated with LHD, suggesting that some kind of shift takes place between infancy and adulthood, with control over these two skills passed from the right hemisphere to the left. This result is (as we noted) compatible with observations by Mills et al. (1997) on the patterns of activation observed in response to familiar words from infancy to adulthood. There are at least two possible explanations for a developmental change, and they are not mutually exclusive.

On the one hand, the early right hemisphere advantage could be explained by hard maturational changes that are exogenous to the learning process itself. For example, Chiron and his colleagues (1997) have provided evidence from PET for a change in resting-state activation across the first 2 years, from bilateral activation that is larger on the right to greater activation on the left. Based on these findings, they suggest that the right hemisphere may mature faster than the left in the first year of development. As it turns out, this is the period in which word comprehension and gesture first emerge in normally developing children. By contrast, word production emerges in the second year and grows dramatically through 30 to 36 months, the period in which (according to Chiron et al., 1997) the left hemisphere reaches the dominant state that it will maintain for years to come. Hence one might argue that the right hemisphere "grabs" control over comprehension and gesture in the first year, and the left hemisphere "grabs" control over the burgeoning capacity for production in the second year, eventually taking over the entire linguistic-symbolic system (including word comprehension and meaningful gestures).

On the other hand, it is also possible that the right-to-left shift implied by our data reflects a qualitative difference between the learning processes required for comprehension and the processes required for production. The first time that we figure out the meaning of a word (e.g., decoding the word "dog" and mapping it onto a particular class of animals), we do so by integrating the phonetic input with information from many different sources, including visual, tactile, and auditory context ("fuzzy brown thing that moves and barks"). It has been argued that the right hemisphere plays a privileged role in multimodal integration and processing of large patterns (Stiles, 1995; more on this below), and for this reason we may expect the right hemisphere to play a more important role when children are learning to comprehend words for the first time. Presumably, this right hemisphere advantage will disappear when words are fully acquired, replaced by a rapid, efficient, and automatic process of mapping well-known sounds onto well-known semantic patterns (more on this below). If this hypothesis has merit, then we might also expect to find evidence for greater participation of the right hemisphere in the early stages of second-language learning in adults, a testable hypothesis and one that has some (limited) support.

It is much less obvious how this shift-in-strategy hypothesis might account for the early right hemisphere advantage in symbolic gesture. Although this is admittedly a speculative answer, this finding may be related to results for normal children showing that comprehension and gesture are highly correlated between approximately 9 and 20 months of age (Fenson et al., 1994). One possible explanation for this correlation may lie in the fact that symbolic gestures are acquired in the context of auditory comprehension (e.g., "Wave bye-bye to grandma," "Hug the baby!"). Hence the two skills may come in together in very small children because they are acquired together in real life.

Deficits in expressive vocabulary and grammar with frontal lesions to either hemisphere from 19 to 31 months

We observed specific effects of lesions involving the frontal lobes in children between 19 and 31 months of age, a brief but dramatic period of development that includes the vocabulary burst and the first flowering of grammar. Contrary to expectations based on the adult aphasia literature, the delays in expressive language associated with frontal lesions were symmetrical, that is, there was no difference between frontal lesions on the left and frontal lesions on the right. There are a number of reasons why we would expect to find specific effects of frontal involvement during this important period in the development of expressive language, including contributions to the planning and execution of motor patterns and contributions from working memory and/or the fashionable array of skills referred to by the term *executive function* (Pennington and Ozonoff, 1996). However, the absence of a left–right asymmetry is more surprising. Nor have we found any evidence for a specific effect of left frontal injury in any of our studies to date, at any age. This difference between infants and adults suggests to us that Broca's area is not innately specialized for language. It becomes specialized across the course of development, after an initial period in which frontal cortex makes a symmetrical contribution to language learning.

Deficits in expressive vocabulary and grammar with left temporal injuries from 10 months to 5 years of age

This is the most robust and protracted finding in our prospective studies, and it is the only evidence we have for an asymmetry that might be systematically related to a left hemisphere advantage for language in the adult brain. Note, however, that the effect only pertains to *expressive* language (contrary to the expectation that temporal cortex is specialized for comprehension), and it applies equally to *both* vocabulary and grammar (contrary to the expectation that temporal cortex is associated with semantics while frontal cortex handles grammar; Zurif, 1980).

We have proposed that a relatively simple bias in style of computation may underlie this left temporal effect, reflecting architectural differences between left and right temporal cortex that are only indirectly related to the functional and representational specializations that are evident in adult language processing. Following a proposal by Stiles and Thal (1993), we note that left and right temporal cortex differ at birth in their capacity to support perceptual detail (enhanced on the left) and perceptual integration (enhanced on the right; see above). These differences are evident in nonverbal processing, but they may have particularly important consequences for language. For example, a number of recent studies have shown that lesions to the right hemisphere lead to problems in the integration of elements in a perceptual array, while lesions to the left hemisphere create problems in the analysis of perceptual details in the same array (e.g., Robertson and Lamb, 1991). Asked to reproduce a triangle made up of many small squares, adult patients with LHD tend to reproduce the global figure (i.e., the triangle) while ignoring information at the local level. Adult patients with RHD display the opposite profile, reproducing local detail (i.e., a host of small squares) but failing to integrate these features into a coherent whole. Stiles and Thal (1993) report that children with focal brain injury behave very much like their adult counterparts on the local–global task, suggesting that the differential contribution of left and right hemisphere processes on this task may be a developmental constant. Interestingly, this double dissociation is most evident in patients with temporal involvement, and the special role of left temporal cortex in processing of perceptual details has also been confirmed in an fMRI study of normal adults engaged in the same local–global task (Martinez et al., 1997).

The same left–right difference may be responsible for the lesion–symptom correlations that we observe in early language development. As I noted earlier, the ability to integrate information within and across modalities may be particularly helpful and important during the first stages of word comprehension and (perhaps) recognition and reproduction of familiar gestures. However, the learning task changes markedly when children have to convert the same sound patterns into motor output. At this point, perceptual detail may be of paramount importance (i.e., it is one thing to recognize the word "dog," but quite another thing to pull out each phonetic detail and construct a motor template). If it is the case that left temporal cortex plays a critical role in the extraction, storage, and reproduction of perceptual detail (visual and/or acoustic), then children with left temporal injuries will be at a greater disadvantage in this phase of learning (see also Galaburda and Livingstone, 1993; Galaburda et al., 1994; Tallal et al., 1991). However, once the requisite patterns are finally constructed and set into well-learned routines, the left temporal disadvantage may be much less evident.

No evidence of lesion–symptom correlations after 5–7 years of age

All of the above lesion–symptom mappings seem to have disappeared when we test children with the same congenital etiology after 5–7 years of age. Although this conclusion is based primarily on cross-sectional findings, the few cases that we have been able to study longitudinally across these periods of development are compatible with the cross-sectional results, providing further evidence for plasticity and compensatory organization across the course of language development. Of course it is entirely possible that we will find a new and improved index of efficiency in language processing that yields information about the subtle deficits that remain, for example, a residual effect of left temporal involvement that shows up in real-time sentence processing and/or in production of complex syntax under certain laboratory conditions. At the very least, however, we may conclude with some confidence that these children have found a form of brain organization for language that works very well, certainly well enough for everyday language use. As a group, children with focal brain injury do tend to perform below neurologically intact age-matched controls. But these differences also tend to disappear when the small group difference in full-scale IQ is taken into account (Bates et al., 1999).

If the familiar pattern of left hemisphere organization for language is not critical for normal language functioning, why does it develop in the first place? To answer this question, we have put forth a "modest proposal" based on the developmental findings and developmental principles listed above, as follows.

Prior to the onset of language development, the infant brain has no innate representations for language, nor does it have a "dedicated language processor" of any kind. However, the initial (prelinguistic) architecture of the infant brain is highly differentiated. The global input–output structure of the brain is well specified (e.g., the retina reports to visual cortex, the cochlea reports to auditory cortex), although there may still be a number of exuberant axons that could (if they are not eliminated in the normal course of development) sustain an alternative form of global architecture if they are needed. There are also innate (experience-independent) variations from region to region in cell density, synaptic density, speed of processing, and the kinds of neurotransmitters that are expressed (Hutsler and Gazzaniga, 1996). Furthermore, even though the infant has little experience in the world, the infant cortex has been inundated with information from the body itself. As Damasio (1994) has noted, the brain is the captive audience of the body, and the body provides the earliest and most reliable input that the growing cortex will ever receive. This includes sensory impressions from the body surface, kinaesthetic feedback from the infant's own movements, and reliable waves of activity from lower brain centers (e.g., bilateral and competitive input from lower-level visual nuclei that, we now know, is critical for the establishment of ocular dominance patterns; Miller et al., 1989; Shatz, 1992). Hence, even though there may be no direct genetic control over synaptic connectivity at the cortical level, the newborn infant starts life with a brain that has been colonized by sensorimotor input from its own body, setting down the basic parameters within which all the rest of behavioral development must take place. These facts combine with the regional differences in cortical architecture described above, setting the stage for the postnatal development of cognition and communication, including the development of grammar (MacWhinney, 1999).

As a result of all these forces, the infant comes to the task of language learning with a heavy set of biases about how information should be processed. Some of these biases are symmetrical (e.g., the role of frontal cortex in control of voluntary movements), and others are asymmetrical (e.g., the local–global biases described above). Following early focal brain injury, these biases show up in the early lesion–symptom mappings that we have described above, but they are eventually overcome by the competitive pressures that define plasticity and development in both the normal and the abnormal case. However, in healthy children without focal brain injury, these biases shape the development of brain organization for language in some highly predictable directions. In particular, left temporal cortex comes to play an increasingly important role in the extraction of the rapid and evanescent linguistic signal—first in the construction of motor templates to match slow and dependable inputs and later in the construction of complex meanings for both comprehension and production (events that we would expect to see in both signed and spoken language; Petitto et al., 1997). In short, under normal conditions (i.e., in the absence of focal brain injury), left temporal cortex wins the language contract. Although there is no asymmetrical bias in favor of left frontal cortex in the early stages of development, the left temporal "winner" recruits its partners in the front of the brain, setting up the familiar ipsilateral circuit that characterizes left hemisphere mediation of language in neurologically intact adults. At this point (and not before), Broca's area has a special job.

This is our proposal for the cascade of events that are responsible for the patterns of brain organization for language that lie behind 200 years of research on adult aphasia and hundreds (going on thousands) of neural imaging studies of language activation in normal adults. No doubt this proposal will have to undergo considerable revision as more information becomes available, but we are convinced that the final story will have to be one in which development and experience play a crucial role. Plasticity is not a civil defense system, a set of emergency procedures that are only invoked when something goes wrong. Rather, the processes responsible for reorganization of the brain following early focal brain injury are the same processes that organize the brain under normal conditions. It is time to exercise the ghost of Franz Gall, trading in the static phrenological view of brain organization for a dynamic approach that reconciles linguistics and cognitive science with developmental neurobiology.

References

Support for the work described here was provided by NIH-NIDCD P50 DC1289-9351 ("Origins of Communication Disorders") and NIH/NINDS P50 NS22343 ("Center for the Study of the Neural Bases of Language and Learning").

Aram, D. M. (1988). Language sequelae of unilateral brain lesions in children. In F. Plum (ed.). Language, Communication, and the Brain. New York: Raven Press, pp. 171–197.

Aram, D. M., Ekelman, B., Rose, D., and Whitaker, H. (1985a). Verbal and cognitive sequelae following unilateral lesions acquired in early childhood. *J. Clin. Exp. Neuropsychol., 7*, 55–78.

Aram, D. M., Ekelman, B., and Whitaker, H. (1985b). Lexical retrieval in left and right brain-lesioned children. *Brain Lang., 28,* 61–87.

Bachevalier, J., and Mishkin, M. (1993). An early and a late developing system for learning and retention in infant monkeys. In M. Johnson (ed.): *Brain Development and Cognition: A Reader.* Oxford: Blackwell, pp. 195–207.

Barkow, J. H., Cosmides, L., and Tooby, J. (eds.) (1992). *The Adapted Mind: Evolutionary Psychology and the Generation of Culture.* New York: Oxford University Press.

Basser, L. (1962). Hemiplegia of early onset and the faculty of speech with special reference to the effects of hemispherectomy. *Brain, 85,* 427–460.

Bates, E., Appelbaum, M., and Allard, L. (1991a). Statistical constraints on the use of single cases in neuropsychological research. *Brain Lang., 40,* 295–329.

Bates, E., Benigni, L., Bretherton, I., Camaioni, L., and Volterra, V. (1979). *The Emergence of Symbols: Cognition and Communication in Infancy.* New York: Academic Press.

Bates, E., and Carnevale, G. F. (1993). New directions in research on language development. *Dev. Rev., 13,* 436–470.

Bates, E., Dale, P. S., and Thal, D. (1995). Individual differences and their implications for theories of language development. In P. Fletcher and B. MacWhinney (eds.): *Handbook of Child Language.* Oxford: Basil Blackwell, pp. 96–151.

Bates, E., and Elman, J. L. (1996). Learning rediscovered. *Science, 274,* 1849–1850.

Bates, E., Elman, J., Johnson, M. C., Karmiloff-Smith, A., Parisi, D., and Plunkett, K. (1998). Innateness and emergentism. In W. Bechtel and G. Graham (eds.): *A Companion to Cognitive Science.* Oxford: Basil Blackwell, pp. 590–601.

Bates, E., Thal, D., and Janowsky, J. (1992). Early language development and its neural correlates. In I. Rapin and S. Segalowitz (eds.): *Handbook of Neuropsychology, vol. 7, Child Neuropsychology.* Amsterdam: Elsevier, pp. 69–110.

Bates, E., Thal, D., and Marchman, V. (1991b). Symbols and syntax: A Darwinian approach to language development. In N. Krasnegor, D. Rumbaugh, R. Schiefelbusch, and M. Studdert-Kennedy (eds.): *Biological and Behavioral Determinants of Language Development.* Hillsdale, NJ: Erlbaum, pp. 29–65.

Bates, E., Thal, D., Trauner, D., Fenson, J., Aram, D., Eisele, J., and Nass, R. (1997). From first words to grammar in children with focal brain injury. *Dev. Neuropsychol. (Spec. Iss.), 13,* 447–476.

Bates, E., Vicari, S., and Trauner, D. (1999). Neural mediation of language development: Perspectives from lesion studies of infants and children. In H. Tager-Flusberg (ed.): *Neurodevelopmental Disorders: Contributions to a New Framework From the Cognitive Neurosciences.* Cambridge, MA: MIT Press (in press).

Bialystok, E., and Hakuta, K. (1994). *In Other Words: The Science and Psychology of Second-Language Acquisition.* New York: Basic Books.

Bishop, D. V. M. (1983). Linguistic impairment after left hemidecortication for infantile hemiplegia? A reappraisal. *Q. J. Exp. Psychol., 35A,* 199–207.

Bishop, D. V. M. (1997). Cognitive neuropsychology and developmental disorders: Uncomfortable bedfellows. *Q. J. Exp. Psychol., 50,* 899–923.

Cappa, S. F., Perani, D., Grassi, F., Bressi, S., Alberoni, M., Franceschi, M., Bettinardi, V., Todde, S., and Fazio, F. (1997). A PET follow-up study of recovery after stroke in acute aphasics. *Brain Lang., 56,* 55–67.

Cappa, S. F., and Vallar, G. (1992). The role of the left and right hemispheres in recovery from aphasia. *Aphasiology, 6,* 359–372.

Caramazza, A. (1986). On drawing inferences about the structure of normal cognitive systems from the analysis of patterns of impaired performance: The case for single-patient studies. *Brain Cog., 5*, 41–66.

Caramazza, A., and Berndt, R. (1985). A multicomponent view of agrammatic Broca's aphasia. In M.-L. Kean (ed.): *Agrammatism.* Orlando: Academic Press, pp. 27–63.

Chiron, C., Jambaque, I., Nabbout, R., Lounes, R., Syrota, A., and Dulac, O. (1997). The right brain hemisphere is dominant in human infants. *Brain, 120,* 1057–1065.

Chomsky, N. (1980a). On cognitive structures and their development: A reply to Piaget. In M. Piattelli-Palmarini (ed.): *Language and Learning.* Cambridge: Harvard University Press, pp. 35–54.

Chomsky, N. (1980b). *Rules and Representations.* New York: Columbia University Press.

Chomsky, N. (1995). *The Minimalist Program.* Cambridge: MIT Press.

Chugani, H. T., Phelps, M. E., and Mazziotta, J. C. (1987). Positron emission tomography study of human brain functional development. *Ann. Neurol., 22,* 487–497.

Clark, R., Gleitman, L., and Kroch, A. (1997). *Science, 276,* 1179.

Courtney, S. M., and Ungerleider, L. G. (1997). What fMRI has taught us about human vision. *Curr. Opin. Neurobiol., 7,* 554–561.

Curtiss, S. (1988). Abnormal language acquisition and the modularity of language. In F. J. Newmeyer (ed.): *Linguistics: The Cambridge Survey: vol. II, Linguistic Theory: Extensions and Implications.* Cambridge, UK: Cambridge University Press, pp. 96–116.

Dall' Oglio, A. M., Bates, E., Volterra, V., Di Capua, M., and Pezzini, G. (1994). Early cognition, communication and language in children with focal brain injury. *Dev. Med. Child Neurol., 36,* 1076–1098.

Damasio, A. R. (1994). *Descartes' Error: Emotion, Reason, and the Human Brain.* New York: G. P. Putnam.

Das, A., and Gilbert, C. D. (1995). Receptive field expansion in adult visual cortex is linked to dynamic changes in strength of cortical connections. *J. Neurophysiol., 74,* 779–792.

Deacon, T. (1997). *The Symbolic Species: The Co-Evolution of Language and the Brain.* New York: Norton.

Dennis, M., and Whitaker, H. (1976). Language acquisition following hemidecortication: Linguistic superiority of the left over the right hemisphere. *Brain Lang., 3,* 404–433.

De Weerd, P., Gattass, R., Desimone, R., and Ungerleider, L. (1995). Responses of cells in monkey visual cortex during perceptual filling in of an artificial scotoma. *Nature, 377,* 731–734.

Dronkers, N. F. (1996). A new brain region for coordinating speech articulation. *Nature, 384,* 159–161.

Dronkers, N. F., Redfern, B. B., and Ludy, C. A. (1999). Lesion localization in chronic Wernicke's aphasia. *Brain Lang.* (in press).

Dronkers, N. F., Wilkins, D. P., Van Valin, Jr., R. D., Redfern, B. B., and Jaeger, J. J. (1994). A reconsideration of the brain areas involved in the disruption of morphosyntactic comprehension. *Brain Lang., 47,* 461–463.

Eisele, J., and Aram, D. (1995). Lexical and grammatical development in children with early hemisphere damage: A cross-sectional view from birth to adolescence. In P. Fletcher and B. MacWhinney (eds.): *The Handbook of Child Language.* Oxford: Basil Blackwell, pp. 664–689.

Elman, J. L., and Bates, E. (1997). *Science, 276,* 1180.

Elman, J. L., Bates, E., Johnson, M., Karmiloff-Smith, A., Parisi, D., and Plunkett, K.

(1996). *Rethinking Innateness: A Connectionist Perspective on Development.* Cambridge: MIT Press/Bradford Books.

Erhard, P., Kato, T., Strick, P., and Ugurbil, K. (1996). Functional MRI Activation pattern of motor and language tasks in Broca's area. *Soc. Neurosci. Abstr., 22,* 260.

Feldman, H., Holland, A., Kemp, S., and Janosky, J. (1992). Language development after unilateral brain injury. *Brain Lang., 42,* 89–102.

Fenson, L., Dale, P., Reznick, J. S., Thal, D., Bates, E., Hartung, J., Pethick, S., and Reilly, J. (1993). *The MacArthur Communicative Development Inventories: User's Guide and Technical Manual.* San Diego: Singular Publishing Group.

Fenson, L., Dale, P. A., Reznick, J. S., Bates, E., Thal, D., and Pethick, S. J. (1994). Variability in early communicative development. *Monogr. Soc. Res. Child Dev., 59(5).*

Fodor, J. A. (1983). *The Modularity of Mind: An Essay on Faculty Psychology.* Cambridge: MIT Press.

Fregnac, Y., Bringuier, V., and Chavane, F. (1996). Synaptic integration fields and associative plasticity of visual cortical cells in vivo. *J. Physiol., 90,* 367–372.

Galaburda, A. M., and Livingstone, M. (1993). Evidence for a magnocellular defect in neurodevelopmental dyslexia. *Ann. N.Y. Acad. Sci., 682,* 70–82.

Galaburda, A. M., Menard, M. T., and Rosen, G. D. (1994). Evidence for aberrant auditory anatomy in developmental dyslexia. *Proc. Natl. Acad. Sci. U.S.A., 91,* 8010–8013.

Geschwind, N. (1965). Disconnexion syndromes in animals and man. *Brain, 88,* 585–644.

Goodglass, H. (1993). *Understanding Aphasia.* San Diego: Academic Press.

Goodman, R., and Yude, C. (1996). IQ and its predictors in childhood hemiplegia. *Dev. Med. Child Neurol., 38,* 881–890.

Gopnik, M. (1990). Feature-blind grammar and dysphasia. *Nature, 344,* 715.

Hernandez, A. E., Martinez, A., Wong, E. C., Frank, L. R., and Buxton, R. B. (1997). *Neuroanatomical Correlates of Single- and Dual-Language Picture Naming in Spanish-English Bilinguals.* Poster presented at the fourth annual meeting of the Cognitive Neuroscience Society, March 1997.

Hirsch, J., Kim, K., Souweidane, M., McDowall, R., Ruge, M., Correa, D., and Krol, G. (1997). FMRI reveals a developing language system in a 15-month-old sedated infant. *Soc. Neurosci. Abstr., 23,* 2227.

Holloway, R., Broadfield, D., Kheck, N., and Braun, A. (1997). Chimpanzee brain: Left–right asymmetries in temporal speech region homolog. *Soc. Neurosci. Abstr., 23,* 2228.

Hutsler, J. J., and Gazzaniga, M. S. (1996). Acetylcholinesterase staining in human auditory and language cortices: Regional variation of structural features. *Cereb. Cortex, 6,* 260–270.

Huttenlocher, P. R., de Courten, C., Garey, L., and van der Loos, H. (1982). Synaptogenesis in human visual cortex synapse elimination during normal development. *Neurosci. Lett., 33,* 247–252.

Isacson, O., and Deacon, T. W. (1996). Presence and specificity of axon guidance cues in the adult brain demonstrated by pig neuroblasts transplanted into rats. *Neuroscience, 75,* 827–837.

Janowsky, J. S., and Finlay, B. L. (1986). The outcome of perinatal brain damage: The role of normal neuron loss and axon retraction. *Dev. Med., 28,* 375–389.

Jenkins, L., and Maxam, A. (1997). *Science, 276,* 1178–1179.

Johnson, J., and Newport, E. (1989). Critical period effects in second language learning: The influence of maturational state on the acquisition of English as a second language. *Cog. Psychol., 21,* 60–99.

Johnson, M. H. (1997). *Developmental Cognitive Neuroscience*. Oxford: Blackwell Publishers.

Just, M. A., Carpenter, P. A., Keller, T. A., Eddy, W. F., et al. (1996). Brain activation modulated by sentence comprehension. *Science, 275,* 114–116.

Karmiloff-Smith, A. (1992). *Beyond Modularity: A Developmental Perspective on Cognitive Science*. Cambridge: MIT Press.

Karni, A., Meyer, G., Jezzard, P., Adams, M. M., et al. (1995). Functional fMRI evidence for adult motor cortex plasticity during motor skill learning. *Nature, 377,* 155–158.

Kempler, D., van Lancker, D., Marchman, V., and Bates, E. (1999). Idiom comprehension in children and adults with unilateral brain damage. *Dev. Neuropsychol.* (in press).

Killackey, H. P. (1990). Neocortical expansion: An attempt toward relating phylogeny and ontogeny. *J. Cog. Neurosci., 2,* 1–17.

Killackey, H. P., Chiaia, N. L., Bennett-Clarke, C. A., Eck, M., and Rhoades, R. (1994). Peripheral influences on the size and organization of somatotopic representations in the fetal rate cortex. *J. Neurosci., 14,* 1496–1506.

Kim, K. H. S., Relkin, N. R., Lee, K. M., and Hirsch, J. (1997). Distinct cortical areas associated with native and second languages. *Nature, 388,* 171–174.

King, M. C., and Wilson, A. C. (1975). Evolution at two levels in humans and chimpanzees. *Science, 188,* 107–116.

Lenneberg, E. H. (1967). *Biological Foundations of Language*. New York: Wiley.

Liu, H., Bates, E., and Li, P. (1992). Sentence interpretation in bilingual speakers of English and Chinese. *Appl. Psycholing., 13,* 451–484.

MacWhinney, B. (1999). The emergence of language from embodiment. In B. MacWhinney (ed.): *The Emergence of Language*. Mahway, NJ: Lawrence Erlbaum (in press).

Marchman, V. (1993). Constraints on plasticity in a connectionist model of the English past tense. *J. Cog. Neurosci., 5,* 215–234.

Marchman, V., Miller, R., and Bates, E. (1991). Babble and first words in children with focal brain injury. *Appl. Psycholing., 12,* 1–22.

Martinez, A., Mosses, P., Frank, L., Buxton, R., Wong, E., and Stiles, J. (1997). Hemispheric asymmetries in global and local processing: Evidence from fMRI. *NeuroReport, 8,* 1685–1689.

Miller, K. D., Keller, J. B., and Stryker, M. P. (1989). Ocular dominance column development: Analysis and simulation. *Science, 245,* 605–615.

Mills, D. L., Coffey-Corina, S. A., and Neville, H. J. (1997). Language comprehension and cerebral specialization from 13 to 20 months. *Dev. Neuropsychol. (Spec. Iss.), 13,* 397–445.

Mueller, R.-A. (1996). Innateness, autonomy, universality? Neurobiological approaches to language. *Behav. Brain Sci., 19,* 611.

Nobre, A. C., Allison, T., and McCarthy, G. (1994). Word recognition in the human inferior temporal lobe. *Nature, 372,* 260–263.

Oyama, S. (1993). The problem of change. In M. Johnson (ed.): *Brain Development and Cognition: A Reader*. Oxford: Blackwell Publishers, pp. 19–30.

Pallas, S. L., and Sur, M. (1993). Visual projections induced into the auditory pathway of ferrets: II. Corticocortical connections of primary auditory cortex. *J. Comp. Neurol., 337,* 317–333.

Pennington, B. F., and Ozonoff, S. (1996). Executive functions and developmental psychopathology. *J. Child Psychol. Psychiatry Allied Disciplines, 37,* 51–87.

Perani, D., Paulesu, N., Sebastian, E., Dupoix, S., Dehaene, S., Schnur, T., Cappa, S.,

Mehler, J., and Fazio, E. (1997). Plasticity of brain language regions revealed by bilinguals. *Soc. Neurosci. Abstr., 23,* 2228.

Pesetsky, D., Wexler, K., and Fromkin, V. (1997). *Science, 276,* 1177.

Petitto, L., Zattore, R., Nikelski, E., Gauna, K., Dostie, D., and Evans, A. (1997). Cerebral organization for language in the absence of sound: A PET study of deaf signers processing signed languages. *Soc. Neurosci. Abstr., 23,* 2228.

Pettet, M. W., and Gilbert, C. (1992). Dynamic changes in receptive field size in cat primary visual cortex. *Proc. Nat. Acad. Sci. U.S.A., 89,* 8366–8370.

Pinker, S. (1991). Rules of language. *Science, 253,* 530–535.

Pinker, S. (1994). *The Language Instincts: How the Mind Creates Language.* New York: William Morrow.

Pinker, S. (1997a). *How the Mind Works.* New York: Norton.

Pinker, S. (1997b). Acquiring language. *Science, 276,* 1178.

Poeppel, D. (1996). A critical review of PET studies of phonological processing. *Brain Lang., 55,* 317–351.

Quartz, S. R., and Sejnowski, T. J. (1997). The neural basis of cognitive development: A constructivist manifesto. *Behav. Brain Sci., 20,* 537.

Raichle, M. E., Fiez, J. A., Videen, T. O., MacLeod, A. M., Pardo, J. V., Fox, P. T., and Petersen, S. E. (1994). Practice-related changes in human brain functional anatomy during non-motor learning. *Cereb. Cortex 4,* 8–26.

Ramachandran, V. S., and Gregory, R. L. (1991). Perceptual filling in of artificial scotomas in human vision. *Nature, 350,* 699–702.

Ramachandran, V. S., Hirstein, W. F., Armel, K. C., Tecoma, E., and Iraqui, V. (1997). The neural basis of religious experience. *Soc. Neurosci. Abstr., 23,* 519.1.

Reilly, J. S., Bates, E., and Marchman, V. (1998). Narrative discourse in children with early focal brain injury. *Brain Lang. (Spec. Iss.), 61,* 335–375.

Reilly, J. S., Stiles, J., Larsen, J., and Trauner, D. (1995). Affective facial expression in infants with focal brain damage. *Neuropsychologia, 1,* 83–99.

Rice, M. (ed.). (1996). *Toward a Genetics of Language.* Mahwah, NJ: Erlbaum.

Robertson, L. C., and Lamb, M. R. (1991). Neuropsychological contributions to theories of part whole organization. *Cog. Psychol., 23,* 299–330.

Shallice, T. (1988). *From Neuropsychology to Mental Structure.* New York: Cambridge University Press.

Shatz, C. J. (1992). The developing brain. *Sci. Am., 267,* 60–67.

Stanfield, B. B., and O'Leary, D. D. (1985). Fetal occipital cortical neurones transplanted to the rostral cortex can extend and maintain a pyramidal tract axon. *Nature, 313,* 135–137.

Stark, R., and McGregor, K. (1997). Follow-up study of a right- and left-hemispherectomized child: Implications for localization and impairment of language in children. *Brain Lang., 60,* 222–242.

Stiles, J. (1995). Plasticity and development: Evidence from children with early focal brain injury. In B. Julesz and I. Kovacs (eds.): *Maturational Windows and Adult Cortical Plasticity. Proceedings of the Santa Fe Institute Studies in the Sciences of Complexity,* vol. 23. Reading, MA: Addison-Wesley, pp. 217–237.

Stiles, J., Bates, E., Thal, D., Trauner, D., and Reilly, J. (1998). Linguistic, cognitive and affective development in children with pre- and perinatal focal brain injury: A ten-year overview from the San Diego Longitudinal Project. In C. Rovee-Collier, L. Lipsitt, and H. Hayne (eds.): *Advances in Infancy Research.* Norwood, NJ: Ablex, pp. 131–163.

Stiles, J., and Thal, D. (1993). Linguistic and spatial cognitive development following early focal brain injury: Patterns of deficit and recovery. In M. Johnson (ed.): *Brain Development and Cognition: A Reader.* Oxford: Blackwell Publishers, pp. 643–664.

Stromswold, K. (1995). The cognitive and neural bases of language acquisition. In M. S. Gazzaniga (ed.): *The Cognitive Neurosciences.* Cambridge: MIT Press.

Sur, M., Pallas, S. L., and Roe, A. W. (1990). Cross-modal plasticity in cortical development: Differentiation and specification of sensory neocortex. *Trends Neurosci., 13,* 227–233.

Tallal, P., Sainburg, R. L., and Jernigan, T. (1991). The neuropathology of developmental dysphasia: Behavioral, morphological, and physiological evidence for a pervasive temporal processing disorder. *Reading Writing, 3,* 363–377.

Thal, D., Marchman, V., Stiles, J., Aram, D., Trauner, D., Nass, R., and Bates, E. (1991). Early lexical development in children with focal brain injury. *Brain Lang., 40,* 491–527.

Thompson-Schill, S., D'Esposito, M., Aguirre, G., and Farah, M. (1997). Role of left prefrontal cortex in retrieval of semantic knowledge: A re-evaluation. *Soc. Neurosci. Abstr., 23,* 2227.

Tovee, M. J., Rolls, E. T., and Ramachandran, V. S. (1996). Rapid visual learning in neurons in the primate temporal cortex. *NeuroReport, 7,* 2757–2760.

Van der Lely, H. K. J. (1994). Canonical linking rules: Forward versus reverse linking in normally developing and specifically language-impaired children. *Cognition, 51,* 29–72.

Vargha-Khadem, F., Carr, L. J., Isaacs, E., Brett, E., Adams, C., and Mishkin, M. Onset of speech after left hemispherectomy in a nine-year-old boy. *Brain, 120,* 159–182.

Vargha-Khadem, F., Isaacs, E., and Muter, V. (1994). A review of cognitive outcome after unilateral lesions sustained during childhood. *J. Child Neurol. 9(Suppl.),* 2S67–2S73.

Weber-Fox, C. M., and Neville, H. J. (1996). Maturational constraints on functional specializations for language processing: ERP and behavioral evidence in bilingual speakers. *J. Cog. Neurosci., 8,* 231–256.

Webster, M. J., Bachevalier, J., and Ungerleider, L. G. (1995). Development of plasticity of visual memory circuits. In B. Julesz and I. Kovacs (eds.): *Maturational Windows and Adult Cortical Plasticity. Proceedings of the Santa Fe Institute Studies in the Sciences of complexity,* vol. 23. Reading, MA: Addison-Wesley, pp. 73–86.

Wernicke, C. (1977). The aphasia symptom complex: A psychological study on an anatomic basis. (N. Geschwind, Trans.) In G. H. Eggert (ed.): *Wernicke's Works on Aphasia: A Sourcebook and Review.* The Hague: Mouton. (Original work published 1874.)

Willmes, K., and Poeck, K. (1993). To what extent can aphasic syndromes be localized? *Brain, 116,* 1527–1540.

Wilson, A. C. (1985). The molecular basis of evolution. In J. Piel (ed.): *The Molecules of Life.* New York: W. H. Freeman, pp. 120–129.

Woods, B. T., and Teuber, H. L. (1978). Changing patterns of childhood aphasia. *Ann. Neurol., 3,* 272–280.

Zurif, E. (1980). Language mechanisms: A neuropsychological perspective. *Am. Sci., 68,* 305–311.

11

Neuroplasticity: Evidence from Unilateral Brain Lesions in Children

DOROTHY M. ARAM

A longstanding issue in developmental neuropsychology has been specialization versus plasticity in the neural substrates for various behavioral functions. Previous reports had suggested that early in life the two hemispheres were equivalent for language functioning (e.g., Marie, 1922), but Lenneberg was the one who was instrumental in developing the commonly held view that language functions were not lateralized early in childhood and that the two hemispheres were comparable in their ability to assume language. Lenneberg's thesis (1967) was that until 2 years of age a perfect equipotentiality existed for language residing in either hemisphere; that until 3 years of age, the right hemisphere "can easily adopt sole responsibility for language"; and that from 3 to 10 years of age when language has become localized predominantly in the left hemisphere "it is possible to re-establish language presumably by reactivating language functions in the right hemisphere" (pp. 180–181). Contrary to Lenneberg and his followers, evidence for anatomical and functional differences between the hemispheres in infants and young children has continued to build, suggesting that the substrate for at least some aspects of language specialization in the left hemisphere exists at a very early age (e.g., Molfese and Segalowitz, 1988).

One approach to studying this issue has been to examine the effects of unilateral brain lesions incurred in early childhood on various aspects of children's development, the approach taken in the study reported here. Our work has yielded evidence on the degree of early specialization versus plasticity of the brain for language in young children and has enabled us to speculate about how reorganization in language functions may occur. We have not directly addressed neuroplasticity. Rather, we have focused on *behavioral plasticity*, the ostensible recovery of behavior following a neural insult, from which *neural plasticity*, the compensatory neural events underlying the reorganization, can only be inferred.

Taken as a whole, our studies demonstrate in many respects a remarkable degree of behavioral plasticity based on the degree of function retained or recovered, presumably accounted for by a significant degree of neural plasticity. Yet there also appear to be limits to recovery, suggesting that equipotentiality does not exist even very early in life. We also present some limited data to suggest that, when recovery occurs, it does not necessarily involve the contralateral hemisphere. Other mechanisms of plasticity must explain the marked degree of development and/or recovery observed for language functions.

The Study

The findings reported here are based on work conducted at Rainbow Babies and Children's Hospital in Cleveland from 1981 to 1994 and supported by the National Institute of Neurological Disorders and Stroke. During that period all children seen as inpatients at Rainbow Babies and Children's Hospital or identified through chart review of the pediatric neurology or cardiology files who met specified criteria and agreed to participate were enrolled and followed for the duration of the study. Except for the presence of a congenital heart disorder in many of the lesioned children, all were developing normally prior to experiencing a unilateral brain lesion, and none presented any additional significant developmental or medical problems. No child was included in the study with a history of premature birth, neonatal complications beyond heart disorders, or identified or suspected genetic abnormalities.

Children with multiple infarcts (e.g., Moya Moya or sickle cell disease) or known or probable bilateral involvement were excluded, including those with lesions secondary to trauma or tumors. No child with an ongoing seizure disorder was included or retained in the study. Clinical neurological examinations and computed tomography (CT) and/or magnetic resonance imaging (MRI) scans were available for all lesioned children indicating the presence of a single unilateral lesion of vascular origin. Over the course of the investigation, the number of children included in any one study varied. This fluctuation occurred because children continued to be added to the study, a few could not be followed due to moving significant distances or death, and some studies required that children be within a certain age range to perform the required tasks. In the studies summarized here, all of the lesioned subjects were tested at least 1 year after lesion onset, thus excluding data from the acute period when ability levels shift rapidly. Over the course of the years we saw well over 100 children with brain lesions. However, many had to be excluded from these studies, usually due to questionable premorbid status or bilateral hemispheric involvement, most commonly the presence of an ongoing seizure disorder. At the conclusion of the study we had enrolled 25 children and adolescents with left hemisphere lesions and 15 with right hemisphere lesions. Age at study termination, age at lesion onset, gender, nature of lesion, and site of lesion are summarized in Table 11-1.

Control subjects were drawn from the population of children with congenital heart disorders seen at our hospital because a majority of lesioned subjects had underlying congenital heart disorders. None of the control subjects had experienced any neurological complications, and all were developing normally with the exception of their cardiac disorder. Each lesioned subject was matched individually to a

Table 11-1. Lesioned children: Subject characteristics and neurological status

	Left Lesioned ($n = 25$)	Right Lesioned ($n = 15$)
Current age (years, months)		
Mean	11.7	8.2
Range	1.3–20.5	0.7–21.2
Lesion onset (years, months)		
Mean	4.3	1.11
Range	0.0–15.11	0.0–9.8
Sex		
Boys	16	7
Girls	9	8
Nature of lesion		
Prenatal	9	7
Cerebral vascular accident	11	8
Arteriovenous malformation	4	0
Other	1	0
Site of Lesion		
Pre- and retrorolandic	2	3
Prerolandic only	6	1
Retrorolandic only	6	1
Subcortical only	5	7

control subject on the bases of age, gender, race, social class as determined by the Hollingshead Four-Factor Index of Social Status (Hollingshead and Redlich, 1958), and arterial blood oxygen saturation level. Lesioned subjects with congenital heart disorders were matched to controls with comparable oxygen saturation levels, while lesioned subjects free of heart disorders were matched to acyanotic controls.

The majority of our studies focused on various aspects of cognitive development, most specifically language and learning disabilities, although we also examined limb growth and the development of auditory functions. We summarize this work in the following sections, beginning with a study of limb growth and progressing to a series of studies addressing language and learning. We then examine the effects of age of lesion onset and site of lesion within a hemisphere on outcome functions and finally present two studies that address more directly the issue of neuroplasticity, a dichotic listening study and an electrophysiological study. The chapter concludes with a summary that pulls these behavioral data together and explores implications for defining the underlying neuroplasticity.

Developmental Outcomes

Limb growth

A study somewhat peripheral to our central interests of language and learning concerned the growth of the hand and foot contralateral to a lesion acquired in early childhood. While we will see that cognitive recovery is for the most part quite impressive, the primary residual functional deficit suffered by the majority of children with acquired lesions involves some degree of hemiparesis or weakness contralateral to the injury. We have shown that there are also changes in limb growth. Previously Satz et al. (1984) demonstrated that, unlike normals who show no systematic differences in foot length asymmetries, epileptic subjects with early onset left-sided foci had significantly shorter right than left feet, while those with early onset right-sided foci had significantly shorter left than right feet. In these earlier studies, however, neither age of lesion onset nor lesion site had been established, variables that were known in our population. Therefore, together with Paul Satz, Aram et al. (1986) reported measurements of foot and hand lengths for 15 neurologically normal children, 17 children with early CT-verified left cerebral lesions, and 12 with right lesions (Table 11-2). For left-lesioned subjects, the length of the left hand and foot significantly exceeded the right, while for right subjects the right hand and foot significantly exceeded the left. No significant foot and hand differences were found for normal controls. While these data suggest that asymmetrical foot and hand growth may serve as a biological marker for early cerebral lesions, they also demonstrate one area of development, limb growth, in which plasticity is limited.

Cognitive development

In contrast to limb growth we have seen very little if any loss of function in overall cognitive development as measured by standard intelligence tests for children with left hemisphere lesions and only minor degrees of impairment for right-lesioned children. In the first of two studies addressing IQ, we reported the level and pattern of performance for 18 left-lesioned and 13 right-lesioned children in comparison with their neurologically normal controls. Table 11-3 summarizes these findings. Verbal IQ (VIQ), performance IQ (PIQ), and full-scale IQ (FIQ) were all well within normal limits for all groups, although right-lesioned children scored significantly lower than did right controls on all three indices. No significant differences between VIQ, PIQ, and FIQ were found within the left-lesioned, right-lesioned, or control groups; thus VIQ and PIQ discrepancies were not found to be related to lesion laterality.

Table 11-2. Hand and foot measurement

Subjects	Mean Left Hand	Mean Right Hand	Mean Left Foot	Mean Right Foot
Left lesioned	14.41 cm ± 2.91	13.93 cm ± 2.87*	18.36 cm ± 3.75	17.86 cm ± 3.90[†]
Right lesioned	12.84 cm ± 1.94	13.56 cm ± 2.38[†]	17.51 cm ± 3.07	18.18 cm ± 3.53[†]
Controls	13.13 cm ± 1.60	13.17 cm ± 1.65	16.56 cm ± 2.65	16.48 cm ± 2.66

Source: Adapted from Aram et al. (1986).

*$p < 0.001$.

[†]$p < 0.01$.

Table 11-3. Intelligence quotients on the *Wechsler Intelligence Scale for Children-Revised* for left- and right-lesioned children compared with controls

	Left (n = 18)		Right (n = 13)		
	Lesioned	Control	Lesioned		Control
Verbal IQ					
M	109.56	116.89	107.08	*	114.54
SD	18.15	14.40	14.59		12.98
Performance IQ					
M	113.78	115.00	102.08	*	116.46
SD	12.27	13.21	12.24		9.03
Full-Scale IQ					
M	112.56	117.61	104.92	*	117.00
SD	15.16	14.53	13.06		12.00

Source: Adapted from Aram and Ekelman (1986).

*$p < 0.05$.

In a second study of intelligence test scores (Aram and Eisele, 1994), we retested the subjects several years later to determine stability of IQ over time. Previous studies (e.g., Banich et al., 1990) had suggested that among children with unilateral brain lesions, intelligence declines over time. Our data (Fig. 11-1) suggest that this is not true for left-lesioned children, although there does appear to be a decrement in IQ over time for the right-lesioned children, especially for verbal intelligence.

Why intelligence quotients for right- but not left-lesioned children show impairment that increases over time is not clear. Some researchers have attributed the differential effects of early left and right hemisphere damage to neuroanatomical differences in the organization and maturation of the two hemispheres (e.g., Corballis and Morgan, 1978; Goldberg and Costa, 1981; Gur et al., 1980). Corballis and Morgan (1978) proposed a *maturation gradient hypothesis* in which the left hemisphere undergoes a more rapid development than the right, leading to a predicted poorer developmental outcome following early right lesions due to the lack of uncommitted neural tissue in homotopic regions of the more mature left hemisphere. There is, however, considerable controversy over whether a hemispheric growth gradient exists and, if so, what direction it takes.

Based on clinical observations we speculated that right-lesioned children may present attentional problems that interfere with optimal learning. Yet our studies of attention thus far have been equivocal (Prather et al., 1999) and do not find consistent differences for the right-lesioned children. Alternatively, verbal intelligence, the area in which the right-lesioned children show the greatest impairment over time, is largely based on lexical knowledge, a linguistic area in which we see, in the following, that right-lesioned children show notable deficits.

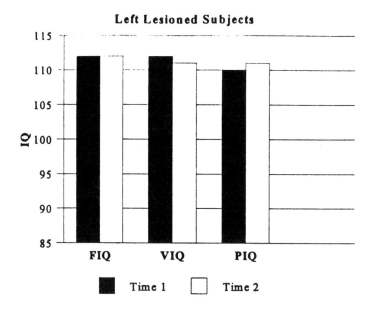

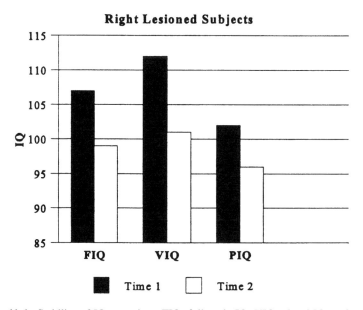

Figure 11-1. Stability of IQ over time. FIQ, full-scale IQ; VIQ, visual IQ; PIQ, performance IQ. (Adapted from Aram and Eisele, 1994.)

Language development

From the numerous studies we have carried out related to language and speech, we have elected to focus on two areas: one, syntactic development, which shows considerable left hemisphere specialization, and a second, lexical development, which appears to be more bilaterally distributed.

Syntactic development. Much of the early debate around language and the degree of hemispheric specialization centered on the role of the left hemisphere in subserving syntax (grammar). For right-handed adults, the left hemisphere has been demonstrated to be primarily responsible for syntactic abilities. Our studies have shown that this is also true for children. Unlike overall intelligence, which was not compromised following left hemisphere lesions, syntax, especially spoken syntax, never fully recovers.

One of our earliest studies compared the spoken syntax of eight left hemisphere–lesioned and eight right hemisphere–lesioned children with that of their controls. Based on analyses of spontaneous language samples, left hemisphere–lesioned subjects performed more poorly than did their controls on most measures of simple and complex sentence structures. In contrast, right-lesioned subjects (despite significantly lower IQs) performed similarly to their controls on these measures (Table 11-4).

We then undertook a study of syntactic comprehension using the Revised Token Test, which analyzes the contribution of verbal memory load as well as specific linguistic structures. Here, too, the left-lesioned children performed significantly poorer than their controls, especially on items that combined syntactic structures and increased memory load. Right-lesioned children did not differ significantly from their controls, although their performance was more erratic than the controls, especially on items that required increased memory, leading us to speculate that attentional limitations may have been a factor for right-lesioned children's performance.

A third study, in which we compared comprehension and production of identical syntactic structures, again evidenced syntactic deficits among the left- but not the right-lesioned subjects. In this study 16 children with early left hemisphere lesions, nine with right hemisphere lesions, and their neurologically normal controls were tested on comprehension (through an Act-Out Task) and production (through an Imitation Task) of several syntactic structures, including complex coordinate, passive, and relative clause structures. Here, too, the left-lesioned children were significantly impaired on the production task while comprehension was relatively preserved. Although right-lesioned subjects performed somewhat below normal controls, their deficits were less pronounced than those of left-lesioned subjects. Taken together, these studies provide substantial evidence for early left hemisphere specialization for syntactic production, with evident limits to the degree of plasticity possible following lesions of the left hemisphere.

Table 11-4. Spoken syntax in children with left or right lesions

	Left Subjects Compared With Left Controls	Right Subjects Compared With Right Controls
Overall Sentences		
Mean length of utterance	*	*
Developmental sentence scores: Complexity score	*	NS
% Total sentences correct	*	*
Simple sentences		
% Attempted	*	NS
% Correct	*	*
Complex sentences		
% Attempted	*	NS
% Correct	*	NS
Embeddings		
Number	*	NS
% Correct		
Conjunctions		
Number	NS	NS
% Correct	NS	NS
Developmental Sentence Scores		
Pronouns		
Mean	NS	NS
Total	NS	NS
Main Verb		
Mean	*	NS
Total	*	*
Interogative reversals		
Mean	*	NS
Total	*	NS
Wh-Questions		
Mean	*	NS
Total	*	NS
Negatives		
Mean	*	*
Total	NS	NS
Grammatical markers number	*	NS
Grammatical markers errors	*	*

Source: Adapted from Aram et al. (1987).

NS, Not significant, randomization test for matched pair.

*Significant at < 0.05.

Lexical development and retrieval. In contrast to syntax, Elizabeth Bates and her colleagues (1997) have provided evidence of the importance of both the left and right hemispheres for the early development of the lexicon. Working with a younger population than most of the children we have followed, Bates (see Chapter 10) has shown that infants and very young children (10–17 months of age) with right hemisphere injury are at greater risk for delays in lexical comprehension. Our studies, generally with somewhat older children extending into adolescence, have substantiated these findings, showing that for lexical learning both hemispheres have a role in recovery/development and that following injury to either hemisphere recovery/reorganization is not complete.

In one of our studies (Eisele and Aram, 1993), the effect of early hemisphere damage on lexical development was investigated with 21 left-lesioned, 12 right-lesioned, and 16 neurologically normal controls. Single-word naming was assessed using the Expressive One-Word Picture Vocabulary Test (EOWPVT) and lexical comprehension was assessed using the Peabody Picture Vocabulary Test–Revised (PPVT-R). Left-lesioned subjects scored comparably to controls in naming, but scored lower than controls on the lexical comprehension task. Right-lesioned subjects scored lower than controls and left-lesioned subjects on both the comprehension and the production tasks. These data led us to suggest that the superiority of the left-lesioned subjects in comparison to the right-lesioned children on both the lexical comprehension and production tasks argued against a simple left hemisphere dominance for early lexical development. Furthermore, the right-lesioned subjects' significant comprehension deficits failed to correlate with more general measures of verbal intelligence, supporting a specialized role of the right hemisphere in mediating the acquisition of word meaning. Our data are in substantial agreement with those of Bates that both hemispheres, but especially the right, serve lexical development and that neither hemisphere, when damaged, can fully compensate for the persistent, albeit mild, deficits that occur.

We also have examined the accuracy and rate of lexical retrieval following lateralized brain lesions in children (Aram et al., 1987). Here we used an experimental measure, the Word-Finding Test, developed by Wiegel-Crump and Dennis (1984). In this task, subjects were asked to retrieve words in three cuing conditions involving semantic, rhyming (phonological), and visual cues. Left-lesioned children were significantly slower than left controls in retrieving words when given semantic and visual cues and made more errors when given rhyming cues. There were no significant differences between the right-lesioned subjects and their controls. On a second measure of lexical retrieval, the Rapid Automatized Naming Test, left-lesioned subjects were significantly slower than left controls in naming all semantic categories, including colors, numbers, objects, and letters. In contrast, right-lesioned subjects responded as or more quickly than did right controls in all access conditions and in naming semantic categories, yet tended to produce more errors than their controls, evidencing a speed-accuracy tradeoff. These findings suggest that the left hemisphere appears to moderate rate of lexical retrieval and is not totally compensated for by other areas of the brain when damaged.

Academic achievement

Reading and spelling. Prompted by the assumption that subtle residual language deficits may well be revealed in more demanding tasks involving reading, we undertook an extensive study of reading and spelling abilities of the children with lesions (Aram et al., 1990). Twenty left hemisphere-lesioned and 10 right hemisphere-lesioned children between 6 and 20 years of age were administered a battery of tests assessing phonological analysis and segmentation, single-word decoding, reading comprehension, and spelling. Although mean performance on all tasks was consistently below that of control subjects, few differences reached statistical significance. These findings demonstrated that the majority of children with early unilateral brain lesions learn to read and spell quite adequately, evidencing considerable functional reorganization of the higher cognitive functions involved in these skills. Contrary to predictions of models based on adults and normal readers, left-lesioned children did not have significantly more difficulty than their controls on tasks of phonological analysis or decoding or spelling of phonologically regular words. Yet five left- and two right-lesioned children did present marked reading deficits in contrast to 1 of 30 control subjects. A family history of reading disorders was implicated in one left-lesioned, one right-lesioned and the control subject, raising the question of the possibility of a genetic basis. All left-lesioned children with involvement of specific subcortical structures did, however, present reading disorders along with other language learning problems, a finding we return to in greater detail.

Mathematics. We then administered a standardized test of mathematic ability (Stanford Diagnostic Mathematics Test) and a battery of experimental tests that examined components of numerical and arithmetic processing to a group of 18 left-lesioned and 9 right-lesioned children and their controls (Ashcraft et al., 1992). We concluded that left lesions during childhood yield more pervasive deficits in mathematics than do right lesions. These deficits were apparent across a broad range of cognitive processes involved in numbers and mathematics, from straightforward oral counting through complex written subtraction. The pattern of deficits by age subgroups suggested that the effect of the lesion was to slow or interfere with a child's mastery of numerical and arithmetic information. That is, younger left-lesioned subjects, and/or subjects with earlier lesion onset, seemed to lag behind their age-matched controls, both in declarative (efficient retrieval of simple math facts) and procedural (e.g., mastery of complex borrowing algorithm in subtraction) knowledge. Right-lesioned subjects demonstrated similar though less pronounced and more limited deficits. Despite the clear and significant deficits demonstrated, very few of the subjects exhibited pronounced or widespread impairments, such as those often observed following lateralized lesions among adults. This finding again demonstrates both a degree of left hemispheric specialization for mathematics early in childhood and a substantial capacity for functional reorganization.

Age of Lesion Onset

One factor thought to be related to level of functioning/recovery following acquired brain lesions in children has been age of lesion onset. It has been assumed in much of the earlier literature that there is a direct relationship between the age of lesion onset and the severity of residual deficit, that is, the later the lesion the greater the deficit. Kennard (1938), for example, advanced this principle to explain the relative sparing of motor functions following ablation of motor and premotor cortex in infant monkeys in comparison to pronounced deficits in adult monkeys. As mentioned earlier, this perspective was also advanced in Lenneberg (1967), who claimed that prior to 2 years of age recovery of language would be complete, attributing the absence of deficits following early lesions to the equipotentiality of the brain thought to exist early in development. Others, however, have suggested that earlier lesions would result in more pervasive deficits than would lesions acquired later (e.g., Basser, 1962). Therefore, throughout our studies we have examined the relationship between age of lesion onset and level of language and learning ability. I will exemplify our findings from two studies and then summarize findings across studies.

Table 11-5 presents our findings for Wechsler Intelligence Scale for Children–Revised IQ scores for children sustaining lesions prior to versus after 1 year of age (Aram and Ekelman, 1986). Performance IQ is significantly lower for left-lesioned children sustaining injury prior to versus after 1 year of age. Other than that, there are no significant differences in verbal, performance, or full-scale IQ between either left- or right-lesioned children sustaining lesion onset before or after 1 year of

Table 11-5. IQ and lesion onset before or after 1 year of age: Mean performance, Mann-Whitney (U), and Results

	Left-Lesioned Children				Right-Lesioned Children			
	Onset <1 Year (n = 7)	Onset >1 Year (n = 11)	U	P	Onset <1 Year (n = 5)	Onset >1 Year (n = 8)	U	P
Verbal IQ								
M	108.14	110.45	36.5	0.8561	105.40	106.83	17.5	0.7140
Mean rank	9.79	9.32			6.50	7.31		
Performance IQ								
M	107.86	117.55	15.0	0.0321*	107.20	97.83	11.5	0.2121
Mean rank	6.14	11.64			8.70	5.97		
Full-Scale IQ								
M	108.57	115.09	35.0	0.7513	106.40	102.67	15.5	0.5071
Mean rank	9.00	9.82			7.90	6.44		

Source: Adapted from Aram and Ekelman (1986).

*$p < 0.05$.

age. If anything, there is a tendency for left-lesioned children with lesions before 1 year of age to perform consistently more poorly than those incurring lesions after 1 year of age. We also see the suggestion of a differential effect of lesion laterality on IQ for children with both left and right lesions after, but not before, 1 year of age. That is, after 1 year of age verbal IQ begins to be impaired to a greater extent than performance IQ for children with left hemisphere lesions, and the converse emerges for children with right hemisphere lesions.

Data from a second study (Table 11-6) reporting findings on the Woodock-Johnson Psycho-Educational Battery compared performances of children sustaining lesions prior to versus after 2 years of age. This study revealed essentially the same findings of no significant difference in performance between children with early and late onset of lesions (Aram and Ekelman, 1988). Again we see a tendency for children with earlier lesions, especially left hemisphere lesions, to perform more poorly than those with later lesion onset, most notably in areas of academic achievement.

Across several studies using different statistical approaches, including examining age as a continuous variable, findings have been essentially the same. We conclude that there is no predictable relationship between age of lesion onset and level of performance on language and learning tasks. If anything, earlier rather than latter lesions are associated with more pronounced deficits. These findings are consistent with findings from other populations of children with more diffuse brain involvement, such as prophylactic central nervous system irradiation for cancer (see Fletcher and Copeland, 1988, for a review), *Haemophilus influenzae* meningitis (Taylor, 1987), and head injury (Levin et al., 1982). These findings also provide at least weak support for Hebb's 1942 "vulnerability hypothesis," which argued for greater susceptibility to injury during early stages of neural maturation, resulting in a greater loss of generalized "intellectual power" necessary for subsequent acquisition of novel information. In contrast, injury sustained in adulthood results in a more selective loss of acquired knowledge.

Site of Lesion

A second factor clearly related to the presence of cognitive deficits in adults has been site of lesion within the hemisphere. Again, throughout our studies we have examined this variable, although we have been severely limited in the conclusions we can draw because of the very low number of children presenting with discrete lesions confined to different parts of the brain. In the early years of this study, findings were based on CT scans, although when MRI emerged all subjects who were eligible (e.g., no surgical clips or pacemakers) were rescanned with MRI. Lesion locations were defined by neuroradiologists blind to the clinical status of the subjects. Initially we categorized subjects as having lesions involving the following areas: prerolandic only, retrorolandic only, cortical only, and subcortical only. Currently, Michael Alexander, at the Boston Veterans Administration, who has studied the relationship between subcortical lesion sites and speech and language

Table 11-6. Age of lesion onset: Woodcock-Johnson Psycho-Educational Battery—mean percentile performance

	Left-Lesioned Subjects				Right-Lesioned Subjects			
	<2 Year (n = 10)	>2 Year (n = 10)	U	Probability	<2 Year (n = 6)	>2 Year (n = 6)	U	Probability
Cognitive								
Verbal ability	54.2	61.2	42.0	0.545	52.8	52.2	16.5	0.810
Reasoning	62.7	57.6	42.5	0.570	41.3	54.3	12.0	0.336
Perceptual speed	57.8	52.4	44.5	0.677	47.7	37.5	15.0	0.631
Memory	53.4	58.2	45.0	0.705	43.8	49.3	17.5	0.936
Scholastic Aptitude								
Reading	58.1	57.9	48.0	0.880	55.8	43.7	14.0	0.522
Math	70.3	61.8	47.5	0.850	55.8	52.3	17.0	0.872
Written language	66.0	70.5	36.5	0.307	48.3	57.8	18.0	1.00
Knowledge	67.8	67.5	44.0	0.650	51.0	60.2	15.0	0.631
Academic Achievement								
Reading	46.3	57.8	37.5	0.540	34.8	53.5	12.0	0.337
Math	55.6	69.5	28.0	0.165	38.2	41.5	17.5	0.936
Written language	52.7	66.8	31.0	0.252	45.2	46.3	17.0	0.872

Source: Adapted from Aram and Ekelman (1988).

U, Mann-Whitney U test.

deficits in adults, is rereading all our scans and refining the classification to specify in greater detail the anatomical sites involved. Here I exemplify our findings
with data drawn from two earlier studies and then draw more general conclusions
relative to the relationship between site of lesion and cognitive deficits among the
children we have studied.

Table 11-7 presents verbal, performance, and full-scale IQ scores for left- and
right-lesioned children according to site of lesion (Aram and Ekelman, 1986). The
small number of children in any one cell precludes statistical treatment of these
data. Examining the mean IQ scores for the left-lesioned children, we see very little difference by site of lesion except for the three subjects with subcortical-only
lesions where a marked lesion laterality effect is apparent with a mean VIQ of 108
and a mean PIQ of 126. Children with left retrorolandic lesions had somewhat lower IQs than those with prerolandic lesions, but the differences are not great and are
based on few children. The small number of right-lesioned children present a more
variable picture. Here, too, however, we see the suggestion of a lesion laterality
effect for those with subcortical-only lesions, with a mean VIQ of 115 and a mean
PIQ of 102. Scores for academic achievement (Table 11-8) also suggest that children with left subcortical lesions are particularly impaired in comparison to children with lesion sites elsewhere in the left hemisphere (Aram and Ekelman, 1988).

Especially for reading and for written language achievement, the four children
with left lesions involving only subcortical areas present notably poorer performance than children with only left cortical involvement. In contrast, right-lesioned
children present the opposite pattern: Those with cortical involvement present substantially lower performance than those with only subcortical involvement. Again,
these observations are based on a very small group of children, and their interpretation is unclear. Nonetheless, one finding that continues to emerge across studies
is that children with left subcortical lesions present the most severe and persistent

Table 11-7. Site of lesion and mean Verbal (VIQ), Performance (PIQ)
and Full-Scale (FIQ) IQ Values

	n	WISC-R Mean IQ		
		VIQ	PIQ	FIQ
Left Lesion				
Prerolandic only	4	115.00	119.75	119.00
Retrorolandic only	6	107.50	104.00	106.33
Cortical only	9	107.89	109.33	109.22
Subcortical only	3	108.00	125.67	118.00
Right Lesion				
Prerolandic only	3	97.00	107.33	101.33
Retrorolandic only	2	103.50	98.00	101.00
Cortical only	5	98.20	102.00	99.40
Subcortical only	5	115.80	102.40	110.20

Source: Adapted from Aram and Ekelman (1986).

Table 11-8. Site of lesion: Woodcock-Johnson Psycho-Educational Battery—Mean percentile performance

	Left-Lesioned Subjects								Right-Lesioned Subjects					
Academic Achievement	Prerolandic (n = 4)	Retrorolandic (n = 6)	U	Probability	Cortical (n = 9)	Subcortical (n = 4)	U	Probability	Prerolandic (n = 3)	Retrorolandic (n = 1)	Cortical (n = 4)	Subcortical (n = 6)	U	Probability
Reading	66.3	61.2	11.0	0.831	61.3	36.5	8.0	0.122	38.3	22.0	34.5	61.0	5.0	0.136
Math	71.8	75.3	10.0	0.670	63.2	57.0	18.0	1.000	26.7	42.0	22.5	56.0	2.0	0.033*
Written language	68.8	71.0	10.0	0.669	69.9	40.3	10.0	0.217	31.3	25.0	36.0	63.2	4.0	0.087†

Source: Adapted from Aram and Ekelman (1988).

U, Mann-Whitney U test.

*Significant at <0.05.

†Significant at <0.10.

deficits. For example, in a study of syntactic comprehension and production (Eisele and Aram, 1994), the two subjects with the most pronounced deficits in both comprehension and production had relatively small lesions involving anterior and posterior subcortical structures. Similarly, in our comprehensive study of reading (Aram et al., 1990), all left-lesioned children with involvement of specific subcortical structures presented significant reading disorders along with other language learning problems. In that study we concluded that, for the left-lesioned group, cortical involvement did not differentiate lesioned subjects with and without reading disorders. All of the left-lesioned subjects with lesions involving the head of the caudate, putamen, and external and internal capsule did present reading disorders along with other language and/or memory disorders. We speculated that these subcortical areas may play a necessary role in the development of higher cognitive functions and may be less capable than cortical areas of reorganizing if damaged at an early age. Our somewhat unexpected findings related to subcortical lesions has lead us to study in greater detail subcortical sites and their relationship to observed deficits, a study currently in progress with Michael Alexander.

Hemispheric Organization

Two of our studies provide more direct evidence of hemispheric reorganization for cognitive functions following unilateral brain lesions. The first of these was a study of auditory processing conducted by Murray (1987). In this study 17 left-lesioned and 11 right-lesioned children were compared with their controls on a battery of linguistic and nonlinguistic central auditory processing measures. Peripheral hearing and speech discrimination for undistorted words were normal for all lesioned and control subjects. All subjects were administered a battery of dichotic and distorted monotic measures. The data revealed that lesioned children experienced greater difficulty centrally processing linguistic auditory stimuli from the ear contralateral to the lesion. Thus left-lesioned children lost the normal right ear preference, and right-lesioned children demonstrated an enhanced right ear advantage. These ear preferences were observed for processing both linguistic and nonlinguistic stimuli and resemble the ear preference patterns typically seen following hemispheric lesions in adults. The findings also demonstrate that functional takeover by the right hemisphere in cases of acquired left lesions is not complete, and the right hemisphere does not fully compensate for the loss of function by the impaired left hemisphere. Furthermore, children with right lesions also demonstrate auditory perceptual deficits for linguistically based stimuli for which the unimpaired left hemisphere is not compensating. This study demonstrates considerable hemispheric specialization for auditory processing and limitations to the degree to which these processes are "transferred" to the contralateral hemisphere.

A second study examined even more directly the hemisphere responsible for recovery of functions following a unilateral brain lesion (Papanicolaou et al., 1990). This study involved the use of the probe evoked potential (EP) paradigm, which consists of recording EPs to a repetitive probe stimulus (e.g., a click for auditory conditions and a strobe flash for visual conditions) presented during a control condition when subjects attend exclusively to this repetitive stimulus and during an experimental condition when subjects are engaged in a cognitive task. The dependent measure was the amplitude of the EPs to the experimental probe stimulus recorded from surface electrodes over left and right hemispheric sites. Normal adults show greater left hemisphere attenuation during language tasks in their auditory probe EPs and greater right hemisphere attenuation during visuospatial tasks. The degree of relative attenuation is interpreted as the degree of hemispheric engagement.

For this study the experimental condition involved a phonological target detection task in which a series of unrelated words spoken at 0.5 words per second was presented through earphones and the subjects were required to signal by raising both index fingers, the presence of a word beginning with *br, p,* or *m.* The visuospatial task consisted of a block rotation task projected on a screen, in which the subject was required to indicate if the block configurations were the same (identified by raising the right index finger) or different (raising the left index finger). Fourteen left-lesioned subjects were compared with their controls. Unlike recovered adult aphasics previously studied with this paradigm who showed a right hemisphere engagement during the phonological detection task, our left-lesioned children displayed the normal pattern of predominant left-hemisphere engagement during the linguistic tasks and right hemisphere engagement during the visuospatial task. Furthermore, the lesioned children's normal right hemisphere attenuation during the mental rotation task did not provide support for an alteration of visuospatial functions subserved by the right hemisphere, as would be expected in accordance with the "verbal sparing" or right hemisphere "crowding" hypotheses. We concluded that these data suggest that language restitution (at least for this phonological detection task) and development following early lesions involves intrahemispheric rather than interhemispheric functional reorganization, that is, reorganization within the same hemisphere rather than transfer to the nondominant hemisphere.

Summary and Conclusions

Across a variety of language and learning tasks, including spoken syntax, syntactic comprehension, lexical development and retrieval, and mathematics, left-lesioned children as a group present mild deficits in abilities in comparison to normally developing peers. Among right-lesioned children, for the abilities studied here, differences in ability level were confined to indices of intelligence and to lexical development. These findings, while suggesting some degree of lateralization of early brain specialization for different aspects of language and learning in young children, also demonstrate the marked recovery and presumed reorganization of language abilities in young children in comparison to adults with similar brain lesions. Interestingly, both limb growth and auditory processing of linguistic and nonlinguistic information evidenced significant residual deficits contralateral to lesions in either hemisphere, suggesting that these more basic sensory and motor aspects of development may be less amenable to reorganization than other higher cognitive functions.

Age of lesion onset was not found to have a consistent relationship to outcome, although there is some suggestion that if anything, earlier lesions may be associated with more pronounced deficits. Lesions involving left subcortical structures were associated with the most persistent and pronounced residual deficits, demonstrating that these structures may play a role in the development of higher cognitive functions and may be less amenable to reorganization following lesions sustained in early childhood. Finally, results of dichotic listening and EP studies suggest that recovery following early lateralized lesions involve predominantly intra- rather than interhemispheric reorganization.

Overall these studies evidence a considerable degree of behavioral plasticity for higher cognitive functions following lateralized brain lesions in children. In the absence of additional complications, children with unilateral brain lesions may anticipate a relatively good prognosis for language and learning. While these studies have detailed outcome for many aspects of language and academic achievement, investigation addressing the differential effect of various sites of lesion and the actual functional reorganization (neural plasticity) that occurs following an acquired lesion has only begun. Studying the effects of site of lesion has been limited by two primary factors: failure of investigators to document site of lesion using sensitive neuroimaging techniques that are now available, such as MRI, and the rare occurrence in children of discrete lesions affecting specified areas of the brain. Future investigators should be encouraged to document site of lesion and analyze findings with respect to contrasting sites of lesion.

Collaborative studies provides one means of amassing a larger number of children with discrete lesions, while detailed case reports of single subjects offer a second alternative. Although several methods have been available for study of central nervous system reorganization for some time, earlier methods were limited in their applicability to children often because of task requirements or the use of radiation. In addition to the use of electrophysiological techniques, functional MRI provides a powerful means for furthering our understanding of the neural plasticity that can account for the considerable behavioral plasticity we and others have reported.

References

Aram, D. M., and Eisele, J. A. (1994). Intellectual stability in children with unilateral brain lesions. *Neuropsychologia, 32,* 85–95.

Aram, D. M., and Ekelman, B. L. (1986). Cognitive profiles of children with early onset unilateral lesions. *Dev. Neuropsychol., 2,* 155–172.

Aram, D. M., and Ekelman, B. L. (1988). Scholastic aptitude and achievement among children with unilateral brain lesions. *Neuropsychologia, 26,* 903–916.

Aram, D. M., Ekelman, B. L., and Satz, P. (1986). Trophic changes following early unilateral injury to the brain. *Dev. Med. Child Neurol., 28,* 165–170.

Aram, D. M., Ekelman, B. L., and Whitaker, H. A. (1987). Lexical retrieval in left and right brain lesioned children. *Brain Lang., 31,* 61–87.

Aram, D. M., Gillespie, L. L., and Yamashita, T. S. (1990). Reading among children with left and right brain lesions. *Dev. Neuropsychol., 6,* 301–317.

Ashcraft, M. H., Yamashita, T. S., and Aram, D. M. (1992). Mathematics performance in left and right brain-lesioned children and adolescents. *Brain Cogn., 19,* 208–252.

Banich, M. T., Levine, S. C., Kim, H., and Huttenlocher, P. (1990). The effects of developmental factors on IQ in hemiplegic children. *Neuropsychologia, 28,* 35–47.

Basser, L. S. (1962). Hemiplegia of early onset and the faculty of speech with special reference to the effect of hemispherectomy. *Brain, 85,* 427–460.

Bates, E., Thal, D., Trauner, D., Fenson, J., Aram, D., Eisele, J., and Nass, R. (1997). From first words to grammar in children with focal brain injury. Special Issue on Origins of Language Disorders. *Dev. Neuropsychol., 13,* 275–343.

Corballis, M., and Morgan, M. (1978). On the biological basis of human laterality: Evidence for a maturational left gradient. *Behav. Brain Sci., 2,* 261–336.

Eisele, J. A., and Aram, D. M. (1993). Differential effects of early hemisphere damage on lexical comprehension and production. *Aphasiology, 5,* 513–523.

Eisele, J. A., and Aram, D. M. (1994). Comprehension and imitation of syntax following early hemisphere damage. *Brain Lang., 46,* 212–231.

Fletcher, J. M., and Copeland, D. R. (1988). Neurobehavioral effects of central nervous system prophylactic treatment of cancer in children. *J. Clin. Exp. Neuropsychol., 10,* 495–538.

Goldberg, E., and Costa, L. D. (1981). Hemisphere differences in the acquisition and use of descriptive systems. *Brain Lang., 14,* 144–173.

Gur, R. C., Packer, I. K., Hungerbuhler, J. P., Reivich, M., Obrist, W. D., Amarnek, W. S., and Sackeim, H. A. (1980). Differences in the distribution of gray and white matter in human cerebral hemispheres. *Science, 207,* 1226–1228.

Hebb, D. O. (1942). The effect of early and late brain injury upon test scores, and the nature of normal adult intelligence. *Proc. Am. Philos. Soc., 85,* 275–292.

Hollingshead, A. B., and Redlich, F. C. (1958). *Social Class and Mental Illness.* New York: Wiley & Sons, Inc.

Kennard, M. A. (1938). Reorganization of motor function in the cerebral cortex of monkeys deprived of motor and premotor areas in infancy. *J. Neurophysiol., 1,* 477–496.

Lennenberg, E. (1967). *Biological Foundations of Language.* New York: Wiley.

Levin, H. S., Benton, A. L., and Grossman, R. G. (1982). *Neurobehavioral Consequences of Closed Head Injury.* New York: Plenum.

Marie, P. (1922). Existe-il dans le cerveau humain des centres innes ou preformes de langage? *Presse Med., 17,* 117–181.

Molfese, D. L., and Segalowitz, S. J. (eds.) (1988). *Brain Lateralization in Children: Developmental Implications.* New York: Guilford Press.

Murray, G. S. (1986). *Auditory Processing of Children With Acquired Unilateral Lesions.* Unpublished Doctoral Dissertation. Cleveland: Case Western Reserve University.

Papanicolaou, A. C., DiScenna, A., Gillespie, L., and Aram, D. M. (1990). Probe-evoked potential findings following unilateral left-hemisphere lesions in children. *Arch. Neurol., 47,* 562–566.

Prather, P., Ebersole, A., and Aram, D. M. (1999). *Attention Abilities in Children With Unilateral Brain Lesions.* Manuscript in preparation.

Satz, P., Yanowitz, J., and Willmore, J. (1984). Early brain damage and lateral development.

In R. Bell, J. Elias, R. Green, and J. Harvey (eds.): *Interfaces in Psychology.* Lubbock: Texas Tech Press, pp. 87–107.

Taylor, H. G. (1987). Childhood sequelae of early neurological disorders: A contemporary perspective. *Dev. Neuropsychol., 3,* 153–164.

Wiegel-Crump, C. A., and Dennis, M. (1984). *The Word-Finding Test.* Toronto: The Hospital for Sick Children. Experimental, unpublished test.

12

Continuity and Change in the Development of Children with Autism

MARIAN SIGMAN AND NORMAN KIM

The extent to which a child with autism continues to develop in the same way during his or her life is of the utmost importance to everyone concerned. Autism is characterized by pervasive impairments in social interactions and communication that are manifested in the first 3 years of life. The most compelling question asked by parents at the time of diagnosis, usually when the child is quite young, is whether the child will be able to have a "normal life." Implicit in this question is the issue of change and continuity—whether the child will ever be able to relate socially to other people, learn to speak and communicate with others, function independently, and abstain from the repetitive and stereotyped behaviors that characterize children with autism. The deficits in social communication that define autism are evidenced to some degree irrespective of intellectual ability (Szatmari et al., 1989). Individual outcomes, however, evince considerable variability, ranging from a very small number of autistic adults who manage to achieve relative normalcy in their level of functioning to the majority who continue to suffer significant impairments throughout their lives. Defining those characteristics of the disorder that tend to remain stable and those that show change represents an initial approach toward identifying the extent and nature of plasticity in the development of children with autism.

The investigation of continuity and change in any individual child is complicated by the enormous developmental transformations that occur in the lives of typically developing children. Unlike height and weight, which can be measured by the same metric across the life span, the abilities and behaviors of most children must be assessed with very different measures across even fairly short periods of time because of the reorganizations in their capacities. In addition, complex skills often build on simpler accomplishments. As an example, nonverbal communicative and symbolic skills may be precursors, or even prerequisites, for the acquisition of language. For this reason, infants who are more capable of nonverbal communication may become more verbally adept in childhood than less communicatively capable infants. As another example, infants who can use detour strategies to reach a blocked goal may be better at vocational planning in adulthood. Although the particular behaviors measured at the initial assessment are qualitatively different from those measured later, and therefore require different methods of measurement, both are presumed to be reflective of the same latent construct (e.g., communicative/symbolic ability and cognitive flexibility in the respective examples). Thus, we are often interested not only in the stability of identical behaviors over time but also in the continuity of processes underlying different but related behaviors (Bornstein and Sigman, 1986).

In this chapter, we review what is known about continuity and change, starting with the issue of the stability of the disorder and its symptoms. Following this, we assess the extent to which there is stability or change in the tested intelligence of children with autism. From there, we examine the extent to which there is stability in the central deficits in verbal and nonverbal communicative skills, representational play, social responsiveness, theory of mind, and executive functioning. Finally, we review what is known about underlying continuity in the development of communicative skills and social relationships.

Definition of the Disorder

We cannot begin to look for continuity and change in the underlying processes of development in children with autism until the disorder has been defined. The goal of the earliest longitudinal studies of children with autism was to describe the disorder of autism and its course (DeMeyer et al., 1973; Eisenberg, 1956; Gittelman and Birch, 1967; Kanner, 1971; Mittler et al., 1966; Rutter and Lockyer, 1967). These investigations accomplished a great deal in terms of both defining the disorder of autism and evaluating the extent to which symptoms that differentiated autistic children from children with other disorders remained stable over time. The results showed that *(1)* individuals with autism do not generally recover from the disorder; *(2)* the ability to use productive language by age 5 years is a major predictor of better outcomes; *(3)* the intelligence scores of most children with autism are significantly below average; *(4)* problems with language and social relations continue even for children with better intellectual performance; and *(5)* childhood autism is very different in symptoms and course from childhood schizophrenia. This information was crucial for determining the pivotal symptoms and establishing the criteria for the diagnosis of the syndrome: significant impairments in social reciprocity and understanding, delay and/or deviance in language use, and stereotyped or circumscribed behavior and interests.

The emphasis in the period of research that followed these studies has been on the identification of central psychological and physiological deficits. With this aim, cross-sectional comparisons of individuals with autism and individuals with other syndromes have dominated the research literature. Using models from developmental psychology and neuropsychology to guide the processes investigated, these studies have provided a clearer picture of some of the psychological disorders of children with autism. This information, along with newly standardized instruments for diagnosis (e.g., the Autism Diagnostic Interview [Le Couteur et al., 1989] and the Autism Diagnostic Observation Schedule [Lord et al., 1989]), can now be used to promote our understanding of continuity and change in the development of children with autism.

Continuity and Change in the Disorder and Symptoms of Autism

A critical issue is the extent to which children diagnosed with autism remain affected throughout their lives. Several investigators have examined a group of autistic children in early childhood and followed them into early or late adolescence. Using diagnoses made by the same clinician, group of clinicians, or diagnostic instrument at two time points, these studies suggest that most individuals with autism remain as severely affected by the disorder in adolescence as in childhood (Cantwell et al., 1989; Chung et al., 1990; DeMeyer et al., 1973; Eisenberg, 1956; Gillberg and Steffenburg, 1987; Kanner, 1971; Lord and Schopler, 1989a,b; Lotter, 1978; Venter et al., 1992). Similarly, using a global classification scheme that categorizes life adjustment from good to very poor (Lotter, 1978), most investigations report that individuals followed into adulthood continue to have very significant handicaps. Taken together, longitudinal studies suggest that 10%–15% of adults with autism have good outcomes; 15%–25% have fair outcomes; 15%–25% have poor outcomes; and 30%–50% have very poor outcomes.

While these studies show that the life adaptation of most individuals with autism does not improve as they age, there have been few studies of the continuity of the diagnosis of autism or the stability of particular symptoms over time. The major reason for the paucity of studies of diagnostic continuity is that, until recently, diagnoses were made by clinicians who frequently used varying criteria for the disorder. Even after diagnostic systems had been formulated and circulated, standardized interviews and observations were lacking so that comparability between diagnosed groups could not be assumed. Observational measures, such as the Childhood Autism Rating Scale (Schopler et al., 1986) and the Autism Behavior Checklist (Krug et al., 1980) did not become available until about 10 years ago and have not been very widely used. Moreover, these systems are appropriate for the diagnosis of young children and do not apply to many older individuals, particularly those who are autistic but not mentally retarded. The recent creation of the Autism Diagnostic Interview (Le Couteur et al., 1989) and the Autism Diagnostic Observation Schedule (Lord et al., 1989), which are designed for diagnoses across the full range of intellectual and chronological development, should facilitate studies of diagnostic and symptom stability.

In our recent longitudinal follow up of a group of 50 children with autism, diagnosed at ages 3–5 years with a variety of procedures,* the Autism Diagnostic Interview–Revised was administered to the parents of subjects about 8–9 years after the original diagnosis (Sigman and Ruskin, 1999). At the time the follow up study was begun, no standardized diagnostic observation was available that was applicable to all of our subjects. The Autism Diagnostic Interview is designed so that a determination can be made as to whether the individual ever met the criteria for diagnosis as well as whether the individual currently meets the criteria. All 50 subjects met the "ever" criteria, while 45 subjects met the "current" criteria for diagnosis. All five subjects who did not meet the current criteria for diagnosis continued to suffer from significant disabilities.

In contrast to the group of subjects originally diagnosed with autism, only 4 of 33 subjects originally diagnosed as developmentally delayed met the current criteria for diagnosis of autism. These four subjects also made the "ever" criteria based on parental recollection of their behavior at younger ages. None of them, however, had been diagnosed as autistic using either the Childhood Autism Rating Scale or the Autism Behavior Checklist at recruitment, and only one appeared autistic currently to clinicians.

These results suggest that most children diagnosed with autism between 3–5 years continue to show all the symptoms of autism later in childhood and adolescence. In contrast, children who do not meet the criteria for diagnosis at 3–5 years do not develop the full range of autistic symptoms later in life. An obvious limitation of this study is that the follow-up diagnosis depended solely on the parental interview. In addition, standardized diagnostic information was only available for part of the sample at intake, and the same diagnostic instruments were not used at both intake and follow up. Furthermore, the results may be generalizable only to children with classic forms of autism because relatively strict diagnostic standards were used at intake. There may be less continuity among children whose diagnosis is less evident.

Even if children continue to be diagnosed as autistic, the nature of their symptoms may change over time. As an example, some cross-sectional studies suggest that older children show less stereotypic behavior than younger children, and this may be particularly true for high-functioning children with autism. However, one investigation of adults with autism noted a very high rate of stereotyped behavior, with some of the high-functioning subjects inhibiting or disguising these behaviors in public (Rumsey et al., 1985). If a child develops language, a lack of verbal skills may be replaced by language that is stilted, lacking in prosody, and marked by pronominal reversals (e.g. saying *you* or *she* instead of *I*). Without longitudinal studies that measure the same symptoms over time, it is difficult to determine how much change there is in the symptoms shown by children as they develop.

*Most initial diagnoses were performed using the *Diagnostic and Statistical Manual* (3rd ed.) (APA, 1980) criteria arrived at by the consensus of having met criteria for a diagnosis of infantile autism on at least two of the following three methods: *(1)* clinical diagnosis by one or more independent clinicians from the UCLA Center for Research on Childhood Psychoses or an inpatient unit in the Neuropsychiatric Institute, *(2)* Childhood Autism Rating Scale (Schopler et al., 1986) scored from a videotaped observation, and *(3)* a parent interview with the Autism Behavior Checklist (Krug et al., 1978).

Continuity and Change in Intelligence Test Scores

A second critical issue for those concerned with autistic children is whether their level of tested intelligence alters as they age. About 75%–80% of individuals with autism are mentally retarded so that they score more than two standard deviations below the mean on intelligence tests compared with individuals of the same age. Individuals with autism who score higher have more interactive social relationships and are more capable of independent functioning at all ages than lower scoring individuals with autism.

Stability in intelligence has been measured in three different ways. First, reliability has been examined with correlations between IQ scores at different ages. Second, changes in mean IQ scores for the sample with autism has been contrasted with changes in samples with other disorders followed over roughly the same time period. Third, the extent of individual change has been compared across diagnostic groups.

The results of several studies suggest that the reliability of IQ scores is about as high for autistic children followed into adolescence as for typically developing, behaviorally disordered, and mentally handicapped groups of children (DeMeyer et al., 1973; Freeman et al., 1985; Lord and Schopler, 1989a,b; Lockyer and Rutter, 1969; Mittler et al., 1966). Correlations from about 4–6 years of age to 10–16 years of age were 0.63, 0.58, and 0.79 in the studies by Lockyer and Rutter (1969), DeMeyer et al. (1974), and Lord and Schopler (1989a), respectively. Like typically developing children, reliability in IQ scores was somewhat lower in children followed from age 3 years than for those followed from later ages (Lord and Schopler, 1989b).

In our longitudinal study (Sigman and Ruskin, 1999), the Cattell Scales were administered at intake to all of the children with autism, aged 3–5 years, except for five who were able to achieve a basal score on the Stanford-Binet (Thorndike, 1972). One year repeat reliability was similar for the children with autism and those with developmental delays, $r\,(21) = 0.62$ and $r\,(28) = 0.66$, respectively, and slightly lower than for the children with Down syndrome and the typically developing children, $r\,(42) = 0.76$ and $r\,(21) = 0.75$, respectively. There is an impression among some researchers and clinicians that the assessment of intelligence in children with autism is fraught with difficulty. However, these results show that test–retest reliability is not so different across groups.

At the long-term follow up, 8–9 years later, 25 subjects with autism were tested with the revised Stanford-Binet (Thorndike et al., 1986). The 18 subjects who were unable to reach basal level on the Stanford-Binet were administered the Bayley Scales. For these children, ratio IQ scores were calculated because their ages were above that of the standardization sample. Reliability for the children who were tested with the Stanford-Binet at outcome was 0.72, similar to that reported by Lord and Schopler (1989a,b), who used either the Bayley or the Merrill-Palmer Scale of Mental Tests at intake with children of about the same age. The cross-age reliability of the children with autism was somewhat higher than that of a group of 25 developmentally delayed children ($r = 0.59$) and a group of 55 children with Down syndrome ($r = 0.55$) followed in our study. Reliability for the 18 children with autism tested with the Bayley Scales at outcome was lower ($r = 0.40$), perhaps because of the very limited variability in scores of the children at such low performance levels. The standard deviation on the Stanford-Binet was five times higher than on the Bayley for the children with autism.

Like other studies, there was little mean change in IQ scores for the autistic group or the developmentally delayed group in contrast to a group of children with Down syndrome. Mean developmental quotient (DQ)/IQ decreased only two to three points, a nonsignificant change for the children with autism and developmental delays, whereas mean DQ/IQ dropped 20 points for the Down syndrome group, replicating many previous studies of children with Down syndrome. The test scores of the Down syndrome group became more homogeneous over time, whereas the scores of the autistic and developmentally delayed groups became much more variable.

In terms of individual change, about half the children with autism (22 of 43) and developmental delays (14 of 32) showed increases in intelligence test scores, whereas only 6 of the 66 children with Down syndrome had higher scores at follow up than at intake. For the six children with Down syndrome whose scores were higher, the increase was only 4.17 points in contrast to 22.38 points for the children with autism and 17.21 points for the children with developmental delays. There were no group differences in the amount of decline for those children whose intelligence scores were lower; the mean drop across diagnostic groups was 23 points.

The most hopeful result of this investigation was that a surprising number of children with autism who tested in the mentally retarded range at intake had scores above that range at follow up some 8–9 years later. Thus, 11 children with autism who had scored in the mentally retarded range on the developmental scale were in the borderline to average range on the follow-up IQ test, with only one child showing a comparable drop. This was in marked contrast to the Down syndrome group, almost half of whom did not test as mentally retarded at intake but all of whom had IQ scores in the retarded range at follow up. In the developmentally delayed group, an equivalent number of children moved in ($n = 4$) and out ($n = 5$) of the mentally retarded range. The improvement in intellectual performance in our group of children with autism is greater than that of previous studies, most of which followed children from older ages. Lord and Schopler (1989b) did report as much change in IQ scores in a sample of comparable age, with 35% of their sample moving from mild retardation to the nonretarded classification.

In summary, there seems to be considerable continuity in both the diagnostic status and the intelligence test scores of children with autism. Most individuals continue to show signs of the disorder, and, for the most part, early assessments of intelligence continue to be valid over time. However, the scores of about one third of very young children with autism rise considerably over time. In a later section, precursors of this phenomenon are considered.

Continuity and Change in the Central Deficits in Autism

As with many other neurodevelopmental disorders, a great deal of research has focused on identifying the core deficits in the syndrome of autism (Sigman, 1995). Certain criteria must be met to establish that a deficit is genuinely a core symptom. These criteria are that the deficit must be specific, universal, and unique to the syndrome.

Specificity refers to the extent of disability. Children who are delayed in all domains equally cannot be said to suffer from any deficits that are specific to the syndrome with which they are diagnosed. To establish specificity, several abilities or behaviors of children with a neurodevelopmental syndrome are compared with the same abilities or behaviors of children who are matched on overall intelligence or language skills. Only in those cases where a single ability or set of abilities is affected can one really speak of specific deficits.

Universality refers to the requirement that all or most of the children who suffer from the syndrome should share the deficit, at least, to some degree. This criterion can only be met by investigations of children who vary in terms of their age, developmental level, and severity of symptoms. For a deficit to be truly characteristic of a syndrome, all children who suffer from the syndrome must be limited in the same skill or characteristic to some extent. If some portion of the sample does not suffer from the same disability, the deficit cannot be considered core to the syndrome unless there is some explanation for the compensation of this subsample for their potential limitations.

Uniqueness refers to the extent to which a deficit or pattern of deficits characterizes one or more than one syndrome. Thus, if executive function deficits are found in children with autism, schizophrenic children, and children with attention deficit hyperactivity disorder, then the executive function deficits are not unique to autism. Uniqueness is the most difficult criterion to establish because an examination of numerous syndromes must be undertaken. Additionally, establishing uniqueness is sensitive to the level at which one chooses to define a particular deficit. Using the earlier example, executive functioning broadly defined may be common to several disorders, but a given disorder may nonetheless be characterized uniquely by a particular pattern of deficits involving subset abilities that comprise executive functioning. Moreover, there are limitations to the number of abilities or characteristics that can be disturbed without threatening the individual's viability. This means that similar disabilities are likely to characterize the functioning of children who suffer from a variety of syndromes. However, if many syndromes involve the same deficit, it cannot be considered core to any individual syndrome.

Obviously, the establishment of a deficit as core to a syndrome is a relative achievement. The investigation of the specificity, universality, and uniqueness of deficits can only be accomplished by the assessment of numerous child abilities as well as diverse groups of children with a variety of syndromes. There is reasonable evidence that most autistic children suffer from core deficits in language, nonverbal communication, representational play, responsiveness to others, theory of mind, and executive function. Evidence from cross-sectional studies suggests that deficits in these functions are found in individuals with autism at most ages. However, there have only been a few studies that have examined the extent to which individual children continue to demonstrate these deficits as they age. In the following section, evidence for continuity and discontinuity in core deficits is discussed.

Language abilities

One of the first areas of function to be identified as deficient in children with autism was the area of language. Many more children with autism fail to acquire language skills than do children with other developmental disorders. Even among children who do acquire language, verbal skills are deficient. The language disorder is specific in that prosody and pragmatics are more impaired than syntax and semantics; universal in that some form of language disability is demonstrated by all individuals with autism who are able to use productive speech and unique in that the same pattern of language disorder is not observed in individuals with other neurodevelopmental disabilities. Thus, a deficit in language does appear to be central to autism, although it can be argued that the language disorder follows from earlier deficits in communication and symbolic representation.

Very few studies have tracked the acquisition of language skills in children with autism. Some research, such as that of Helen Tager-Flusberg (1986), has involved longitudinal observations of a few children with autism to elucidate the developmental progression in their language acquisition. Using a more psychometric approach, a gradual increase in mean receptive and expressive language ages was demonstrated in one study carried out at the University of California, Los Angeles (Freeman et al., 1985). In their extensive follow up (to a mean age of 12 years) of the 126 children with autism referred to their Clinical Research Center from 1954 to 1969, DeMeyer et al. (1973) found that 49% of their sample eventually developed useful speech, a proportion comparable to the 46% reported by Rutter and Lockyer (1967) and the 51% reported by Eisenberg (1956). At initial evaluation at about 5.5 years of age, only 40 of their 126 subjects had communicative speech. Those children whose speech had some communicative features at initial evaluation were more likely to develop true conversational speech at follow up than those who were either mute or had noncommunicative echolalic speech. Thus, children with autism are able to acquire verbal skills over time, but about half do not. Moreover, the children who do become capable of conversational speech are more likely to have used at least a few word communicatively at younger ages.

In a study of the stability of intelligence (Lord and Schopler, 1989a), test scores were compared in three groups of children with autism *(1)* those who could understand language at both 4 and 10 years of age; *(2)* those who gained an understanding of language after 4 years; and *(3)* those who never demonstrated an understanding of language. The criterion for understanding language was a basal score (equivalent to 23 months) on the Peabody Picture Vocabulary Test. Children who gained language after 4 years and those who understood language by 4 years had higher intelligence test scores at 10 years than did children who never understood language. At age 4 years, however, children who were to gain language in the subsequent years scored no better on intelligence tests than did children who failed to do so. Thus, intelligence test scores did not predict which group of children would ultimately gain language skills.

In our longitudinal study (Sigman and Ruskin, 1999), the stability of language skills could be assessed in very much the same way as described above for intelligence because similar language measures were used at intake and follow up. Correlations between initial and follow-up language ages were calculated for the three groups of children. As would be expected, early language age predicted later language age. The correlations (with initial chronological age covaried) were $r(39) = 0.56$, $r(59) = 0.49$, and $r(29) = 0.71$ for the children with autism, Down syndrome, and developmental delay, respectively. These correlations cannot be compared with those for the stability of intelligence scores because the latter are age adjusted, which increases stability (see Francis et al., 1994, for a discussion of this issue).

The stability of receptive language was slightly higher than for expressive language for the autistic and developmentally delayed groups. For the children with Down syndrome, the predictions were very different for receptive and expressive language. The correlation between early and later receptive language ages was $r(57) = 0.55$ in contrast to $r(57) = 0.10$ for early and later expressive language. Thus, early expressive language skills in no way predicted later expressive language skills for the children with Down syndrome. These findings point to an instability in the acquisition of expressive language skills among children with Down syndrome that is not demonstrated by children with autism or other developmental disorders.

In terms of change over time, all the groups showed increases in mean language ages, although very much less than would be expected for typically developing children. At follow up, some 8–9 years after intake, the mean gain in language age was 28 months for the children with autism, 23 months for the children with Down syndrome, and 36 months for the children with developmental delays.

The third way of looking at continuity of language skills was in terms of the acquisition of some understanding of language assessed in terms of receptive language skills. Using a receptive language age of 23 months as the criterion for beginning language understanding in our study, following the practice of Lord and Schopler (1989a), 9 of 41 children with autism demonstrated some understood language at recruitment and follow up, 23 children did not understand language at recruitment but did so at follow up, and 9 children never demonstrated understanding of verbal labels. Replicating the findings of Lord and Schopler (1989a), the children who gained an understanding of language did not differ in initial intelligence from the children who never came to understand language. The findings were similar for the two studies despite the fact that the earlier study used a nonverbal measure of intelligence whereas the later study used a general measure of intelligence. It is also worth noting that, in our study, the subdivision of the sample was identical using receptive language abilities of 23 months and expressive language abilities of 18 months, which might be seen as the inception of communicative language usage. Thus, early assessments of intelligence do not seem to be predictive of later language skills.

In summary, both receptive and expressive language abilities are fairly stable over time. Children with autism, as a group, make very slow progress in acquiring language skills. In our longitudinal sample, the mean change in language age was only 28 months over a period of almost 9 years. However, individual children are able to change much more than this. Only 1 of the 11 children with autism who moved out of the mentally retarded group started this study with receptive language capacities over 23 months at initial testing, but all gained a receptive language age equivalent to 6–9 years olds. The children who showed this kind of advance were aged 3–5 when tested originally, and instability in language skills may characterize younger children more than older children.

Nonverbal communication and play skills

Children with autism, as a group, have specific and unique deficits not only in language but also in nonverbal communication and play skills (Sigman and Ruskin, 1999). The deficit in nonverbal communication is specific to joint attention skills—the ability to share attention with another person—and it is unique to autism. Children with autism are more like other developmentally delayed children in their use of nonverbal behavior regulation, behaviors used to elicit aid in obtaining a desired object or action, and dyadic interaction behaviors in structured situations, whereas only children with autism fail to share gaze with others. The deficit in representational play skills is also specific and unique in that children with autism do not show deficits in their use of other object concepts, such as sensorimotor and object categorization skills. Other developmentally delayed children demonstrate a greater variety of functional and symbolic play behaviors than mental-age–matched children with autism. The evidence as to whether these deficits are universal in children with autism is not clear. For high-functioning adolescents and adults, nonverbal communication and representational play are subsumed by verbal activities. With low-functioning adolescents and adults, administration of infant procedures seems inappropriate.

Continuity in nonverbal communication and play skills cannot be evaluated in the same way as continuity in intelligence and language skills because there are no standardized measures that take into account the developmental transformations that normally occur in communicative and symbolic activities during childhood. As part of our longitudinal study, we assessed individual stability in joint attention and behavior regulation skills (Sigman and Ruskin, 1999). For this purpose, we used a modified version of the Early Social Communications Scales (Mundy et al., 1996), a measure that had been used as an index of nonverbal communication in the initial sample of children between 3 and 5 years of age. The new version substituted toys that seemed more appropriate for older children and eliminated the social interaction tasks.

Similar to their behavior when younger, the older children with autism initiated joint attention behaviors much less than the comparison groups of children with Down syndrome and developmental delays. In addition, the children with autism also initiated behavior regulation less than the children in the comparison groups. While this was also true when the children were younger, the difference in behavior regulation was larger at the older age. Thus, older children with autism continued to show profound deficits in nonverbal communication. Moreover, there was stability in the extent to which the children with autism and the children with developmental delays (but not the children with Down syndrome) initiated joint attention. Children who initiated joint attention frequently continued to initiate joint attention more frequently at older ages than children who had initially engaged in less joint attention. There was no individual continuity in initiating requests or responding to bids for joint attention in any of the groups. Thus, the tendency to initiate joint attention with others seems to be a stable trait for children with autism.

Responsiveness to other people

Similar to joint attention and language skills, there is individual stability in responsiveness to others. In several studies, we have shown that, in contrast to comparison groups, children with autism attended less to other people whether they were showing strong emotions or were more subdued (Corona et al., 1998; Dissanayake et al., 1996; Sigman and Ruskin, 1997; Sigman et al., 1992). In these studies, both 3–5-year-old and school-aged children with autism looked less at an experimenter pretending to feel pain, fear, anger, or amusement than children with other developmental disabilities. This was not only because of the emotion that the person was displaying. The children with autism also attended less than comparison children to a person showing more neutral affect. In fact, the children with autism looked more at the experimenter and showed more interest and concern when she pretended to have hurt herself badly than when she was less distressed. Those 3–5-year-old autistic children who were more responsive and attentive to the experimenter in the original study were more attentive and empathic in the follow up conducted 8–9 years later (Dissanayake et al., 1996). Thus, there was both group stability and individual continuity in social responsiveness among children with autism.

Theory of mind

The limited social responsiveness of individuals with autism is considered by some theorists to be attributable to a deficit in "theory of mind" -the attribution of mental states to another; the understanding that others' beliefs, thoughts, and perspectives are different from one's own; and the ability to use this understanding to interpret and predict another person's behavior (Baron-Cohen and Swettenham, 1997; Leslie, 1987).

Deficits in this form of social understanding seem unique, specific, and universal in autism. Early studies of theory of mind used false belief tasks to ascertain whether autistic children could attribute different states of mind, or different beliefs, to another and whether this inability was specific to the disorder or indicative of general cognitive dysfunction. Normal children were able to master such tasks at about 4 years of age, whereas a majority of even mildly mentally handicapped autistic children were unable to pass simple, first-order theory of mind tasks (Baron-Cohen and Swettenham, 1997). These are false belief tasks where the child's answers are based on a character's point of view that is different from the child's own. In contrast, comparison groups of children with various neurodevelopmental disorders, such as Down syndrome and language impairment, performed as well as normal children (Baron-Cohen, 1989; Perner et al., 1989). However, some evidence suggests that deficits in theory of mind abilities may also be present in other disorders (Yirmiya and Shulman, 1996; Yirmiya et al., 1996; Zelazo et al., 1996).

In testing the specificity of theory of mind deficits in autism, Baron-Cohen (1991) performed three experiments to examine whether this deficit was due to a specific failure in understanding mental states or due to more general deficits in other areas of social cognition. In comparison to nonautistic controls, autistic children did not show deficits in the recognition of simple social relationships (such as parent and child), simple reciprocity, or animate–inanimate distinctions, while they did show deficits in theory of mind tasks. In another study, individuals with autism demonstrated awareness of false *representations,* recognizing as wrong a photograph of a doll that showed her wearing a dress of a color different from that of the actual dress of the doll, but did not demonstrate understanding of false *belief,* which required the ability to adopt the perspective of another and answer questions based on that perspective, which was different from the child's own (Leekam and Perner, 1991).

It is difficult to demonstrate that theory of mind deficits are universal in autism because only a small proportion of autistic individuals, those with good verbal skills, can perform correctly on these tasks. Within this subsample of autistic individuals, there is some consistency across studies. Stability in theory of mind deficits has rarely been investigated. In the one study of which we are aware, performance did not improve much over a 3-year time span (Ozonoff and McEvoy, 1994).

Executive function

Another class of deficits has been proposed involving the individual's drive to attempt to abstract meaning from the complex array of information received, to integrate information to select an appropriate response, and to organize goal-directed behaviors (Bailey et al., 1996). The construct used to describe the abilities necessary to do such problem-solving is termed *executive function,* and individuals with autism are seen as limited in these capacities (Ozonoff, 1995).

In addressing the question of the specificity and uniqueness of executive function deficits in autistic individuals, Pennington and Ozonoff (1996) found some evidence of executive dysfunction in a number of disorders—Tourette syndrome, conduct disorder, ADHD, and autism—but the evidence was consistent only for ADHD and autism. The deficits were more severe in the autistic samples, and the autistic individuals had more difficulty with tasks requiring the ability to plan and shift response set, like the Wisconsin Card Sort and the Tower of Hanoi, while the individuals with ADHD had difficulties with tasks requiring inhibition. Similarly, individuals with Turner syndrome exhibit deficits in tasks measuring distractibility (Temple et al., 1996), visuospatial skills, and working memory (Romans et al., 1997) aspects of executive functioning, which have not proven to be particularly deficient in autistic individuals.

Impairments in planning and cognitive flexibility appear to be universal, remaining throughout development. In one longitudinal study, the autistic sample evinced significantly more problems on executive function tasks than a learning-disabled comparison group at both the original and follow-up assessments (Ozonoff and McEvoy, 1994). The literature from cross-sectional studies supports this view, showing early evidence of executive functioning deficits in young autistic children (McEvoy et al., 1993) as well as older individuals. In terms of individual stability, the autistic subjects' performance on executive functioning tasks did not improve over the course of 3 years, while the learning-disabled cohort's performance did improve over the same time period.

Continuity in Underlying Processes

As discussed earlier in this chapter, an important form of continuity is heterotypic, marked by qualitative differences in the manifestation of a skill through the course of development, rather than homotypic, in which there are no qualitative changes in the skill. Developmental research suggests that nonverbal communicative skills and symbolic representational abilities are precursors, and perhaps even prerequisites, for language acquisition. In other words, children have to be aware that social communication is possible and beneficial to be motivated and capable of developing the understanding and use of language. In addition, language as a symbolic system builds on simpler representational systems. For this reason, children may not be able to acquire linguistic skills in the absence of some elementary capacity to symbolize nonverbally. The deficits described above in nonverbal communication and symbolic play of children with autism may result in their limited verbal capacities.

To investigate the role of nonverbal communication and play in the verbal development of children with autism, the associations between these skills were measured in our longitudinal study (Sigman and Ruskin, 1999). Autistic children who initiated and responded to joint attention and responded more to social interactions had better language skills than autistic children who showed less joint attention and response to social interactions. Moreover, gains in language skills 8–9 years later were predicted by the proportion of time that the children with autism responded to bids for joint attention at 3–5 years of age.

Representational play skills were also concurrently associated with language abilities. In addition, the diversity of functional play acts predicted the gain in language over the 8–9-year period.

Another possible consequence of early communicative and representational skills might be seen in the social domain. Children with more interest and ability to communicate nonverbally at young ages might also be more able to form relationships with others. Representational play skills might also be an index of social capacities in that young children have to observe social acts and interactions to represent these activities in play. Findings from our longitudinal study support these conjectures in that both the frequency of initiating joint attention in interaction with the experimenter and the number of different representational play acts with toys were predictors of the level of social engagement on the playground. These early behaviors were correlated with later peer engagement even when early level of intelligence was statistically controlled.

In summary, heterotypic continuity existed in the communicative/symbolic domain. Young children with autism who were more engaged with both people and toys were more verbally adept and subsequently more socially engaged with peers. Thus, there is considerable individual continuity in the development of children with autism in intelligence, language abilities, nonverbal communicative and play skills, responsiveness to others, theory of mind, and executive functions. Moreover, the development of language and social relatedness appears to depend on the acquisition of communicative and symbolic skills that underlie these capacities in normal children.

Predictors of Change

While we have identified major continuities in the development of autistic children, we have also found that a sizeable number of children with autism improve in terms of their language abilities and intellectual performance. To identify the predictors of change in intelligence, nonverbal communication and play skills were compared for those children who remained in the mentally retarded range with those children who moved out of the mentally retarded range. The two groups differed in terms of their initial intelligence level as well as the frequency with which they responded to joint attention, requested objects or assistance with objects, and demonstrated different play acts. When the groups were compared and initial intelligence was covaried, there were still significant group differences in nonverbal communication skills. The children who remained retarded were less likely than those who became high functioning to follow the pointing gestures of others and to request assistance or objects when they were 3–5 years of age.

A similar comparison was conducted between the nonverbal communication and play skills of children who gained an understanding of language and those who never demonstrated this understanding using the criterion described above. These two groups did not differ in initial intelligence, as discussed earlier, but they did differ in terms of the diversity of functional play. Children who were to gain language understanding engaged in a greater number of different functional play acts than children who did not demonstrate this understanding at any age point. In summary, nonverbal communication and play acts do seem to be precursors to the acquisition of language skills and the increase in intelligence test scores shown by a portion of the children with autism.

Role of the Environment in Continuity and Change

In this chapter, we have demonstrated that there is considerable continuity in the development of children with autism, but that some children with autism do improve in their linguistic and intellectual functions. Some of the bases for these improvements seem to stem from the children's own abilities and may, therefore, have neurological origins. Identifying the individual, neurological variances that underlie such differential outcomes may serve as a first step toward discerning the neurological underpinnings of the disorder. The investigation of the substrates of nonverbal communication and play skills through functional magnetic resonance imaging would seem to be a worthwhile endeavor.

In addition, it is possible that certain environmental conditions may help to advance the nonverbal communication and representational skills of young children with autism and thereby enhance their language and intellectual abilities. Transformations in behavior are assumed to occur because of both neurological maturation and learning experiences. Studies of neural plasticity have demonstrated that these factors are related so that experience with a particular environment leads to changes in developing neural systems (Fox et al., 1994; Greenough and Sirevaag, 1991; Rosenzweig and Bennett, 1996). There have been virtually no studies investigating the effects of environmental variations on the behavioral or neurological development of children with autism. For this reason, we have no idea of the extent to which environments may play a part in either sustaining continuity or promoting change in children with autism. While the disorder of autism is undoubtably caused by biological dysfunctions, the intellectual strengths and weaknesses of children with autism may be modified to some extent by environmental factors. There is a need for research into the associations between environmental factors and neurological and behavioral development to determine the extent to which plasticity is possible in the life course of individuals with autism.

References

Some of the research reported in this chapter was supported by grant NS25243 from the National Institute of Neurological Disorders and Stroke and grant HD17662 from the National Institute of Child Health and Development.

American Psychiatric Association. (1980). *Diagnostic and statistical manual of mental disorders (3rd ed.)*. Washington, DC: American Psychiatric Association.

Bailey, A., Phillips, W., and Rutter, M. (1996). Autism: Towards an integration of clinical, genetic, neuropsychological, and neurobiological perspectives. *J. Child Psychol. Psychiatry, 37,* 89–126.

Baron-Cohen, S. (1989). The autistic child's theory of mind: A case of specific developmental delay. *J. Child Psychol. Psychiatry, 3,* 285–297.

Baron-Cohen, S. (1991). The theory of mind deficit in autism: How specific is it? *Br. J. Dev. Psychol., 9,* 301–314.

Baron-Cohen, S., and Swettenham, J. (1997). Theory of mind in autism: Its relationship to executive function. In D. J. Cohen and F. R. Volkmar (eds.): *Handbook of autism and pervasive developmental disorders* (2nd ed.). New York: John Wiley & Sons, pp. 880–894.

Bornstein, M. H., and Sigman, M. D. (1986). Continuity in mental development from infancy. *Child Dev., 57,* 251–274.

Cantwell, D. P., Baker, L., Rutter, M., and Mawhood, L. (1989). Infantile autism and developmental receptive dysphasia: A comparative follow-up into middle childhood. *J. Autism Dev. Disord., 19,* 19–33.

Chung, S. Y., Luk, S. L., and Lee, W. H. (1990). A follow-up study of infantile autism in Hong Kong. *J. Autism Dev. Disord., 20,* 221–232.

Corona, R., Dissanayake, C., Arbelle, S., Wellington, P., and Sigman, M. (1999). Is affect aversive to children with autism? Behavioral and cardiac responses to experimenter distress. *Child Development, 69,* 1494–1502.

DeMeyer, M. K., Barton, S., DeMeyer, W. E., Norton, J. A., Allen, J., and Steele, R. (1973). Prognosis in autism: A follow-up study. *J. Autism Childhood Schizophrenia, 3,* 199–246.

Dissanayake, C., Sigman, M., and Kasari, C. (1996). Long-term stability of individual differences in the emotional responsiveness of children with autism. *J. Child Psychol. Psychiatry, 37,* 461–467.

Eisenberg, L. (1956). The autistic child in adolescence. *Am. J. Psychiatry, 112,* 607–612.

Fox, N. A., Calkins, S. D., and Bell, M. A. (1994). Neural plasticity and development in the first two years of life: Evidence from cognitive and socioemotional domains of research. *Devel. Psychopathol., 6,* 677–696.

Francis, D. J., Shaywitz, S. E., Stuebing, K. K., Shaywitz, B. A., et al. (1994). The measurement of change: Assessing behavior over time and within a developmental context. In G. Reid Lyon (ed.): Frames of reference for the assessment of learning disabilities: New views on measurement issues. Baltimore: Paul H. Brookes Publishing, pp. 29–58.

Freeman, B. J., Ritvo, E. R., Needleman, R., and Yokota, A. (1985). The stabilty of cognitive and linguistic parameters in autism: A five-year prospective study. *J. Am. Acad. Child Psychiatry, 24,* 459–464.

Gillberg, C., and Steffenburg, S. (1987). Outcome and prognostic factors in infantile autism and similar conditions: A population-based study of 46 cases followed through puberty. *J. Autism Dev. Disord., 17,* 273–288.

Gittelman, M., and Birch, H. G. (1967). Childhood schizophrenia: intellect, neurological status, perinatal risk, prognosis, and family pathology. *Arch. Gen. Psychiatry, 17,* 16–25.

Greenough, W. T., and Sirevaag, A. M. (1991). A neuroanatomical approach to substrates of behavioral plasticity. In H. N. Shair, G. A. Barr, and M. A. Hofer (eds.): *Developmental Psychobiology.* New York: Oxford University Press, pp. 255-270.

Kanner, L. (1971). Follow-up study of 11 autistic children originally reported in 1943. *J. Autism Childhood Schizophrenia, 1,* 119–145.

Krug, D. A., Arick, J. R., and Almond, P. J. (1980). *Autism Screening Instrument for Education Planning.* Portland, OR: AISEP Educational Company.

Le Couteur, A., Rutter, M., Lord, C., Rios, P., Robertson, S., Holdrafer, M., and McLennan, J. (1989). Autism diagnostic interview: A standardized investigator-based instrument. *J. Autism Dev. Disord., 19,* 363–387.

Leekam, S., and Perner, J. (1991). Does the autistic child have a metarepresentational deficit? *Cognition, 40,* 203–218.

Leslie, A. M. (1987). Pretense and representation: The origins of "theory of mind." *Psychol. Rev., 94,* 412–426.

Lockyer, L., and Rutter, M. (1969). A five-to-fifteen year follow-up study of infantile psychosis. III. Psychological aspects. *Br. J. Psychiatry, 115,* 865–882.

Lord, C., Rutter, M., Goode, S., Heemsbergen, J., Jordan, H., Mawhood, L., and Schopler, E. (1989). Autism diagnostic observation schedule. A standardized observation of communicative and social behavior. *J. Autism Dev. Disord., 19,* 185–212.

Lord, C., and Schopler, E. (1989a). Stability of assessment results of autistic and non-autistic language-impaired children from preschool years to early school age. *J. Child Psychol. Psychiatry, 30,* 575–590.

Lord, C., and Schopler, E. (1989b). The role of age at assessment, development level, and test in the stability of intelligence scores in young autistic children. *J. Autism Dev. Disord., 89,* 483–499.

Lotter, V. (1978). Follow-up studies. In M. Rutter and E. Schopler (eds.): *Autism: A Reappraisal of Concepts and Treatment.* New York: Plenum Press, pp. 475–495.

McEvoy, R. E., Rogers, S. J., and Pennngton, B. F. (1993). Executive function and social communication deficits in young autistic children. *J. Child Psychol. Psychiatry, 34,* 563–578.

Mittler, P., Gilles, S., and Jukes, E. (1966). Prognosis in psychotic children: Report of a follow up study. *J. Ment. Defic. Res., 10,* 73–83.

Mundy, P., Hogan, A., and Doehring, P.(1996). *A Preliminary Manual for the Abridged Early Social Communication Scale* (ESCS).

Ozonoff, S. (1995). Executive functions in autism. In E. Schopler and G. B. Mesibov (eds.): *Learning and Cognition in Autism.* New York: Plenum Press, pp. 199–219.

Ozonoff, S., and McEvoy, R. E. (1994). A longitudinal study of executive function and theory of mind development in autism. *Dev. Psychopathol., 6,* 415–431.

Pennington, B. F., and Ozonoff, S. (1996). Executive functions and developmental psychopathology. *J. Child Psychol. Psychiatry, 37,* 51–87.

Perner, J., Frith, Y., Leslie, A. M., and Leekman, S. R. (1989). Exploration of the autistic child's theory of mind: Knowledge, belief, and communication. *Child Devel., 60,* 689–700.

Romans, S. M., Roeltgen, D. P., Kushner, H., and Ross, J. L. (1997). Executive function in girls with Turner's syndrome. *Dev. Neuropsychol., 13,* 23–40.

Rosenzweig, M. R., and Bennett, E. L. (1996). Psychobiology of plasticity: Effects of training and experience on brain and behavior. *Behav. Brain Res., 78,* 57–65.

Rumsey, J. M., Rapoport, J. L., and Sceery, W. R. (1985). Autistic children as adults: Psychiatric, social, and behavioral outcomes. *J. Am. Acad. Child Psychiatry, 24,* 465–473.

Rutter, M., and Lockyer, L. (1967). A five to fifteen year follow-up study of infantile psychosis. I. Description of sample. *Br. J. Psychiatry, 113,* 1169–1182.

Schopler, E., Reichler, R. J., amd Renner, B. R. (1986). *The Childhood Autism Rating Scale.* New York, New York: Irvington Publishers.

Sigman, M. (1995). What are the core deficits in autism? In S. H. Broman and J. Grafman (eds.): *Atypical cognitive deficits in developmental disorders: Implications for brain function.* Hillsdale, NJ: Lawrence Erlbaum Associates, Inc., pp. 139–157.

Sigman, M., and Ruskin, E. (1999). Continuity and change in the social competence of children with autism, Down syndrome, and developmental delays. *Monograph of the Society For Research in Child Development.*

Sigman, M. D., Kasari, C., Kwon, J., and Yirmiya, N. (1992). Responses to the negative emotions of others by autistic, mentally retarded, and normal children. *Child Dev., 63,* 796–807.

Szatmari, P., Bartolucci, G., Bremner, R., Bond, S., and Rich, S. (1989). A follow-up study of high-functioning autistic children. *J. Autism Dev. Disord., 19,* 213–225.

Tager-Flusberg, H. (1986). Constraints on the representation of word meaning: Evidence from autistic and mentally retarded children. In S. Kuczaj and M. Barrett (eds.): *The Development of Word Meaning.* New York: Springer-Verlag, pp. 139–166.

Temple, C. M., Carney, R. A., and Mullarkey, S. (1996). Frontal lobe function and executive skills in children with Turner's syndrome. *Dev. Neuropsychol., 12,* 343–363.

Thorndike, R. (1972). *Stanford-Binet Intelligence Scale: 1972 Norm Tables.* Boston: Houghton Mufflin.

Thorndike, R. L., Hagen, E. P., and Sattler, J. M. (1986). *The Stanford Binet Intelligence Scale.* Chicago, IL: Riverside Publishing Company.

Venter, A., Lord, C., and Schopler, E. (1992). A follow-up study of high-functioning autistic children. *J. Child Psychol. Psychiatry, 33,* 489–507.

Yirmiya, N., and Shulman, C. (1996). Seriation, conservation, and theory of mind abilities in individuals with autism, individuals with mental retardation, and normally developing children. *Child Dev., 67,* 2045–2059.

Yirmiya, N., Solomonica-Levi, D., Shulman, C., and Pilowsky, T. (1996). Theory of mind abilities in individuals with autism, down syndrome, and mental retardation of unknown etiology: The role of age and intelligence. *J. Child Psychol. Psychiatry, 37,* 1003–1014.

Zelazo, P. D., Burack, J. A., Benedetto, E., and Frye, D. (1996). Theory of mind and rule use in individuals with Down's Syndrome: A test of the uniqueness and specificity claims. *J. Child Psychol. Psychiatry, 37,* 479–484.

13

Biological and Behavioral Heterogeneity in Autism: Roles of Pleiotropy and Epigenesis

ERIC COURCHESNE, RACHEL YEUNG-COURCHESNE,
AND KAREN PIERCE

Infantile autism stands as one of the most common neurobiological disorders of infancy and early childhood, occurring in 1 of 1,000 individuals (Bresnahan et al., 1998). Among the different developmental disorders, autism is one of the most severe, involving abnormalities in sensory, motor, attention, memory, speech, language, social, and affective functions (Table 13-1).

Schain and Freedman (1961) were the first to identify a biological abnormality—elevation of whole blood serotonin levels (hyperserotonemia)—in formal experimental studies of patients with autism. This finding was followed by a long period filled with conflicting and nonreplicating reports. Current evidence confirms that hyperserotonemia occurs in at least 25% of patients with autism (Cook and Leventhal, 1996). This means that 75% of the autistic patients tested did not exhibit hyperserotonemia, making this the first clear example of heterogeneity of biological abnormality in this disorder. Affected autistic subjects have elevated serotonin transport into platelets and decreased serotonin 5-HT$_2$ receptor binding. Treatments based on this finding are not beneficial for all autistic patients with hyperserotonemia; while some symptoms in some patients may not change or may worsen, a substantial number who are treated with serotonin transporter inhibitors have a reduction in ritualistic behavior and aggression (Cook and Leventhal, 1996; McDougle et al., 1996). In sum, the first known biological feature to be discovered as abnormal in autistic patients is not present in all autistic individuals, and studies of treatments based on this finding show heterogeneous symptom outcomes with a mixture of benefit and failure to benefit.

Following this early promising, if somewhat puzzling, beginning in the study of the biological bases of autism, decades of research would pass before scientists

Table 13-1. Anomalies observed in individuals with autism

Behavioral and Psychological

Deficits in joint attention
Lack of social responsiveness
Reduced or inappropriate affect
Abnormal language development
Unusual preoccupations and interests
Self-stimulatory behaviors
Frequent mental retardation
Self-injurious behavior
Poor eye contact
Literal memory
Tactile defensiveness

Neurobehavioral

Deficits in shifting attention
Deficits in adjusting the spatial distribution of attention
Deficits in orienting attention
Deficits in arousal and attention modulation
Deficits in stimulus selectivity
Deficits in sensory modulation
Deficits in executive functions
Deficits in metacognition
Deficits in visual filtering

Neurological

Gait and other motor control abnormalities
Abnormal EEG patterns
Oculomotor dysfunction
Vestibular functioning abnormalities

Neuroanatomical

Cerebellar neuron loss and hypoplasia in majority of patients; vermis hyperplasia in small subset
Parietal lobe volume loss in a subset of patients
Thinning of posterior corpus callosum
Increased cell packing density in the limbic system
Increased brain size in a small subset of patients
Dysgenesis of superior olive and agenesis of facial motor nucleus in one patient
Frontal lobe gray matter size correlated with cerebellum abnormality

Neurochemical

Elevated whole blood serotonin levels
Monoaminergic system functioning abnormalities
Opioid functioning abnormalities
Abnormal plasma β-endorphin levels
Elevated T_3 and T_4 levels
Unmodulated plasma growth hormone responses to insulin-induced hypoglycemia

discovered sites of neuroanatomical abnormality; obtained evidence pointing to the timing of biological (as opposed to behavioral) onset, and identified neural substrates correlated with specific functional deficits. In the last decade, much progress has been made on all fronts of autism research.

A valuable message from the multiple-front biological research on autism has been confirmation that autism is a biologically heterogeneous disorder, as first indicated by the studies of hyperserotonemia. It is becoming clear that the disorder is heterogeneous at both the intraindividual and interindividual levels. Within an autistic person, the symptoms are heterogeneous and diverse across multiple systems; among a group of patients diagnosed with autism, the array and severity of symptoms within the syndromic spectrum are also heterogeneous and diverse from one patient to the next. The more focused and magnified the biological examination, the more evidence of biological heterogeneity is seen. These biological details will prove essential to discovery of the causes and biological and behavioral consequences in this disorder.

A Summary of Biological Findings in Autism

Discovery that neuroanatomical abnormalities exist

The neocerebellar vermis (Courchesne et al., 1994b, 1988) and the cerebellar hemispheres (Gaffney et al., 1987; Murakami et al., 1989) were the first neural structures demonstrated to be anatomically abnormal in large samples of autistic patients. Up to that time, only single autopsy case reports had provided provocative evidence. Williams et al. (1980) reported diffuse Purkinje neuron loss throughout the cerebellum in the one case in their study with the clearest symptoms of autism (the remaining three cases displayed autism-like characteristics likely due to Rett syndrome, phenylketonuria [PKU], and head injury). Ironically, Williams et al. (1980) dismissed the importance of their own finding, concluding that autism is not associated with any definite neuropathological defect. In a study of four autism cases, the first quantitation of Purkinje neuron loss was by Ritvo et al. (1986), whose data showed that this defect was greater in the vermis, including the anterior and neocerebellar vermis, than in the neocerebellar hemispheres. Bauman and Kemper (1994) also reported reduction of Purkinje neuron numbers in a group of six autistic autopsy cases, with the reduction in neocerebellar hemispheres being especially marked. Fehlow et al. (1993) reported one male autism case with Purkinje loss in the neocerebellar vermis, but Guerin et al. (1996) reported no Purkinje neuron abnormality in one female whose symptoms leave open the possibility of a Rett syndrome rather than an autism diagnosis. Finally, Bailey et al. (1998) reported Purkinje neuron pathology in the vermis and hemispheres in each of their six autism cases. In five of the six cases, the pathology observed was loss of Purkinje cells in the vermis and hemispheres; the final case displayed abnormality as well in the form of cytoplasmic inclusions in Purkinje cells, with this abnormality most prominent in the vermis. These new observations by Bailey et al.

(1998) bring the grand total number of postmortem accounts of cerebellar Purkinje loss or cellular pathology in autism to 18 out of a total 19 reported cases. Bailey et al. (1998) thus solidify the notion that the cerebellum is the most consistently documented location of abnormality in autism. This study also cites cortical abnormalities (primarily frontal) in four of the six cases as well as developmental abnormalities of the brain stem (e.g., presence of ectopic neuron clusters; abnormal inferior olives, a structure intimately connected with Purkinje neurons).

Recent magnetic resonance imaging (MRI) studies have supported the original MRI studies of the cerebellum as well as the autopsy findings. They have also identified additional sites and types of neuroanatomical abnormalities in patients with autism. For instance, in living autistic patients, there is MRI evidence of hypoplasia of the neocerebellar vermis in the majority of patients (Fig. 13-1), as well as hyperplasia in a small subgroup (Fig. 13-2). In the brain stem, MRI studies have reported hypoplasia (Gaffney et al., 1988; Hashimoto et al., 1995) as well as normal size (Hsu et al., 1991; Piven et al., 1992). In the cerebrum, there is thinning in posterior subregions of the corpus callosum in most, but not all, patients (Egaas et al., 1995); similarly, there is reduced volume in parietal lobes in a subset of patients (Fig. 13-3) (Courchesne et al., 1993). Frontal lobe growth changes have been linked to indices of cerebellar size in most, but not all, patients (Fig. 13-4) (Carper and Courchesne, 1999), demonstrating an inverse relationship between measures of the neocerebellar vermis and frontal lobe volumes (i.e., decreased vermal measures related to increased frontal gray matter). This finding is interesting in light of the thickening of frontal gray matter recently reported in four autopsy cases (Bailey et al., 1998). Additionally, postmortem examinations have found reduced neuron counts and/or arrest of growth or undergrowth in the cerebellum (Arin et al., 1991; Bauman and Kemper, 1985, 1994; Fehlow et al., 1993; Ritvo et al., 1986; Williams et al., 1980), limbic system (Bauman and Kemper, 1985, 1994; Raymond et al., 1996), and brain stem (Rodier et al., 1996). Postmortem (Bailey et al., 1998) and MRI studies (Courchesne et al., 1999b) have also identified several autistic individuals with macroencephaly, although the great majority of patients have a brain size within the normal range (Fig. 13-5) (Courchesne et al., 1999a,b).

While some anatomical defects (i.e., cerebellar maldevelopment) appear to be common across the great majority of autistic patients and others are not, apparently all autistic individuals have multiple anatomical abnormalities. These observations naturally raise questions as to what factors cause the *intra*individual heterogeneity as well as the *inter*individual heterogeneity.

Discoveries of time of biological onset

Currently, the strongest evidence addressing the question of the time of biological onset comes from postmortem and MRI evidence showing that cerebellar (Bailey et al., 1998; Courchesne, 1995; Hashimoto et al., 1995; Ritvo et al., 1986) and brain stem (Rodier et al., 1996) anatomical abnormalities most likely have a prenatal onset. Reduction in Purkinje neuron numbers is typically present without accompanying gliosis (e.g., Ritvo et al., 1986), a finding indicative of an early—pre-

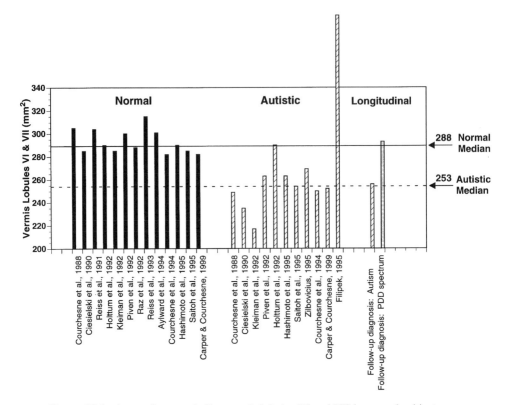

Figure 13-1. Areas of neocerebellar vermis lobules VI and VII in normal subjects compared with autistic patients. The horizontal line at 290 mm² is the median normal value across the studies with normal subjects. For most of the studies, medians are graphed. Note that Piven et al. (1992) originally concluded that their autistic patients did not significantly differ from normal volunteers. That conclusion was in error; in 1995 Piven and Arndt wrote, "in the study by Piven et al. (1992), we detected significant differences in neocerebellar [vermis lobules VI and VII] size when we compared autistic individuals with age-, sex-, and social class-comparable 'normal, healthy' volunteers." The list of the Piven et al. (1992) original vermis measurement values is available upon request. Note also that Kleiman et al. (1992) also originally reported that their autistic patients did not differ from control subjects. That conclusion was in error because they made arithmetical and statistical reporting errors on their own data. Examination of their original raw measurement values (see Yeung-Courchesne [1997] and Courchesne [1997] for the entire list of their original measurement values) shows that their autistic subjects had the most extreme and statistically significant hypoplasia of any autism report to date. The data values for Piven et al. (1992) and Kleiman et al. (1992) in the bar graph are the medians of all of their autistic subjects, and so-called hyperplasia cases were included in this bar graph calculation. Different, independent samples of autistic subjects are reported in Courchesne et al. (1994c), Saitoh et al. (1995), and Carper and Courchesne (1998); the 18 original autistic subjects of Courchesne et al. (1988) are among the 51 autistic subjects reported by Courchesne et al. (1994c), who also report the results from the new sample separately. (Adapted from Courchesne, 1997.)

natal or early postnatal—onset for this defect (Fig. 13-6). In the first prospective MRI study of autism, Hashimoto et al. (1995) found cerebellar vermis hypoplasia in infants who were subsequently confirmed to be autistic. Regression analyses of growth curves for the neocerebellar vermis in autistic patients indicates a perinatal or prenatal onset of the vermis hypoplasia (Courchesne, 1995). Supporting evidence also comes from animal model research that has found that exposure to an anticonvulsant medication during embryogenesis caused Purkinje neuron loss throughout the posterior cerebellum (Ingram et al., 1996). Additionally, evidence from a single postmortem autism case has been interpreted as an indication that maldevelopment in the brain stem may begin as early as the first trimester (Rodier et al., 1996; for review, see Courchesne, 1997). While the onset appears to be quite early, certainly by infancy in the majority of cases, the developing neural system remains plastic, and opportunities to effect changes in structure and function continue into childhood (see later section on epigenesis). Nonetheless, the fact that the biological time of onset is early highlights the need to discover biobehavioral techniques that prompt compensatory neuroplastic changes as early as possible.

Autism: Vermian Lobules VI-VII

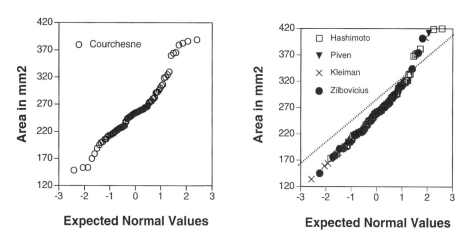

Figure 13-2. Dotted lines in plots show normal expected mean values for neocerebellar vermis lobules VI and VII based on over 200 normal subjects. Compared with this normal expected value, the majority of autistic patients from five different laboratories (Hashimoto, Piven, Kleiman, Zilbovicius, and Courchesne; see Courchesne [1997] for references) have reduced neocerebellar vermis area; this is consistent with the data in Figure 13-1. The plot also shows that a small percentage of autistic patients have a neocerebellar vermis area larger than the normal expected mean values. This is evidence of heterogeneity in cerebellar anatomy in autistic patients: The majority have hypoplasia of the neocerebellar vermis, while a small minority may possibly have hyperplasia of that same subregion. (Adapted from Courchesne et al., 1994b,c.)

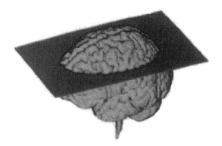

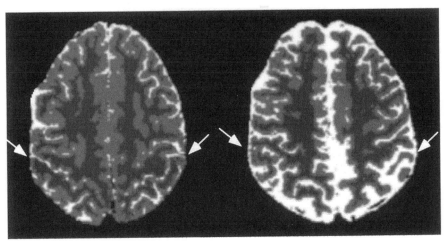

Figure 13-3. *(Right)* Example of segmented MRI from one autistic patient with substantial parietal volume loss. *(Left)* One autistic patient with no evidence of parietal volume loss. Central sulcus marked by arrows. The plane through the three-dimensional brain reconstruction at the top shows the approximate position for these images. (Adapted from Courchesne et al., 1993.)

Anatomical and functional correlations and associations

Research in the field of autism is replete with claims of brain–behavior associations (e.g., deficits in executive function are claimed to be associated with frontal abnormalities, deficits in emotion perception are claimed to be associated with amygdala dysfunction, deficits in shifting attention are claimed to be associated with cerebellar abnormalities, and so on). It is important, however, to make the distinction between brain–behavior *correlations* and brain–behavior *associations.* Correlations represent the direct mapping of the degree of a behavior (e.g., rate of emotion identification) to the morphology of a particular structure (e.g., temporal lobe volume) or degree of functioning of that structure (e.g., reduced hemodynamic responding during functional imaging). As such, they can be described as linear relationships (e.g., as X increases, Y increases to a similar degree). Associations, on the other hand, merely suggest a possible relationship (e.g., subgroup A corresponds to structural abnormality A), though neither correlation nor associations are definitively causational.

Understanding the relationship between brain structure, function, and behavior in autism is significant because it provides a foundation for the development of individualized treatments for this disorder (as well as the development of animal models testing hypothesized causes or effective treatments; see below). The high level of detail provided by brain–behavior correlations, and not associations per se, may in fact be the critical ingredient when developing treatment interventions *for a particular child.* That is, knowing that a particular individual has a specific amount of cell loss in a particular area, and this, in turn, yields a particular degree of behavioral abnormality, will surely be more informative for treatment decisions than knowing that a particular individual falls within a *range* of possible anatomical abnormalities and a *range* of related behavioral outcomes.

Despite the importance of such work, the first report of statistically significant correlations between measures of neuroanatomical and functional abnormalities in autistic patients was not made until recently (Townsend et al., 1996a). In adult autistic patients, greater parietal gray matter volume loss was correlated with greater behavioral deficits in deployment of visuospatial attention. Understanding brain–behavior associations, although not as informative for individualized treatment decisions, still plays a valuable role in dissecting possible subgroups and underlying pathologies involved in autism, as well as providing insights and theories that may, in turn, lead to significant correlational findings. Townsend and Courch-

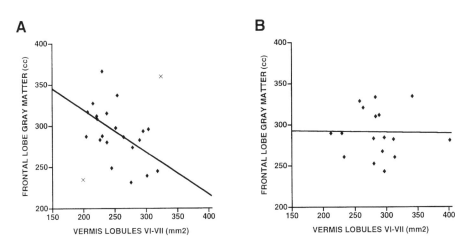

Figure 13-4. In autistic patients, the greater the abnormality in neocerebellar vermis lobules VI and VII, the greater the volume of frontal lobe gray matter. *(A)* Autism patients. ♦, Twenty-one of 23 male patients show a significant correlation ($r = 0.532$; $p = 0.01$); line indicates regression for these subjects; x, Two male outliers. *(B)* Control subjects. ♦, Male subjects; line indicates regression for these subjects ($r = 0.019$; $p = 0.94$). (From Carper and Courchesne, 1998.)

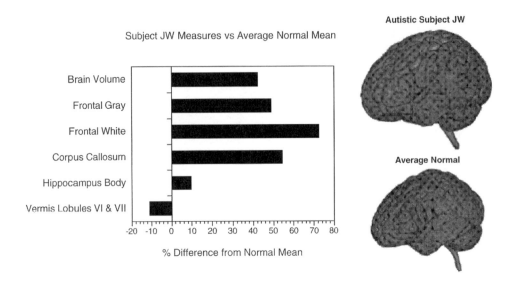

Figure 13-5. *(Top)* Three-dimensional MRI of 3.4-year-old autistic child, Subject J. W. (brain volume = 1,816 ml). *(Center)* MRI of a normal subject. (brain volume = 1,366 ml). *(Bottom)* Quantitative brain measures for Subject J. W. compared with quantitative normative measures; measures of his brain volume—frontal gray (387 ml) and white (170 ml) matter volumes, corpus callosum area (823.7 mm^2), mean posterior hippocampal body area (53.9 mm^2), and cerebellar vermis lobules VI and VII area (264.1 mm^2)—are graphed as percent differences from the average values for each of these structures in young normal children. Normal values are from Courchesne et al. (1999a) for brain volume; Carper and Courchesne (1998) for frontal lobe volumes; Egaas et al. (1995) for the corpus callosum area; Saitoh et al. (1995) for the hippocampal body area; and Courchesne et al. (1994) and Saitoh et al. (1995) for vermis lobules VI and VII area.

esne (1994) also obtained the first associations linking specific anatomical abnormalities to specific physiological and behavioral abnormalities in autistic patients. In their P1 event related potential (ERP) study, they demonstrated "neglect-like" visuospatial attention abnormality ("spotlight attention") in autistic patients with parietal volume loss (Fig. 13-7). Specifically, this subset of autistic individuals engaged in faster button presses to targets as well as earlier and more enhanced (i.e., increased amplitude) electrophysiological responding during a task of selective visual attention. This "spotlight of attention" effect has been clearly documented in the autism literature for over three decades, beginning with the idea of "stimulus overselectivity" in the 1970s (Lovaas et al., 1971), "tunnel vision" in the 1980s (Rincover and Ducharme, 1987), spatial neglect in the early 1990s (Bryson et al., 1990), and, currently, a related idea—"weak central coherence" (Frith and Happé, 1994). Furthermore, a preference for a narrow attentional focus in autism has been noted in a variety of contexts, including overselective responding to multiple sensory stimuli (Lovaas et al., 1971; Kolo et al., 1980), complex visual stimuli (Koegel and Wilhelm, 1973; Koegel and Rincover, 1976), social stimuli (Pierce et al., 1997), verbal instructions (Burke and Cerniglia, 1990), and object identification (Schreibman and Lovaas, 1973). This pattern of responding has also been suggested as a contributing factor to superior performance on the Block Design tasks (Shah and Frith, 1993) and Embedded Figures Tasks (Shah and Frith, 1983) in individuals with autism. Despite the abundant documentation of this type of responding in autism, until now no relationship with anatomy had been demonstrated. Interestingly, Townsend and Courchesne (1994) also report an abnormally wide and apparently nonselective visuospatial attention in other autistic patients

Boy without CNS pathology

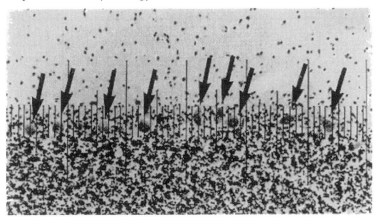

Autistic boy

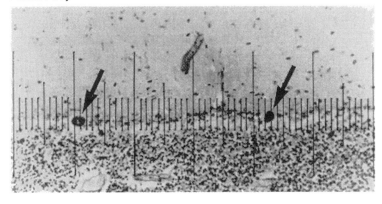

Figure 13-6. In autism, reduction in cerebellar Purkinje neuron numbers is a common finding across postmortem cases examined to date. *(Top)* Control case. *(Bottom)* Autism case. There is a comparable span of cerebellar cortex in the control case and the autism case. Arrows point to Purkinje cell bodies in these Nissel-stained sections. There also appears to be fewer granule neurons in the autism case. (Adapted from Ritvo et al., 1986.)

P1 ATTENDED vs UNATTENDED

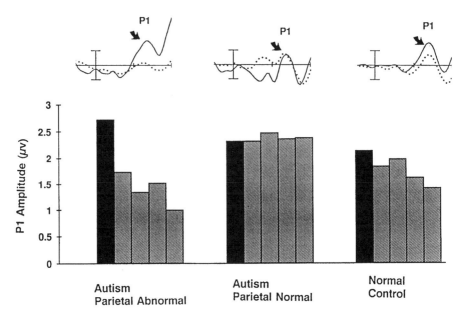

Figure 13-7. Event-related brain potential (ERP) evidence that autistic patients with parietal lobe volume loss have an extremely narrow "spotlight" of visuospatial attention. Bar graphs are shown for autistic patients with and without parietal abnormalities and normal control subjects. P1 peak amplitude ERP responses at occipital scalp sites to visual stimuli at an attended location (dark bar) are compared with P1 ERP responses at that location when attention was focused one, two, three, and four locations away (lighter bars in order left to right). Visuospatial locations were separated by 2.7° of visual angle. Waveforms at the top show P1 ERP responses at occipital sites to attended (solid line) compared with average of all unattended (dotted line) locations. (From Townsend and Courchesne, 1994.)

who do not have parietal volume loss (Fig. 13-7; also see Fig. 13-3), exemplifying once again the wide range of heterogeneity found in this disorder.

The second set of studies ever to demonstrate specific anatomic–behavior correlations in autism were those by Harris et al. (1998, 1999) and Townsend et al. (1999). They found in young autistic children (Singer-Harris, 1997) and in autistic adults (Townsend et al., 1999) that neocerebellar vermal abnormality is significantly correlated with orienting attention deficits (Fig. 13-8).

Brain–behavior associations, though not correlations, have been shown in other studies: Cerebellar anatomic abnormality has been associated with shifting attention deficits (Courchesne et al., 1994d). Quantitative behavioral examinations have found signs of abnormal cerebellar and parietal neurologic functioning in some but not all children with autism (Haas et al., 1996). Haznedar et al. (1997) found the anterior cingulate to be anatomically smaller in a small sample of autis-

tic patients than in normal controls, and, when the same autistic and normal subjects performed the California Verbal Learning task, PET activation in that region
was lower in the autistic subjects: however, Haznedar et al. (1997) did not find correlations between the size of cingulate anatomic abnormality and PET activation
levels or between either of these and task performance.

Some studies have shown abnormal frontal lobe metabolism or blood flow in
autism (George et al., 1992; Minshew et al., 1993; Rumsey et al., 1985; Zilbovicius et al., 1995), but the type of abnormality varies among the different reports
and is not uniform among all patients. PET imaging detects evidence of abnormal
dentato-thalamo-frontal serotonergic function in males but not females with
autism (Chugani et al., 1997). Others have shown behavioral impairment on "executive function" tasks, which is often interpreted as an indication of frontal lobe
damage (McEvoy et al., 1993; for review, see Pennington and Ozonoff). However, no study has found a significant correlation between the degree of abnormal
"executive function" and a measure of frontal lobe anatomical defect.

Another area of debate in the field of autism research surrounds the origin,

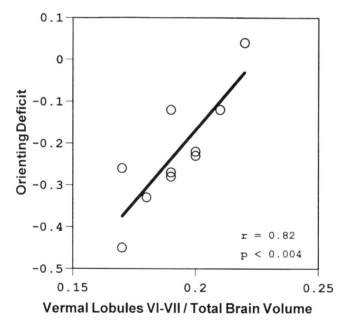

Figure 13-8. Correlation of orienting attention deficit with neocerebellar vermis lobules
VI–VII in 10 autism subjects. Data are from autistic patients performing in a Posner-type
attention task (Posner et al., 1984; Townsend et al., 1996a). Orienting Deficit is an index of
time to orient attention computed from response at the cued location as follows: (% correct
with 100 msec cue-to-target interval) − (% correct with 800 msec cue-to-target interval)/
(% correct with 100 msec cue-to-target interval). Vermal lobule VI–VII area measures in
each subject were normalized by that subject's total brain volume to control for overall size
of brain. (From Townsend et al., 1999.)

as well as degree, of social deficits found in this disorder. At a global level, abnormalities in the ability to maintain interactions and initiate with peers (Pierce and Schreibman, 1995, 1997) and to recognize faces (Boucher and Lewis, 1992) and emotions (Hobson et al., 1988) persist. More subtle social abnormalities such as deficits in joint attention (Lewy and Dawson, 1992) and the ability to follow a speaker's gaze (Leekam et al., 1997) have also been clearly documented. Neuroscience research points to limbic structures (e.g., amygdala; Adolphs et al., 1994) and face sensitive areas of temporal cortex (e.g., fusiform gyrus; Kanwisher et al., 1997) as involved in the aforementioned social behaviors, but there are as yet no reports on neurobiological research on autism that demonstrate either associations or correlations between social processing deficits and these structures in autism. This paucity, however, has not prevented interesting theoretical discussions regarding the potential role of temporal lobe structures in the symptomology of autism (Bachevalier, 1994; Barth et al., 1995; Waterhouse and Fein, 1997).

As discussed in a later subsection, detailed knowledge of brain–behavior relationships may point the way to elucidating how developmental experiences can be tailored to affect successful compensatory responses in the autistic child.

Contribution of autism research to basic science

For more than a century, neurologists and neuroscientists alike have held the view that the singular function of the human cerebellum is to help coordinate movement (Ito, 1984). Although autism research has, historically, not contributed significantly to elucidating issues in the basic cognitive neurosciences, evidence of cerebellar involvement in autism has prompted new basic science experiments and theories on the role of the human cerebellum. For instance, a new study (Allen et al., 1997) has shown that the cerebellum is active during visual attention and that motor and attention functions activate different localized regions within the cerebellum, inferring regional specialization for motor and cognitive functions (Fig. 13-9). Reviews of recent literature on animals and humans point out that the cerebellum is involved in a wide range of functions, including sensory, motor, attention, memory, speech, language, social, and affective functions (Table 13-2) (Courchesne and Allen, 1997; Leiner et al., 1995; Schmahmann and Sherman, 1997). For instance, the cerebellum is activated during language association learning tasks (Color Plate II) (Raichle et al., 1994). The evidence is now overwhelming that the cerebellum is not exclusively a motor-control device. The evidence is also overwhelming that it is critically involved in association learning. From this information, we proposed that the cerebellum provides a critical role in learning predictive associations that allow it to send anticipatory signals to many different functional systems within the brain (Courchesne and Allen, 1997). We suggest that this theory may contribute to the understanding of many neuropsychiatric disorders (Allen and Courchesne, 1998) and to the understanding of how developmental experiences (behavioral treatment programs) can best effect successful compensatory responses in the autistic brain (see later).

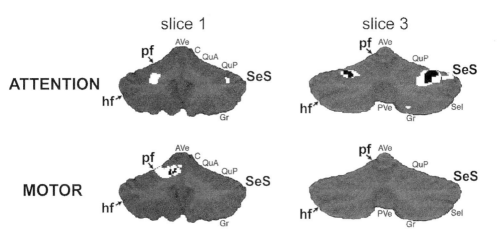

Figure 13-9. Cerebellar activation during an attention-only task and during a motor-only task in normal subjects. Functional maps show that attention alone was sufficient to activate the normal human cerebellum and did so independently of motor involvement. Attention and motor activation sites were located in different regions within the cerebellum. Maps show the most common sites of activation across subjects. Yellow indicates overlap of three or more subjects; Blue indicates any two subjects; hf is horizontal fissure; pf is primary fissure; gr is gracile lobule; pve is posterior vermis; and sel is semilunar lobule. *(Top)* During the attention task, the most common site of activation was in the left superior posterior cerebellum (the posterior portion of the quadrangular lobule [QuP] and the superior portion of the semilunar lobule [SeS]). *(Bottom)* During the motor task, the most common site was in the right anterior cerebellum (the anterior portion of the quadrangular lobule [QuA], the central lobule [C], and the anterior vermis [AVe]). (Adapted from Allen et al., 1997.)

Lessons from biological findings and next steps

As is evident from the above list of neuroscience discoveries in the autistic population, abnormal biological features in autism span many systems (see Table 13-1). As a population, autistic individuals share a wide array of heterogenous phenotypic features. As individuals, each autistic person has multiple biological and behavioral abnormalities. Additionally, as individuals, no two autistic persons are completely alike. Heterogeneity of symptoms is a fact in autism as it is in many mental disorders. In the behavioral domain, this is recognized and accepted by the psychiatric professional community. The *Diagnostic and Statistical Manual of Mental Disorders* (DSM-IV) lists as diagnostic criteria for autistic disorder a dozen behavioral features from which a total of six items across three behavioral domains is sufficient to fulfill diagnostic criteria. This acknowledges the fact that, under the diagnostic umbrella of autistic disorder, not all persons who meet diagnostic criteria exhibit all of the same behavioral phenotypic features; the corollary is that not all behavioral phenotypic features for autism are found in all autistic individuals.

Table 13-2.   PET and fMRI studies show that the cerebellum is active during

Attention
Allen et al. (1997), Le and Hu (1996)

Sensory Discrimination
Gao et al. (1996)

Semantic Association
Martin et al. (1995), Peterson et al. (1989)

Working Memory
Awh et al., Fiez et al. (1995), Klingberg et al. (1996)

Associative Learning
Blaxton et al. (1996), Logan and Grafton (1995), Molchan et al. (1994)

Practice-Related Learning
Raichle et al. (1994)

Procedural Learning
Flament et al. (1996), Grafton et al. (1994), Jenkins et al. (1994), Rao et al. (1995)

Motor Skill Acquisition
Friston et al. (1992), Seitz et al. (1994)

Problem Solving
Kim et al. (1994)

Concept Formation
Berman et al. (1996), Nagahama et al. (1996)

Spatial Memory
Moscovitch et al. (1995)

Object Memory
Moscovitch et al. (1995)

Verbal Memory
Andreasen et al. (1995), Grasby et al. (1993)

Episodic Memory
Andreasen et al. (1995)

Semantic Memory
Andreasen et al. (1995)

Speech
Artiges et al. (1995)

Motor Imagery
Decety et al. (1994), Parsons et al. (1995)

Motor Preparation
Deiber et al. (1996)

Motor Control
Allen et al. (1996), Ellerman et al. (1994), Fox et al. (1985)

Adapted from Courchesne and Allen (1997). See original work for citations.

In the biological domain, however, heterogeneity of anatomical and neural functional phenotypes does not receive the same acceptance. There is an unspoken *expectation* among the clinical research community that biological findings have to be unanimous (homogeneous) across the entire autistic population to be valid. This, perhaps, stems from an assumption that all the heterogeneous behavioral symptoms can be accounted for by one unifying explanation. All would agree that behavioral features are the most downstream manifestations of a developmental cognitive disorder such as autism. Because it is clear that all biological research efforts are directed at identifying markers further *up*stream in the anomalous developmental pathways, it is often assumed that any finding in the biological domain *claims* to provide that explanation or that it *should* provide that explanation. In reality, very nearly all biological findings are only a few more steps upstream than behavioral manifestations. They are, themselves, outcomes of deviant developmental pathways that began either at the genetic or cellular level. Just as behavioral outcomes are heterogeneous, so are biological outcomes; and biological outcomes are as much phenotypic features for the disorder as are behavioral outcomes.

A different approach is to learn from the lessons taught by the hyperserotonemia story begun by Schain and Freedman (1961)—biological heterogeneity in autism is inevitable. As autism research evolves, it will be the very idea of heterogeneity that will provide scientists the support to take the next important steps.

Heterogeneity in Autism: A Biological Inevitability

Two biological mechanisms and conditions that are designed to create efficiency and adaptive neuroplasticity during development—*pleiotropy* and *epigenesis*—simultaneously and inevitably open the door to many different possible developmental outcomes. In this way, biological mechanisms of efficiency and plasticity leave the system vulnerable to abnormal perturbations (i.e., genetic or environmental conditions outside the normally expected biological trajectory). Furthermore, each site of abnormal perturbation can, in its turn, trigger still further abnormal development in other sites. These two mechanisms, we believe, are the reasons for the intra- and interindividual heterogeneous symptom outcomes we see in autism, as well as in many other developmental disorders.

In the following sections, we elaborate on the mechanisms of pleiotropy and epigenesis in both normal and abnormal development, gleaning support from animal research. We extend the hypothesis of how the mechanism of pleiotropy can magnify and multiply the effects of a single genetic mutation to result in a wide range of seemingly unrelated phenotypes within an autistic individual. We additionally hypothesize on how the process of epigenesis—by which internal and external influences impinging on a developing organism mediate its developmental outcome—can explain the interindividual heterogeneity of phenotypic symptoms within a group of persons with autism. Finally, on the basis that external epigenetic influences such as nutritive factors, sensory and social experiences, and learning mediate cell differentiation effects through neural activity (Kandel et al., 1991), we propose that early and biologically informed intervention is likely to be effective in optimizing the developmental outcome of autistic individuals.

The Pleiotropy Hypothesis of Autism

Pleiotropy is defined as the "diverse effects of a single gene or gene pair on several organ systems and functions" (Gelehrter and Collins, 1990, p. 306). It is an evolutionary adaptation that may partially alleviate the problem of "poverty of the genome" because it is a mechanism for genetic coding efficiency: The same gene code can accomplish multiple developmental tasks in multiple cell types at different times. This remarkable efficiency is the Achilles heel of genetic control mechanisms because *mutations in a gene's code can cause multiple developmental jobs to fail.*

This phenomenon supports the hypothesis that, at least in principle, a single gene mutation could be sufficient to account for the heterogeneous phenotypes seen in autism, which is among the most heritable neuropsychiatric disorders (Plomin et al., 1994). On the other hand, statistical models predict multigene liabilities in autistic individuals (Pickles et al., 1995). Whether autism is due to a single gene mutation in some cases or to the combined action of variants of several genes in other cases, we argue that pleiotropy is very likely to explain the *intra*individual heterogeneity, that is, the seemingly unrelated array of anatomical, physiological, psychological, and behavioral abnormalities within a person with autism.

There are, in fact, many examples of single-gene defects that produce a heterogeneous array of biological and behavioral abnormalities in animals and in humans, including phenylketonuria (PKU), fragile-X syndrome, Lesch-Nyhan syndrome, and adenylosuccinate lyase deficiency (ASL). We argue that the following such examples should be a reminder that autism could well prove to be another example of a pleiotropic disorder.

Examples of pleiotropy from the animal literature

In the animal literature, many examples of pleiotropy can be found, but recent autism research (Cook et al., 1997b, 1998) makes opportune the discussion of pleiotropic effects involving the $GABA_A$ beta-3 subunit gene. This gene is on the proximal arm of chromosome 15 in the critical region (15q11–13) for Prader-Willi syndrome and Angelman syndrome. Duplication of this region has been reported in a number of autistic patients by several laboratories (Cook et al., 1997b, 1998; Gillberg et al., 1991; Hotof and Bolton, 1995; Schroer et al., 1998). This duplication appears in about 3% of the autistic patients tested from our laboratory (unpublished data: E. Courchesne and R. Yeung-Courchesne in collaboration with E. Cook and C. Lord), a rate higher than any other type of chromosome defect that has been reported in the literature for autism cases. Most recently, in a study of 140 families with an autistic child, Cook et al. (1998) found linkage disequilibrium and association between autistic disorder and a marker location within this 15q11–13 subregion; the marker location was within the GABA$_A$ beta-3 subunit gene.

This gene controls production of the beta-3 subunit of GABA$_A$ receptors. Normally, it plays different roles in the developing brain and the mature brain. In the mature brain GABA$_A$ receptors mediate rapid inhibitory neurotransmission, and the beta-3 subunit is a major constituent of a substantial percentage of these receptors. In contrast, in the developing brain, changes in the distribution of expression of GABA$_A$ receptor subunits indicate that it may function as a neurotrophic factor affecting neural differentiation, growth, and circuit organization. Additionally, its peak expression occurs in different cell types at different times during brain development. In the prenatal murine brain, it reaches peak expression in the cerebral cortex, hippocampus, and thalamus and postnatally in the cerebellar cortex (Laurie et al., 1992; Nadler et al., 1994). After peak expression, rapid down-regulation occurs in the murine thalamus (Laurie et al., 1992) and inferior olive (Chang et al., 1995), whose climbing fibers constitute a major functional input to Purkinje neurons. While cerebral cortex and, to a lesser extent, hippocampus have lower levels of expression of the beta-3 subunit by adulthood, expression in the cerebellum does not change during postnatal maturation (Laurie et al., 1992; Nadler et al., 1994). In the mature murine brain, the beta-3 subunit is most intensely expressed in the cerebellum (Purkinje and granule cells), hippocampus, and pyriform cortex (Wisden et al., 1992).

In mice, defects in the same GABA$_A$ beta-3 subunit gene can cause a wide array of neural and behavioral abnormalities during development as well as craniofacial defects (e.g., Homanics et al., 1997) (Fig. 13-10). At the molecular level, mice with a knockout of the GABA$_A$ beta-3 subunit have a marked deficit in the GABA$_A$ receptor levels in the brain and a greater reduction of benzodiazepine binding relative to muscimol binding; this molecular evidence suggests that other GABA$_A$ subunits depend on the presence of the beta-3 subunit for normal functional development. At the neurophysiological level, these GABA$_A$ beta-3 subunit knockout mice have EEG abnormalities and seizures; abnormal EEG patterns stop when the animal becomes maximally alert or aroused. At the neurobehavioral level, these mice have motor, sensory, and social communication abnormalities: They display hyperactivity and often run in tight circles; they have difficulty with some skilled movements (e.g., walking on grids), but do not have a grossly jerky gait; they are hyperresponsive to human contact and other sensory stimuli; and mothers with GABA$_A$ beta-3 subunit knockout fail to show normal nurturing behavior even when their pups are normal. Additionally, these mice may have cleft palate (57%), and so a defect in the GABA$_A$ beta-3 subunit gene may be one factor in multiple pathways involved in the formation of cleft palate. Lastly, these mice have reduced longevity.

The rough resemblance between the neurophysiological and behavioral developmental consequences in the GABA$_A$ beta-3 subunit gene knockout mouse and some of the characteristics seen in some autistic individuals is certainly interesting (see Table 13-1, Fig. 13-11). Autistic individuals are often seen as having insufficient inhibitory control; having EEG abnormalities including seizures; be-

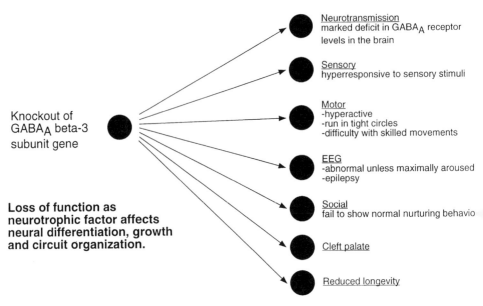

Figure 13-10. The GABA$_A$ beta-3 subunit gene exerts pleiotropic effects. When this single gene is knocked out in the mouse, the developmental outcomes (listed at the right) include multiple biological and behavioral abnormalities. (Based on Homanics et al., 1997.)

ing hyperactive and doing repetitive movements such as walking around and around; being hypersensitive especially to contact with other living beings; and having deficits in affiliative species-normal social behavior. Additionally, in the mature mouse brain, the GABA$_A$ beta-3 subunit is most intensely expressed in the cerebellum (Purkinje and granule cells), hippocampus, and pyriform cortex (Wisden et al., 1992), all three regions being consistently reported as anatomically abnormal in autistic patients in either quantitative magnetic resonance imaging or autopsy studies (Bauman and Kemper, 1994; Courchesne, 1997).

Nonetheless, words of caution are needed here. Linkage disequilibrium with markers in this region may be pointing *not* to the GABA$_A$ beta-3 subunit gene but, instead, may be alerting us to a defect in a yet to be identified *neighboring* gene. Moreover, the linkage disequilibrium between autism and a marker located within the GABA$_A$ beta-3 subunit gene in our single study (Cook et al., 1998) needs to be replicated, and functional variants within that gene need to be shown to have differential biological consequences. Furthermore, even if this finding is frequently replicated, it would still most likely reflect genetic mechanisms important in one subgroup of autistic patients and not reflect mechanisms universal in the autistic population—the etiology of autism is certainly heterogeneous.

The important point here is that animal model studies in recent years have shown that single genes often play different functional roles in different cell types at different times during development. So defects in such genes trigger a cascade of changes that are not confined to narrow channels of particular neural structure, functional system, or behavioral domain, but instead, sweep across multiple structures, systems, and domains. In doing so, they produce complex abnormal biological and behavioral phenotypes.

Examples of pleiotropic effects in human developmental disorders

Evidence from rare human developmental disorders leaves no doubt that single gene mutations are capable of creating in each affected individual a heterogeneous array of biological and behavioral abnormalities (Table 13-3). For example, mutation in single genes underlies a number of rare human neurodevelopmental disorders (e.g., the PAH gene in PKU [Eisensmith and Woo, 1991; Folling, 1971]; the FMR-1 gene in the fragile-X syndrome [Verkerk et al., 1991; Yu et al., 1991]; the HPRT gene in Lesch-Nyhan syndrome [Stout and Caskey, 1985]; and the ASL gene in adenylosuccinate lyase syndrome [Stone et al., 1992]). Every one of these single-gene mutation disorders is characterized by multiple neural and behavioral abnormalities as well as by non-neural ones. In fact, even though each disorder is due to completely different gene mutations affecting completely different molecular mechanisms, there is considerable overlap among them in the domains of neural and behavioral abnormality. Moreover, domains of defect in one or another of these disorders are also abnormal in autism, including cerebellar, cerebral, and limbic system anatomical abnormalities; self injurious behavior; speech and language maldevelopment; and abnormal social communication skills. It seems to us that some subgroup of autistic patients will be discovered who, likewise, have a single gene mutation that is completely different from each of these other rare developmental disorders, that affects completely different molecular mechanisms, but that produces the same array of domains of neural and behavioral abnormality.

Another illustration of pleiotropy is found in fragile-X syndrome. The physical and behavioral phenotype of this disorder is caused by an absence of function of the FMR-1 gene. When the CGG trinucleotide repeat number expands beyond 200 (full mutation), the FMR-1 gene becomes methylated and is essentially turned off. There is no RNA message produced in a fully methylated full mutation of FMR-1. Without a message, the cell is unable to produce the FMR-1 protein FMRP. FMRP is a binding protein for messenger RNA; it binds and carries both its own message and the messenger RNA from approximately 4% of brain proteins. The phenotype in fragile-X syndrome may be related to FMRP's role in carrying the message of other genes so that, when FMRP is absent, the other genes are not expressed, and so the different functions needed at different sites at different developmental phases that are mediated by these genes are compromised. This may, in part, explain why the fragile-X syndrome phenotype involves so many different manifestations in different tissues (Hagerman, 1996).

Table 13-3. Anomalies observed in individuals with phenylketonuria

Genetic Abnormalities

Multiple (eight) restriction fragment length polymorphism (RFLP) sites in or near the coding
    region of the PAH gene on chromosome 12 (12q22–q24.1)
Six haplotypes with varying phenotypes and severity of impairment

Behavioral and Psychological Abnormalities

Social retardation
Abnormal emotional reactivity
Sensorimotor deficits
Speech deficits or failure
Hyperactivity
Irritability
Erratic aggressive behavior
Clumsiness in motor skills
Rocking
Mental retardation

Neurological Abnormalities

Abnormal EEG; epileptiform seizures
Disturbed sleep patterns
Stooped posture
Muscular hypertonicity

Neuroanatomical Abnormalities

Microcephaly (about 10% less brain weight than normal)
Decreased ratio of white to gray matter in central nervous system
Reduced cerebral cortical thickness
Reduced neuron size
Dendritic development
Reduced number of synaptic spines
Increased cell packing density
Abnormal myelination
Fibrous gliosis, may indicate loss of axis cylinders and myelin sheaths
Loss of pigment in usually pigmented brain regions
Lamellar-type inclusion bodies in oligodendroglial cells in the brain

Neurochemical Abnormalities

Reduced serotonin and catecholamine levels

Biochemical Abnormalities

Virtual absence of hepatic phenylalanine dehydroxylase (98%–99% of patients)
Virtual absence of dihydropteridine reductase (1%–2% of patients)
Phenylalanine is not converted to tyrosine → hyperphenylalaninemia
Increased blood levels of aromatic acids (abnormal metabolites of phenylalanine)
Phenylketonuria

Systemic Abnormalities

Mousy odor
Hypopigmentation
Dry skin, eczema, and other nonspecific skin lesions
Reduced sperm count and semen volume in males
Other: untreated phenylketonuria mothers give birth to children with irreversible brain damage

Conclusion

If there is one overriding lesson from the study of rare human developmental disorders, it is that surprisingly often, they are initially triggered by mutations in single genes that cause a wide variety of neurobiological and behavioral abnormalities, often involving sensory, motor, attention, memory, speech, language, affective, and social functions. It would not be unexpected, then, for the heterogeneous biological and behavioral abnormalities present in each autistic person, to be explained—at least in a subgroup of autistic patients—by the presence of mutations in one or more genes each of which has pleiotropic effects. A phenotypic outcome as diverse and complex as is seen in autism, however, is most assuredly the result of not only pleiotropic mechanisms but also those that take into account the multitude of environmental contingencies surrounding an individual as they emerge from cell to adulthood.

The Epigenesis Hypothesis of Autism

Epigenesis is the process by which an organism develops from an undifferentiated cell through successive formation and development of organs and parts that do not pre-exist in the fertilized egg (as opposed to the erroneous concept of preformation). In each instant of this process of development, growth outcome is impacted by the microenvironment surrounding the cells, such as the presence, absence, or concentration of trophic factors, neurotransmitters, enzymes, metabolites, toxic agents such as medication, viruses, and end products of trauma and immune responses. All of these conditions surrounding the proliferating, migrating, aggregating, differentiating, and synapsing cells can alter the structural and functional outcomes of the organs or systems undergoing development, resulting in variant forms of the "normal" organs or systems, with varying efficiency and efficacy of function. The interplay among internal *contingent events or conditions* as well as between those and external environmental events and conditions determines the precise developmental path taken (Cicchetti and Rogosch, 1996; Courchesne et al., 1994a; Yeung-Courchesne and Courchesne, 1997).

In autism, epigenetic processes, when perturbed by abnormal events or conditions, will produce many different possible developmental outcomes including novel and abnormal ones. Furthermore, as predicted from the results of numerous animal model experiments, in autism the neural reorganization caused by abnormal perturbation in one site or system will not remain neatly confined to this primary site. Instead it will, in turn, trigger still further abnormal development in other sites and systems, thus increasing the extent of biological and behavioral outcome heterogeneity in each individual with autism. Moreover, because each autistic individual will experience individual-specific contingent events or conditions, the precise path taken will not be identical between two autistic individuals (indeed, even cloned animals that experience different, individual-specific conditions may not have identical neural configurations [Macagno et al., 1973]; Fig. 13-11).

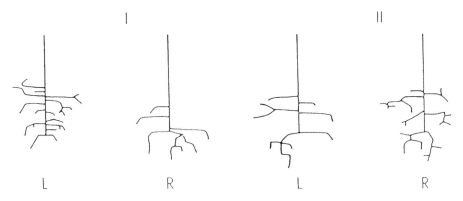

Figure 13-11. Even cloned insects that experience different, individual-specific conditions do not have identical neural configurations. Drawing of computer reconstructions of the branching pattern of the same retinal axon on left (L) and right (R) sides of the brain of two *Daphnia* specimens (I and II) to show the considerable variability experienced. The two specimens are isogeneic members of a single parthenogenetic clone. (After Macagno et al., 1973. From Lund, 1978.)

Epigenetic responses to abnormal events and conditions

From the epigenetic point of view (Quartz and Sejnowski, 1997), the developing neural system is, in fact, *biologically designed to be perturbable,* to be pushed down different paths in order to best learn from and adapt to information delivered by the intrinsic and extrinsic milieu. In the words of Quartz and Sejnowski (1997, p. 537), in "neural constructivism, the representational features of cortex are built from the dynamic interaction between neural growth mechanisms and environmentally derived neural activity," and, most importantly, "the representational properties of cortex *[are] built by the nature of the problem domain confronting it"* (italics added). In normal development, mechanisms involving many factors (tropic factors; competitive and cooperative neural activity) come into play to ensure *(1)* that the number of neurons in one location matches that in its target location; *(2)* that the initial exuberant axon connectivity is followed by selective sparing of some connections and the elimination of others; *(3)* that the rapid period of synapse production is followed by the selective stabilization of those that are functionally adaptive; *(4)* that functional neural activity gradually and optimally shapes the geometry and size of axonal and dendritic arbors during a prolonged period of growth; and, finally *(5)* that representation maps have a spatially orderly relationship to one another (for reviews, see Courchesne et al., 1994a,d; Cowan et al., 1984; Kandel et al., 1991; Quartz and Sejnowski, 1997).

We theorize that in autism, where the developing brain has already suffered the adverse effects of mutations in one or more pleiotropic genes, those very epigenetic properties that make the normally developing brain so exquisitely adaptive and malleable make the autistic brain highly *vulnerable* to unusual functional reorganization, which may or may not be beneficial. This view is supported by a wealth of studies examining neuroplasticity following abnormal perturbations to the developing brain. In such experiments, the otherwise normally developing nervous system is presented with abnormal contingent events or conditions such as sensory deprivation, a focal lesion, a viral infection, abnormal levels of neurotropic factors, abnormal neural activity, or exposure to toxins (Courchesne et al., 1994a,d; Cowan et al., 1984; Kandel, 1991; Quartz and Sejnowski, 1997). Such experiments show that loss of neurons in one location can trigger remote loss in secondary or tertiary locations. Changes in neuron numbers in one target location can cause aberrant axon connections to form or to be retained when normally they would have been pruned back. Abnormal activity reaching a site that might otherwise have been normal can produce abnormal overgrowth or undergrowth of axonal and dendritic arbors, abnormal representational maps, and behavioral dysfunction. Through epigenetic processes, therefore, a single defect can set off a domino effect propagating maldevelopment to still other structures and functions; the result is heterogeneity of abnormality beyond the point of initial etiological impact. As discussed in the next section, we theorize that each of these types of abnormal events and conditions occurs in the developing autistic brain, triggering an analogous cascade of maldevelopment.

Cortical development may be particularly vulnerable

Cerebral cortex appears to be particularly vulnerable to abnormal instructions from sensory systems and readily constructs abnormal representations—representations that might be enlarged, shrunken, absent, novel, underresponsive, or nonselectively overresponsive. For instance, during fetal growth in rats, elimination of the neural signals from the facial whiskers causes both a reduction in the cerebral cortical "map" representing the facial whisker area and an excessive enlargement of its cortical map representing facial structures—the lower lip and jaw—that remained normally neurally active. Different forms of early abnormal neural activity produce different forms of structural and functional abnormalities. The malleability and vulnerability of cerebral cortex may be developmentally inevitable: Initially cerebral cortex is a "protocortex" that is "undifferentiated . . . composed of a large number of vertically oriented basic units or columns that have the same potential for processing capabilities" (Killackey, 1990, p. 13), and dependent on intrinsic cues from the thalamus for further organization (Killackey, 1990; O'Leary, 1989, 1992). So, on the one hand, in early stages of development the removal of a section of protocortex leaves the remaining protocortex to differentiate normally, while on the other hand the mis-instruction of protocortex due to abnormal intrinsic cues (e.g., from abnormal thalamus, cerebellum, or sensory systems) or the *mis-registration* of normal intrinsic cues by a defective protocortex (e.g., one lacking a functional $GABA_A$ beta-3 subunit) will actively create abnormal cortical organization. In general, the earlier the onset of abnormality and the longer the period of abnormality, the greater the neural and behavioral deficits, the longer the recovery time, and the poorer the final level of recovered neural and behavioral function.

Cerebral cortex may not be alone in this duality of developmental malleability and vulnerability. Cerebellar cortex might also begin as a protocortex. The cerebellum possesses key properties analogous to the cerebrum: Its cortex is also initially undifferentiated; is composed of a large number of vertically oriented basic units that have the same potential for processing capabilities, but in this case the units are Purkinje neuron-defined; and its dependent on intrinsic cues, but in this case from the pons for further functional organization. Cerebellar cortex has become a unique model site for identifying molecular, cellular, and system basis learning, and the Purkinje neuron is a key feature (Lisberger, 1998). Based on such new evidence and a reformulation of the role of the cerebellum (Allen et al., 1997; Courchesne and Allen, 1997), it is possible that cerebellar protocortex learns its specialized functional representations not only via information received from the periphery but also via intrinsic cues from the cerebrum and other subcortical structures (e.g., limbic, hypothalamic). Based on these properties, its size, and its connections, its role in development may be significant: For instance, in terms of the number of neurons it contains, the cerebellum is the largest structure in the human brain (Williams and Herrup, 1988). This tremendous number of neurons coupled with the high input-to-output axon ratio (cerebellar afferents-to-efferents: 40:1; Carpenter, 1991) suggests that its function must be massively integrative. It is also one of the most widely connected structures, having physiological connections with all major divisions of the central nervous system (for review, see Courchesne and Allen, 1997). Experiments are needed to test the idea that cerebellar cortex, like the cerebral cortex, is vulnerable during early development to abnormal inputs from sensory systems and readily constructs abnormal representations.

The pathological pleiotropic effect in the epigenesis of autism

The pleiotropic hypothesis of autism says that, whether autism results from one or more genes, the key genes will be ones that normally accomplish multiple developmental assignments, act in multiple cell types, and do so at different times. Defects in such a gene or genes will produce abnormality in each developmental assignment, in each cell type, and at each time for which it normally plays a role. Each and every such abnormal effect will trigger still further abnormal development. These additional abnormalities will not necessarily be in structures or functions whose development is normally mediated by the gene or genes in question. These secondary and tertiary effects of the original pleiotropic points of pathological impact may be felt at one or more genetic, molecular, cellular, and system levels. The net result is that the system is pushed down multiple, novel developmental paths. Because of these pathological epigenetic effects, the pleiotropic effects exerted by a gene when it is mutated are not completely predictable from what that gene influences when it is normal. That is, the biological and behavioral outcome heterogeneity in each individual will quantitatively and qualitatively exceed what would be expected solely from knowledge of the specific functions *normally* mediated by that gene or genes.

Such pathological pleiotropic effects are evident in rare human neurodevelopmental disorders such as fragile-X and PKU. In fragile-X as noted earlier, when FMRP is absent other genes that depend on it for their own normal functional expression fail to be normally expressed, and so these failures in turn compromise still other different functions dependent on them, and those in turn are also compromised, and so forth. An analogous story can be told for PKU, where the multiple abnormal defects in social behavior, language development, emotional reactivity, aggressive behavior, memory, attention, and sensorimotor functions are due to the pathological epigenetic transformations arising from the effects of excess phenylalanine and not due to the specific role of the PAH gene or phenylalanine in each and every one of these particular functions—because, of course, neither has any such specific role in any of those functions.

When gene mutations are found that cause autism, it is hypothesized that such pathological pleiotropic effects will eventually be described and that many of the outcome abnormalities will not be directly predictable solely from knowledge of the specific functions normally mediated by that gene or genes. To fully account for all outcome abnormalities, experiments will be necessary to identify the pathological paths of epigenetic transformation.

The need for studies of specific epigenetic paths in autism

Important though it is in explaining developmental outcome, at present nothing is known with certainty about epigenetic paths in autism. Speculations about psychological and behavioral outcomes have been posed; for instance, there are speculations that hippocampus and amygdala abnormalities affect social and emotional development (Waterhouse et al., 1996); that serotonergic abnormalities underlie repetitive/compulsive behaviors and oxytocin-related abnormalities underlie social deficits (Modahl et al., 1998); that frontal lobe abnormalities affect executive functions (Ozonoff, 1995); and that parietal and cerebellar abnormalities impair attention operations that are needed during the acquisition of social and nonsocial information (Courchesne et al., 1994c; Townsend and Courchesne, 1994; Townsend et al., 1996a).

Due to the consistent findings of developmental cerebellar abnormalities in autism (see beginning of this chapter), this structure serves as an appropriate choice for elucidating the concept of epigenesis in this disorder. In a typically functioning cerebellum, inputs are received from either climbing fibers (originating from inferior olivary nuclei) or mossy fibers (originating from brain stem and spinal cord nuclei). In the normal mature cerebellar cortex, each Purkinje cell receives monosynaptic inputs from just one climbing fiber, and each climbing fiber projects to multiple Purkinje cells. Mossy fibers synapse on granule cells, which in turn form parallel fibers that make excitatory contacts on numerous Purkinje cells. The results of cerebellar cortical computations are sent via Purkinje axons to the deep cerebellar nuclei, which in turn signal multiple brain regions via monosynaptic or multisynaptic pathways (Schmahmann, 1997; Courchesne and Allen, 1997). As the only output source from cerebellar cortex, the Purkinje neuron thus plays a vital role in efficient functioning, and epigenetic suggestions have been made about the consequence of early loss of these cells (see Courchesne et al., 1988, 1994a,d; Courchesne, 1995; Yeung-Courchesne and Courchesne, 1997). If the reduction in Purkinje neuron numbers occurs early in development, as we see in autism, then a series of predictions can be made based on known epigenetic principles and the large amount of empirical data on cerebellar development accumulated over the last 25 years. The reduction in Purkinje numbers will cause a reduction in other cell types in cerebellar cortex, including granule, basket, and stellate neurons. Reduction of granule neurons in turn reduces the number of parallel fibers and so the number of possible combinations of information reaching each surviving Purkinje neuron, which reduces the possibilities of adaptive learning in the cerebellum. Reduced numbers of neurons alters the physical distances traveled by parallel fibers between different Purkinje neurons and so can disturb critical cerebellar timing functions.

The combined loss of Purkinje and other cerebellar cortical neurons also causes a mis-construction of neural circuits within the cerebellum. For instance, reduced Purkinje numbers results in the aberrant retention of multiple climbing fibers on individual surviving Purkinje neurons, which in turn confounds the normally precise one-to-one climbing fiber input that instructs each Purkinje neuron during cerebellar learning. Unstable and conflicting climbing fiber instructions might slow or prevent learning because each climbing fiber provides different, perhaps even contradictory, information. Additionally, in the face of significant reduction in granule cells, mossy fibers make connections directly with Purkinje neurons, something they normally never do and something that bypasses the cerebellar learning path from mossy fiber to granule cell to Purkinje neuron.

As mentioned earlier, Purkinje neurons normally provide the only cortical inhibitory control over output of neural activity from deep cerebellar neurons. Their loss, therefore, reduces effective inhibitory control over the neural activity of the deep cerebellar nuclei, such as the dentate nuclei, in the autistic brain. There are two possible consequences. First, with fewer Purkinje neurons present and competing for synaptic space on neurons in the dentate nucleus, climbing and mossy fibers might establish more than their normal number of excitatory synapses on these cerebellar output neurons. Alternately, the surviving Purkinje neurons successfully compete for and make connections with more than the normal number of output neurons. That is, with fewer Purkinje neurons competing for synaptic space on dentate neurons, each surviving one can grab more than its normal share of synaptic connections. In autistic patients with extreme reduction in Purkinje neuron numbers, such as a case described by Bauman and Kemper (1985), the former abnormal circuit is most likely. In autistic patients with much less Purkinje reduction, the latter abnormal circuit is more likely.

Patchy Purkinje neuron loss in cerebellar cortex will act like small focal lesions would in cerebral cortex: Local representational maps will be abnormal and regional specialization abnormal, perhaps with some representations and regional functions absent or shrunken, others mis-located, and so on. If cerebral and cerebellar cortices have reciprocal interactions that lead to the coherent development and specification of cortical representations, then abnormal cerebellar maps may drive aberrant formation of cerebral cortical maps.

Mis-constructed cerebellar circuits and abnormal representational maps not only compromise the prime learning function of the cerebellum, but these abnormalities will cause a failure in the regulation of output signals from deep cerebellar nuclei, which are normally spontaneously excitatory. In autistic patients who have extensive reduction in Purkinje numbers, there would be excessive excitatory output activity from the deep nuclei in response to any single input signal because these nuclei experience too little Purkinje inhibitory control and too much climbing and mossy fiber excitation. In autistic patients who have much less Purkinje neuron loss, the beam of Purkinje inhibition might be much too broad, causing an abnormally broad reduction of output activity in response to any single input signal. Thus, variation in the quantity of Purkinje numbers might create not only *qualitatively* different cerebellar circuits in different autistic patients, but *opposite types of abnormal output activity* from the deep nuclei.

Abnormal cerebellar output activity produces abnormal cerebral and subcortical metabolic activity, according to neuroimaging studies on adults with acquired focal cerebellar lesions (e.g., Attig et al., 1991; Botez et al., 1991; Kimura et al., 1989; Rousseaux and Steinling, 1992). From the standpoint of autism, it is of particular interest that cerebellar to frontal cortical connections have been recently confirmed via new anatomical techniques (Middleton and Strick, 1994); cerebellar to limbic functional connections have been long known (Newman and Reza, 1979). In the autistic brain, abnormal cerebellar output activity might likewise produce abnormal cerebral and limbic metabolic activity, and, according to the hypothesis outlined above, abnormal cerebellar activity during development might alter growth and functional specification of cerebral cortex. In fact, neuroimaging evidence is suggestive of abnormal metabolic activity in frontal cortex in young children and adults with autism (George et al., 1992; Rumsey et al., 1985; Zilbovicius et al., 1995), abnormal cerebello-thalamo-frontal serotonergic function in autistic males (Chugani et al., 1997), and abnormal task-related cerebellar activations during nonverbal auditory stimulation and language performance (Müller et al., 1999a,b in press). A new study finds that the greater the cerebellar anatomic abnormality, the greater the frontal cortical volume (Carper et al., 1997), a result consistent with the idea mentioned above that excessive loss of Purkinje neuron control may allow excessive cerebellar excitation to drive excessive growth in frontal cortex.

Mis-constructed cerebellar circuits and defective cerebellar learning functions will interfere with the normal development and performance of the many language, affective, cognitive, memory, autonomic, motor, and sensory functions that involve the cerebellum (Table 13-2). Certainly cerebellar damage in children and adults can lead to mutism; emotional lability; dysprosody; expressive language deficits; impaired orienting and shifting attention; impaired executive functioning (planning, set-shifting, verbal fluency, abstract reasoning, working memory); impaired visuospatial and constructive organization and memory; and blunted affect or disinhibited affect (Akshoomoff and Courchesne, 1992, 1994; Schmahmann and Sherman, 1997; Townsend et al., 1996a). Autistic patients have abnormalities in each of these areas, and it is not much of a stretch to hypothesize that if damage to the normal cerebellum in the young child or adult produces these types of abnormalities, damage to the early developing cerebellum will do likewise.

A new theory of the role of the cerebellum is that it affects so many functions because it performs a unique function in preparatory learning (Allen et al., 1997; Allen and Courchesne, 1998; Courchesne and Allen, 1997). According to this theory, the fundamental purpose of the cerebellum is to *learn to predict and prepare internal conditions* needed to facilitate the efficient and timely responses of a wide variety of motor and nonmotor systems. Such learned associative responses provide *automatic,* moment-to-moment signaling. So, this cerebellar preparatory function is neither a sensory nor a motor activity, but rather a general one that prepares whichever neural systems (e.g., sensory, motor, autonomic, memory, attention, affective, speech, language) may be needed in upcoming moments. Depending on its prediction of whatever information acquisition, analysis, or action is about to be needed, it may, for example, reposition sensory receptors; alter cerebral blood flow levels; enhance neural signal to noise; enhance neural responsiveness in hippocampus, thalamus, and superior colliculus; and modulate motor control systems.

To perform this precise temporally dependent preparatory function, the cerebellum must learn the predictive relationships among temporally ordered multidimensional sequences of exogenously derived (e.g., sensory events) and endogenously derived (e.g., signals from frontal and parietal cortex, hippocampus, hypothalamus, and so forth) neural activities including those derived from the consequences of its own output—preparatory signaling. This is an expansion on previous models showing the role of the cerebellum in predictive learning (e.g., Courchesne et al., 1994c; Miall et al., 1993). Miall et al. (1993, p. 214), state that "it is tempting to suggest that the cerebellum may be involved in more complex predictions, linking it to more cognitive processes." Paulin (1993) proposed that the cerebellum improves the efficiency of motor control through the process of state estimation, which might involve prediction.

In our theory, complete knowledge of upcoming events is not necessary to trigger specific preparatory actions. Simple exposure to aspects of a sequence of activities (even a single internal or environmental event) predictive of events that will soon arrive may be sufficient to trigger preparatory responding by the cerebellum. To be maximally adaptive to real world variability, the cerebellum must be a "pattern extractor" capable of getting the "gist" of what has been happening and what is likely to happen next and then flexibly deciding what internal conditions are needed to prepare for a particular predicted up-coming operation, be it acquisition, analysis, or action.

If one were to name a single characteristic of the cognitive style of patients with autism, it would be that they are literal minded and unable to get the "gist of things" (e.g., see the very first description of an autistic child, Kanner [1943]). In autism, impairment of preparatory learning might give rise to reliance on unusual and consciously controlled strategies for anticipating up-coming events, such as an insistence on sameness. Temporal accuracy would be reduced in high-demand temporal–spatial sequencing problems. Flexibility in association learning and rapidly and unconsciously altering associations would be reduced. Repetitive and redundant sequences of information would be favored over high-speed, variable, and precisely ordered spatiotemporal sequences of information that demand rapid predictive and preparation computations. Given the type of aberrant cerebellar learning circuits that are likely to arise in the autistic Purkinje neuron–deficit cerebellum (see above), odd associations would be expected, unlikely and erroneous predictions would be made on a moment-to-moment basis, and maladaptive and unusual combinations of anticipatory or preparatory reactions would be a common developmental consequence.

This, of course, represents only a brief sketch or outline of what a full epigenetic account involving just the cerebellum might look like. Our pleiotropy hypothesis of autism argues that, in those autistic persons with a genetic etiology, multiple original points of pleiotropic impact will occur, not just one in the cerebellum, and thus a more complete sketch or outline of epigenesis in autism would require the above sort of outline for each and every point of pleiotropic impact in neural and non-neural systems—and the epigenetic interactions among them! As a handy example, an epigenetic account of the outcome behaviors in the $GABA_A$ beta-3 knockout mouse would require examination of epigenetic consequences of a $GABA_A$ beta-3 receptor defect in cerebrum, cerebellum, limbic system, and thalamus, along with a description of interactions among them, and then, for instance, we might know why these animals have social nurturing deficits (it is certainly not because the $GABA_A$ beta-3 is a social nurturing–specific receptor). This biological view of developmental disorders makes clear why notions of diagnostic specificity (i.e., only individuals with a particular disorder should possess a specific abnormality) may, in fact, hinder research progress in this field.

The divergence effect in the epigenesis of autism

While the pleiotropy and epigenetic hypotheses explain why an autistic person with a genetic etiology has multiple types of biological and behavioral abnormalities, it would not explain the *differences* in types or severities of abnormalities between any two persons with autism who have identical genetic defects. We propose that such differences are due to the fact that each autistic person will experience *individual-specific* contingent events or conditions so that the precise path taken will not be identical between any two persons with autism. Divergence effects occur because genes operate in continuous interaction with extrinsic as well as intrinsic conditions and events, not in isolation. Even cloned insects that experience different, individual-specific conditions do not have identical neural configurations (Macagno et al., 1973) (Fig. 13-11). The terms *multifinality* and *divergence heterogeneity* also refer to this phenomenon wherein two individuals with similar or even identical biological beginnings may take divergent developmental paths and end with some degree of dissimilar biological and/or behavioral outcome (Cicchetti and Rogosch, 1996; Courchesne et al., 1994a,d; Yeung-Courchesne and Courchesne, 1997). In short, from a common starting point, individual-specific contingency effects push development down one path or another leading to different outcomes. Individual-specific contingent conditions may strongly alter epigenetic outcome such that, in two individuals with the same gene defect, one might have a more favorable outcome, while the other has a distinctly unfavorable outcome.

Among all rare neurodevelopmental disorders, PKU (Eisensmith and Woo, 1991) offers the best illustration of the power of individual-specific contingency conditions to drive development down favorable or unfavorable paths. Normally PAH codes for phenylalanine hydroxylase, an enzyme that metabolizes phenylalanine. If two newborn infants have the same PAH gene mutation, the baby who stays on a diet with *abnormally low levels* of phenylalanine (an amino acid normally found in many foods) will have a normal developmental outcome, but the baby who has a diet with *normal levels* of phenylalanine will develop severe neural defects and retardation (Table 13-3). The single difference in dietary experience is a key contingency or deciding factor—not the gene defect alone.

In the infant who has the diet with normal levels of phenylalanine, *abnormal sequences* of biochemical, neural, and behavioral events are initiated, and once this developmental path of neural "mis-construction" and functional "mis-organization" has been taken, there is no known way to "de"-misconstruct and "de"-misorganize abnormalities. In the words of Blau (1979), the importance of this enzyme "was not realized until it became apparent how serious its absence could be." Fortunately, knowledge of the sequence of biochemical changes initiated by the PAH mutation led to the realization that the path of devastating neural and cognitive development can be averted by an unusual contingent condition—the dietary restriction of phenylalanine intake beginning at the first postnatal month. Thus, in PKU, the single contingent condition of typical amounts of phenylalanine in the diet pushes development down a path of neurobehavioral disaster, and, conversely, the *unusual* contingent condition of a diet abnormally low in phenylalanine will *avert* this disaster. PKU, therefore, epitomizes what is the central goal of studies of autism: the identification of the sequences of key biological contingency effects that push development down a path toward a more favorable outcome.

Another example of different outcomes from the same genetic mutation is seen in fragile-X syndrome: In a study involving 250 fragile-X males (Hagerman et al., 1994), 7 patients maintained a long-term nonretarded IQ. Of these, 4 demonstrated a full mutation (over 200 repeats of CGG) that was unmethylated. The other 3 demonstrated a mosaic pattern, which is a mixture of some cells with a full mutation and some cells with a lower repeat number, between 50 and 200 repeats, which is unmethylated. For the fragile-X group as a whole, a full mutation that lacked methylation or had incomplete methylation had a higher IQ than individuals with a full mutation that was fully methylated. The methylation process appears to turn off the gene and cause a more severe form of the fragile-X syndrome than is seen in those with methylation variation (Hagerman et al., 1994).

There is reason to think that some behavioral differences between some autistic individuals is divergence heterogeneity. The best available recent example comes from a family with two siblings who have the identical 15q11–13 duplication (see child III-1 and child III-2 in Figure 1 in Cook et al., 1997a).* Child III-1 had a much poorer clinical outcome than did Child III-2 (see p. 929 and Table 1 in Cook et al., 1997a), with dysmorphic features, a communication age equivalence of 3 years 1 month, and all the signs and symptoms fitting the DSM–IV, Autism Diagnostic Interview, and Autism Diagnostic Observation Schedule criteria for autism. In contrast, Child III-2 did not have dysmorphic features; had a much higher communication age equivalence of 6 years 8 months; and was not as severely clinically affected—meeting DSM–IV criteria for PDD-NOS, atypical autism, rather than autism because he had better eye contact and coordinated use of gesture than most children with autism. Though both siblings began life with the identical chromosomal defect, for the second sibling intervening contingent events or conditions lead to a more advantageous clinical outcome. Did the second sibling have variants of other genes that were relatively protective, or conversely did the more severely affected sibling have variants of other genes whose effects amplify the deleterious effects of the duplicated gene(s); or did the two siblings encounter different extrinsic conditions (viruses, toxins, behavioral treatment modalities, and so forth)? It is clearly important to discover the key "disadvantageous" contingencies and the "protective" or "beneficial" contingencies.

The convergence hypothesis of autism

While the pleiotropy and epigenetic hypotheses speak to the questions of why each person with autism has multiple abnormalities and why no two autistic persons have exactly the same types and/or severity of abnormalities, it is additionally possible that more than one etiology can trigger the development of autism. That is, it is possible that many of the most common biological and behavioral outcomes— cerebellar abnormalities, limbic system abnormalities, attention abnormalities, reciprocal social interaction and communication abnormalities, and ritualistic and repetitive behaviors and interests—might be caused by different and unrelated etiologies, such as virus infections, exposure to toxins, and different gene mutations. If this proves true, then autism would be an example of convergence heterogeneity.

Convergence, or *equifinality,* refers to the idea that heterogeneous biological beginnings (unrelated genetic, viral, or toxin etiologies) can lead to overlapping or common biological or behavioral outcomes (Cicchetti and Rogosch, 1996; Courchesne et al., 1994a,d; Yeung-Courchesne and Courchesne, 1997).

If heterogeneous etiologies do cause autism in different patients, then they may do so because they produce a final and common neurostructural and/or neurofunctional outcome. For instance, in patients with autism, cerebellar Purkinje neuron loss is the single most commonly reported neuronal defect. Although it is not known what causes Purkinje loss in patients with autism, it is a possibility that dif-

---

*A third sibling without this duplication was normal; as noted above, duplication of 15q11–13 has been found in a number of autistic patients and suggests—though does not prove—that this defect is capable of causing autism or many autistic-like symptoms.

ferent etiologies lead to Purkinje loss in different patients. Animal studies show that during brain development a variety of etiologies can cause the common outcome of Purkinje neuron loss, including genetic defects (e.g., in the EN-2 gene), viral infections (e.g., lymphocytic choriomeningitis virus), exposure to toxins (e.g., the anticonvulsant medication valproate), and physical trauma (e.g., via nitric oxide–mediated mechanisms) (see Yeung-Courchesne and Courchesne, 1997). Purkinje neurons appear to be one of two key sites of learning in the cerebellum (Lisberger, 1998), and their loss would radically alter the learning function of the cerebellum. Because the cerebellum may be important in learning novel language, cognitive, and sensorimotor skills and in using that learned information to prepare neural systems throughout the brain to optimally acquire, analyze, or act on a moment's notice (Allen and Courchesne, 1998; Courchesne and Allen, 1997), loss of the *function* of this key neuron might have far-reaching developmental consequences (even in adults, newly acquired cerebellar damage can compromise executive functions and affect expression; Schmahmann and Sherman, 1997).

It is important to note, however, that distinctive biological dissimilarities may signal etiological differences. For instance, autistic patients with cerebellar hypoplasia and Purkinje neuron loss most likely have a different etiology than autistic patients with posterior cerebellar vermis hyperplasia. Another possible example comes from studies of brain size in autism. In the largest study of its kind, brain size in 60 of 61 living autistic patients was undistinguished from an equally large sample of normal subjects (Courchesne et al., 1999a); however, the one deviant autistic patient was a 3.44 year old boy with a brain size (1,999 gm) larger than any normal adult brain reported in the literature over the last 100 years (and 9% larger than the largest autistic adult male brain reported in the literature). At autopsy, brain size in three other autism cases were found to be nearly the size of this one (Bailey et al., 1998; Courchesne et al., 1999b). The enormously deviant overgrowth of the brain (primarily the cerebrum) in these four autism cases very likely reflects genetic abnormalities not shared by other autistic patients with a normal brain size. In designing studies of the genetic bases of patients with autism, such biological phenotypic differences may be as important as behavioral phenotypic differences.

Experience and brain development in autism

Understanding the role of developmental mechanisms such as epigenesis and the concept of convergence in autism is central not only to theoretical discussions of the disorder but also to the implication that it is possible to alter *the developmental course* of the disorder. Animal research provides substantial evidence on the effects of epigenetic factors, such as an enriched environment, on the development of brain structure, including increased neuron size (Diamond et al., 1967), neuron density (Turner and Greenough, 1985), dendritic branching (Volkmar and Greenough, 1972), number of synapses (Turner and Greenough, 1985), and percentage of total tissue volume (Sirevaag, 1988). Research with humans is equally provocative (see related chapters in this volume) and provide convincing evidence that neural circuits in humans are not constant but, rather, dynamic. If the epigenesis theory of autism is valid and neuroplasticity can in fact occur in the autistic brain, then the ultimate goal of intervention efforts would be to provide environmental stimulation that pushes the child down the most beneficial developmental pathway. That is, the aim should be to present environmental contingencies that optimize functional development and in so doing potentially avert or prevent subsequent abnormal circuitry. Issues related to *what, how,* and *when* contingent events might stimulate optimal functional neural reorganizations in autism are key variables in the discussion of neuroplasticity in this disorder.

Perusal of the autism literature suggests that plasticity may in fact be occurring in the autistic brain after exposure to structured environmental stimulation. Unlike the decades following Leo Kanner's original description of autism in 1943, which suggested that improvement was unlikely, recent research has demonstrated that *some* individuals with autism can undergo positive phenotypic alterations with intervention (Lovaas, 1987; Pierce and Schreibman, 1996, 1997). The convergence hypothesis of autism (above) states that even when two autistic patients *seem* to have similar behavioral outcome symptoms, the underlying neural circuitry and mechanisms, as well as the developmental paths to those outcomes, need not be the same. If not the same, their dissimilar abnormal neural circuitry may not respond to the same drug or behavioral treatment in the same way. The most efficacious treatments must be tailored to fit, in each child, the specific biological and brain bases leading to that child's clinical manifestation of autism. In other words, with regard to treatment of autism, "one size does not fit all."

This conclusion is in accordance with treatment studies using systematic manipulation of environmental variables (e.g., Discrete Trial Training, Pivotal Response Training) that report variance in behavior outcomes across individuals. For example, Lovaas (1987) reported that 47% of children with autism receiving high-intensity behavioral treatment (i.e., 40 hours per week) were placed in mainstreamed academic environments after treatment, while the remaining 53% were not. These differential rates of treatment success cannot be explained by single behavioral phenotypic characteristics (e.g., severity of autistic symptoms, IQ, language ability) in that no significant differences in initial behavioral symptoms were found between treatment "high responders" and treatment "low responders." The explanation for the variable responses to common treatment might be found if one takes into account *biological substrates that distinguish these two outcome groups.*

In order to optimize compensatory neuroplasticity in the autistic nervous system, experiences and learning-based treatment efforts can be built on brain–behavior research that provides information regarding the most fruitful starting point form which to intercede *for each particular child.* Although brain-based treatments of this type have yet to occur, current evidence now supports the conclusion that available experimental and analytic methods can be used to sort patients into biologically distinct groupings on which to test whether different treatment approaches have reliably different efficacies in prompting beneficial compensatory neuroplasticity. However, to succeed, it is necessary to first establish direct experimental associations and correlations between specific behavioral and psychological dysfunctions on the one hand and specific underlying physiological, anatomical, and other biological abnormalities on the other. Recent studies have, in fact, succeeded in doing so (e.g., Haas et al., 1996; Townsend and Courchesne, 1994; Townsend et al., 1996a,b). These studies suggest, and new studies may further specify (Allen et al., 1997), the distinctly different compensatory mechanisms used by different autistic individuals. Furthermore, such brain–behavior findings will identify specific neurobehavioral operations (e.g., deployment of visuospatial attention; shifting attention; others) that may be pivotal to the normal development of still more complex, higher cognitive, linguistic and social functions. The validity of treatment efforts based on epigenetic theories can thus be easily tested: The strength of brain–behavior correlations (e.g., overly focused visuospatial attention correlated with parietal abnormalities) should decrease over the course of treatment as compensatory mechanisms are enhanced in the autistic brain.

It is interesting that, perhaps more so than with any other disorder, treatment efforts in autism rely on the *repetition* of contingent environmental events to enhance learning functions. During Discrete Trail Training, for example, a child may be exposed to the same environmental contingency (e.g., saying the word *car* in the presence of a toy car is paired with reinforcement) dozens or more times per day. This form of repeated contingencies or associations is a common method for initiating plasticity in animals (e.g., Greenough et al., 1985) and may be particularly needed in autism because it targets a function—associative learning—mediated by the cerebellum, a structure consistently cited as abnormal in autism (for review, see Courchesne, 1997). The importance of the cerebellum in associative learning has been well documented (for review, see Courchesne and Allen, 1997). For example, Logan and Grafton (1995) compared activity during the presentation of random unpaired tones and air puffs to that during paired conditioning trials. Relative to the unpaired condition, increased glucose metabolism was evident during the paired associative conditions in various cerebellar regions. In autism, perhaps, substantial changes in behavioral phenotypes can be more readily achieved by deliberately employing sensory and learning experiences that specifically compensate for deficient mechanisms (e.g., impaired associative learning mechanisms) and that trigger functional reorganization using residual intact circuits.

In addition to the implications of *what* central mechanisms should be targeted for intervention and *how* such interventions might operate, *when* such efforts are instituted is of equal importance. Animal models of developmental abnormality show the importance of critical periods or "windows of opportunity" for effective treatment. In the kitten, the longer the period of abnormal neural activity caused by monocular deprivation from birth, the more abnormal the neural structural and functional outcome. Abnormality compounds gradually, and, correspondingly, the possibility for recovery declines gradually. Thus, the longer one waits before starting treatment, the poorer the chances for neural structural and functional recovery, and eventually an age is reached when treatments are not effective (Kandel et al., 1991; Mitchell, 1988; Movshon and Kiopes, 1990). Fortunately, the human cerebral cortex has an exceptionally long period of continued growth, providing the opportunity for change. Therefore, assuming the biological etiologies causing autism begin prenatally or early in infancy, the lesson from developmental biology is to take advantage of these windows of epigenetic opportunity by intervening as early as possible.

Two important questions, then, are how to identify individuals at risk for autism as early as possible and how to decide which specific type of treatment might be most efficacious for each case. First, while no definitive biological "markers" have been found that are universal in all autistic patients, some important and specific *in vivo* biological characteristics have been found in subgroups (e.g., unusually small cerebellum, unusual thinning of the posterior subregions of the corpus callosum, unusually large cerebrum, unusually small brain stem). In *combination* with early behavioral features (Adrien et al., 1993; Baron-Cohen et al., 1996; DiLavore et al., 1995; Osterling and Dawson, 1994), biological features may help to identify infants and toddlers at significant risk for autism. Preliminary results from prospective, longitudinal neuroanatomical studies support this hope (Courchesne and colleagues, in preparation). Second, as suggested above, brain–behavior findings in autistic children, adolescents, and adults (Chugani et al., 1997; Courchesne et al., 1994c; Harris et al., 1999b; Townsend and Courchesne, 1994; Townsend et al., 1996a,b) offer the new opportunity to develop treatments that are specific to these neurobehavioral deficits. If such future efforts are successful, then such brain–behavior-based treatments, when begun early, may significantly help infants and toddlers who are identified to be at high risk for autism because they have a characteristic combination of biological and behavioral features.

Early and biologically informed treatments are especially critical when rare human neurodevelopmental disorders are due to mutations of genes with pleiotropic effects. Theoretically, if initiated early enough, a single, biologically precise treatment may prevent the cascade of multiple paths of maldevelopment (see above), but, if not, then multiple types of treatment may be needed to address each of the distinct and unrelated biological and behavioral outcomes that characterizes such gene mutations. PKU is an example. When left untreated in infants, the pleiotropic effects resulting from mutation in the PAH gene are irreversible and devastating, and the multiple and diverse biological and behavioral problems confronting each afflicted PKU patient require diverse and continuous forms of treatment none of which fully restores normality of function. Fortunately, such devastating developmental outcomes and complex treatment regimes can be averted by a single contingent condition (a diet low in phenylalanine) *if begun at the biologically critical time.* The $GABA_A$ beta-3 gene knockout mouse is an animal model example of the treatment challenge faced when pleiotropic effects of a gene mutation are not stopped early in development. In this model, once it has developed its biological and behavioral abnormalities (see Fig. 13-11), treatment of the cause (absence of the normal beta-3 subunit protein and thus abnormal $GABA_A$ receptor function) will not remove that mouse's facial dysmorphology; will not re-fashion all of its many neural circuits that were misconstructed during development; will not reverse all of its abnormal learning; and so on. Instead, effective treatment would likely require multiple specific drugs and behavioral training with each tailored to a particular aspect of the mouse's disorder (e.g., to the seizure abnormality; to the hypersensitivity; to the motor hyperactivity; to the lack of maternal nurturing responses). Thus, for genes with pleiotropic effects, once the chain reaction of maldevelopment in multiple and unrelated systems has proceeded to its conclusion, a single treatment is highly unlikely to restore normality.

Not surprisingly, then, a major goal of autism research is to devise specific biological or behavioral countereffects that avert or significantly mitigate the disorder *before* they are fully manifested and require multiple, marginally effective treatments. Early intervention research efforts (e.g., Lovaas, 1987; Sheinkopf and Siegel, 1998; Anderson et al., 1987) have embraced this idea, with treatment often beginning as early as 14 months of age (Green et al., 1997). What are missing from this approach, however, are child-specific, biologically grounded facts to guide treatment curricula. In short, current efforts, although somewhat effective, still operate under the misguided "one size fits all" model. For example, in the Discrete Trial Training methodology advocated by Lovaas and colleagues, all children progress through the intervention in the same manner: Skill A must be mastered before skill B can be introduced, and skill B must be mastered before skill C can be introduced, and so on. This strategy, which ignores underlying neuropathology for each child, may miss the critical "window of opportunity" by failing to intensely treat underlying pivotal mechanisms.

Conclusions

In a recent lecture to the neuroscience community in San Diego, Sir Francis Crick argued that, unlike the state in physics, overarching theories in biology are difficult to achieve, and good ideas are often, surprisingly, quite wrong: "In biology, just because an idea is elegant, does not mean it is right" (Francis Harry Compton Crick in a speech at the San Diego neuroscience retreat in Sante Fe, CA, in 1998). He gave an anecdote about a world famous physicist who did his best work while soaking in his bath, working out physics problems in his head. Eventually, the scientist turned to solving problems in biology. Sometime later the physicist-turned-biologist complained that since taking up biology he could no longer take working-baths because as soon as he began to reason through a biological problem he would have to jump out of his tub to check a relevant fact. Unlike the physical world in which all objects and their interactions are governed by invariant physical laws and can be predicted by calculations based on these laws, the biological world is not governed by such orderly rules or logic. Events involving biological systems are based on adaptation for survival and propagation, and events that do occur are often opportunistic. There are as many ways for a system to develop as there are elements with which to interact and to which it must adapt for continued living. One cannot predict or generalize from logical and reasonable extrapolation how a system should operate. Instead, one must discover the facts of the actual design solution in each case. Evolution is often capricious and solutions, fortuitous.

In autism research over the last decade, the more closely one looks at the underlying biology, the greater the heterogeneity observed. It is a safe prediction that in the coming decade the variety and complexity of underlying biological features of interest in autism will multiply. No current, seemingly reasonable or even "elegant" theory is likely to succeed in explaining the heterogeneous collection of biological and behavioral characteristics of autism that are currently known or will later be known. We must stick to finding the facts about how the system is *actually* designed and let them speak for themselves.

Rather than unrealistically expecting some particular finding to account for all of the known or to-be-known variability, a biologically realistic aim would be to develop more precise and "local" minihypotheses about the facts and factors that may explain parts of that heterogeneity. New technologies in molecular genetics now allow inducible animal models in which a gene's expression is knocked out at selected developmental times or allow cell-type–targeted knockouts such as recently done by Susumu Tonegawa and colleagues to demonstrate the crucial role of NMDA-mediated neural plasticity in hippocampal pyramidal cells in spatial learning and memory (McHugh et al., 1996). No doubt, when genes with pleiotropic effects are found that are involved in the development of autism, it may very well be possible to determine the specific developmental contribution of that gene factor in each local site where it is expressed. We predict that this would be done by using inducible animal models with gene knockouts targeted at critical developmental time windows and at selected cell types.

To evaluate whether a "local" minihypothesis is worth pursuing, its popularity or elegance—or its lack thereof—should play no part. One test is to observe whether the hypothesis translates into fact regardless of how unexpected, unwanted, or puzzling that fact may be; for good biology is about good fact, not good fiction. Another test of a worthwhile idea is whether it leads to discovery of etiological beginnings; and still another is whether it in some way leads to treatments that avert or mitigate adverse clinical outcomes.

Although biological and behavioral heterogeneity in autism poses obvious challenges, more importantly, it provides fresh opportunities for research into possible etiologically distinct subgroupings and novel treatment approaches. Wherever there are biological and behavioral nonuniformities in autism, there are opportunities to identify and tease apart different etiologies and/or different epigenetic mechanisms. For instance, distinctly different biological features (those with normencephaly versus those with macrenphaly; those with vermis hypoplasia versus those with hyperplasia; those with cerebral volume loss versus those without) may mark possible subgroups of patients who have corresponding differences in etiological origins or epigenetic mechanisms. Such differences might prompt specific and testable hypotheses about underling origins or mechanisms. Certainly, such biological phenotypic subgroups may inform design and analysis strategies in genetic studies. Also, identification of those biological phenotypes associated with more favorable clinical outcome and those with a less favorable one may trigger research that uncovers differences in biological and/or behavioral steps leading to better and worse clinical outcome; and, in turn, these findings might then suggest treatments that push development down a more favorable path. Even though all behavioral, psychological, physiological, and anatomical abnormalities described in autistic patients are outcomes, they mark what must be explained by studies of candidate etiological and epigenetic factors, and they also mark what must be changed by candidate treatment procedures. Moreover, they also define the phenotypic standard against which the success or failure of animal models are judged; and so knowledge of the distinctly different biological and behavioral phenotypes in the autistic population is absolutely necessary. In the search for etiologies, epigenetic explanations, and treatments for autism, the biological and behavioral differences will make all the difference in the world.

References

This work was supported by funds from NINDS (2-R01-NS-19855) and NIMH (1-R01-MH-36840) awarded to Eric Courchesne. We thank Ralph-Axel Müller and Pamela Moses for helpful comments on the manuscript.

Adrien, J. L., Lenoir, P., Martineau, J., Perrot, A., Hameury, L., Larmande, C., and Sauvage, D. (1993). Blind ratings of early symptoms of autism based upon family home movies. *J. Am. Acad. Child Adolescent Psychiatry, 32,* 617–626.

Akshoomoff, N. A., and Courchesne, E. (1992). A new role for the cerebellum in cognitive operations. *Behav. Neurosci., 106,* 731–738.

Akshoomoff, N. A., and Courchesne, E. (1994). ERP evidence for a shifting attention deficit in patients with damage to the cerebellum. *J. Cog. Neurosci., 6,* 388–399.

Allen, G., Buxton, R. B., Wong, E. C., and Courchesne, E. (1997). Attentional activation of the cerebellum independent of motor involvement. *Science, 275,* 1940–1943.

Allen, G., and Courchesne, E. (1998). The cerebellum and non-motor function: Clinical implications. *Mol. Psychiatry, 3,* 207–210.

Anderson, S. R., Avery, D. L., DiPietro, E. K., Edwards, G. L., et al. (1987). Intensive home-based early intervention with autistic children. *Educ. Treat. Children (Spec. Iss.), 10,* 352–366.

Arin, D. M., Bauman, M. L., and Kemper, T. L. (1991). The distribution of Purkinje cell loss in the cerebellum in autism. *Neurology, 41(Suppl. 1),* 307.

Attig, E., Botez, M. I., Hublet, C., Vervonck, C., Jacquy, J., and Capon, A. (1991). [Cerebral crossed diaschisis caused by cerebellar lesion: Role of the cerebellum in mental functions]. *Rev. Neurol., 147,* 200–207.

Awh, E., Smith, E. E., and Jonides, J. (1995). Human rehearsal processes and the frontal lobes: PET evidence. *Annals of the New York Academy of Sciences, 769,* 97–117.

Aylward, E. H., Reiss, A., Barta, P. E., Tien, A., Han, W., Lee, J., and Pearlson, G. D. (1994). Magnetic resonance imaging measurement of posterior fossa structures in schizophrenia. *American Journal of Psychiatry, 151,* 1448–1452.

Bachevalier, J. (1994). Medial temporal lobe structures and autism: A review of clinical and experimental findings. *Neuropsychologia, 32,* 627–648.

Bailey, A., Luthert, P., Dean, A., Harding, B., Janota, I., Montgomery, M., Rutter, M., and Lantos, P. (1998). A clinicopathological study of autism. *Brain, 121,* 889–905.

Baron-Cohen, S., Cox, A., Baird, G., Swettenham, J., Nightingale, N., Morgan, K., Drew,

A., and Charman, T. (1996). Psychological markers in the detection of autism in infancy in a large population. *Br. J. Psychiatry, 168,* 158–163.

Barth, C., Fein, D., and Waterhouse, L. (1995). Delayed match-to-sample performance in autistic children. *Dev. Neuropsychol., 11,* 53–69.

Bauman, M. L., and Kemper, T. L. (1985). Histoanatomic observations of the brain in early infantile autism. *Neurology, 35,* 866–874.

Bauman, M. L., and Kemper, T. L. (1994). *The Neurobiology of Autism.* Baltimore: Johns Hopkins University Press.

Blau, K. (1979). Phenylalanine hydroxylase deficiency: Biochemical, physiological, and clinical aspects of phenylketonuria and related phenylalaninemias. In M. B. H. Youdim (ed.): *Aromatic Amino Acid Hydroxylases and Mental Disease.* New York: John Wiley & Sons, pp. 77–139.

Botez, M. I., Laeveillae, J., Lambert, R., and Botez, T. (1991). Single photon emission computed tomography SPECT in cerebellar disease: Cerebello-cerebral diaschisis. *Eur. Neurol., 31,* 405–412.

Boucher, J., and Lewis, V. (1992). Unfamiliar face recognition in relatively able autistic children. *J. Child Psychol. Psychiatry, 33,* 843–859.

Bresnahan, M., CDC, and NAAR co-sponsored conference. (1998). Autism: Emerging issues in prevalence and etiology, November 6–7, Atlanta. *NAARrative, 11,* 1–24.

Bryson, E. E., Wainwright-Sharp, J. A., and Smith, I. M. (1990). Autism: A developmental spatial neglect syndrome? In J. T. Enns (ed.): *The Development of Attention: Research and Theory.* North-Holland: Elsevier Science, pp. 405–427.

Burke, J. C., and Cerniglia, L. (1990). Stimulus complexity and autistic children's responsivity: Assessing and training a pivotal behavior. *J. Autism Dev. Disord., 20,* 233–253.

Carpenter, M. D. (1991). *Core Text of Neuroanatomy.* Baltimore: Williams & Wilkins.

Carper, R. A., Chisum, H. J., and Courchesne, E. (1997). Brain and frontal lobe volumes do not differ between autistic subjects and normal controls. *Fourth Annual Meeting of the Cognitive Neuroscience Society.* Boston, MA, p. 39.

Carper, R. A., and Courchesne, E. (1999). Frontal lobe volume in children with autism. Submitted for publication.

Chang, C. C., Luntz-Leybman, V., Evans, J. E., Rotter, A., and Frostholm, A. (1995). Developmental changes in the expression of gamma-aminobutyric acid A/benzodiazepine receptor subunit mRNAs in the murine inferior olivary complex. *J. Comp. Neurol., 356,* 615–628.

Chugani, D. C., Muzik, O., Rothermel, R. D., Behen, M. E., Chakraborty, P. K., Mangner, T. J., da Silva, E. A., and Chugani, H. T. (1997). Altered serotonin synthesis in the dentato-thalamo-cortical pathway in autistic boys. *Ann. Neurol., 14,* 666–669.

Cicchetti, D., and Rogosch, F. A. (1996). Equifinality and multifinality in developmental psychopathology. *Dev. Psychopathol., 8,* 597–600.

Ciesielski, K. T., Allen, P. S., Sinclair, B. D., Pabst, H. F., Yanofsky, R., and Ludwig, R. (1990). Hypoplasia of cerebellar vermis in autism and childhood leukemia. *5th International Child Neurology Congress.* Tokyo: Karger, p. 650.

Cook, E. H., Jr., Courchesne, R. Y., Cox, N. J., Lord, C., Gonen, D., Guter, S. J., Lincoln, A., Nix, K., Haas, R., Leventhal, B. L., and Courchesne, E. (1998). Linkage-disequilibrium mapping of autistic disorder, with 15q11–13 markers. *Am. J. Hum. Genet., 62,* 1077–1083.

Cook, E. H., Jr., Courchesne, R., Lord, C., Cox, N. J., Yan, S., Lincoln, A., Haas, R., Courchesne, E., and Leventhal, B. L. (1997a). Evidence of linkage between the serotonin transporter and autistic disorder. *Mol. Psychiatry, 2,* 247–250.

Cook, E. H., and Leventhal, B. L. (1996). The serotonin system in autism. *Curr. Opin. Pediatr., 8,* 348–354.

Cook, E. H., Jr., Lindgren, V., Leventhal, B. L., Courchesne, R., Lincoln, A., Shulman, C., Lord, C., and Courchesne, E. (1997b). Autism or atypical autism in maternally but not paternally derived proximal 15q duplication. *Am. J. Hum. Genet., 60,* 928–934.

Courchesne, E. (1995). Infantile autism. Part 1: MR imaging abnormalities and their neurobehavioral correlates. *Int. Pediatr., 10,* 141–154.

Courchesne, E. (1997). Brainstem, cerebellar and limbic neuroanatomical abnormalities in autism. *Curr. Opin. Neurobiol., 7,* 269–278.

Courchesne, E., and Allen, G. (1997). Prediction and preparation, fundamental functions of the cerebellum. *Learning Memory, 4,* 1–35.

Courchesne, E., Chisum, H., and Townsend, J. (1994a). Neural activity-dependent brain changes in development: Implications for psychopathology. *Dev. Psychopathol., 6,* 697–722.

Courchesne, E., Chisum, H. J., Cowles, A., Egaas, B., Lincoln, A. J., Schreibman, L., Haas, R. H., Saitoh, O., and Yeung-Courchesne, R. (1999a). The size of the brain in infantile autism: In vivo and autopsy evidence. Manuscript in submission.

Courchesne, E., Press, G. A., and Yeung-Courchesne, R. (1993). Parietal lobe abnormalities detected with MR in patients with infantile autism. *Am. J. Roentgenol., 160,* 387–393.

Courchesne, E., Müller, A., and Saitoh, O. (1999b). Brain weight in autism: Five new postmortem autism cases compared to all previously published autism cases and 8,000 normative cases in the literature. Manuscript in submission.

Courchesne, E., Saitoh, O., Yeung-Courchesne, R., Press, G. A., Lincoln, A. J., Haas, R. H., and Schreibman, I. (1994b). Abnormality of cerebellar vermian lobules VI and VII in patients with infantile autism: Identification of hypoplastic and hyperplastic subgroups with MR imaging. *Am. J. Roentgenol., 162,* 123–130.

Courchesne, E., Townsend, J., Akshoomoff, N. A., Saitoh, O., Yeung-Courchesne, R., Lincoln, A. J., James, H. E., Haas, R. H., Schreibman, L., and Lau, L. (1994c). Impairment in shifting attention in autistic and cerebellar patients. *Behav. Neurosci., 108,* 848–865.

Courchesne, E., Townsend, J., and Chase, C. (1994d). Neurodevelopmental principles guide research on developmental psychopathologies. In D. Cicchetti and D. Cohen (eds.): *A Manual of Developmental Psychopathology.* New York: John Wiley, pp. 195–226.

Courchesne, E., Yeung-Courchesne, R., Press, G. A., Hesselink, J. R., and Jernigan, T. L. (1988). Hypoplasia of cerebellar vermal lobules VI and VII in autism. *N. Engl. J. Med., 318,* 1349–1354.

Cowan, W. M., Fawcett, J. W., O'Leary, D. D., and Stanfield, B. B. (1984). Regressive events in neurogenesis. *Science, 225,* 1258–1265.

Diamond, M. C., Londer, B., and Raymond, A. (1967). Extensive cortical depth measurements and neuron size increases in the cortex of environmentally enriched rats. *J. Comp. Neurol., 131,* 357–364.

DiLavore, P. C., Lord, C., and Rutter, M. (1995). The pre-linguistic autism diagnostic observation schedule. *J. Autism Dev. Disord., 25,* 355–379.

Egaas, B., Courchesne, E., and Saitoh, O. (1995). Reduced size of corpus callosum in autism. *Arch. Neurol., 52,* 794–801.

Eisensmith, R. C., and Woo, S. L. (1991). Phenylketonuria and the phenylalanine hydroxylase gene. *Mol. Biol. Med., 8,* 3–18.

Fehlow, P., Bernstein, K., Tennstedt, A., and Walther, F. (1993). [Early infantile autism and excessive aerophagy with symptomatic megacolon and ileus in a case of Ehlers-Danlos syndrome]. *Padiatr. Grenzgebiete, 31,* 259–267.

Filipek, P. A. (1995). Quantitative magnetic resonance imaging in autism: The cerebellar vermis. *Current Opinion in Neurology, 8,* 134–138.

Folling, A. (1971). The original detection of phenylketonuria. In H. Bickel, F. P. Hudson, and L. I. Woolf (eds.): *Phenylketonuria and Some Other Inborn Errors of Amino Acid Metabolism: Biochemistry, Genetics, Diagnosis, Therapy.* Stuttgard: G. Thieme Verlag, pp. 1–3.

Frith, U., and Happé, F. (1994). Autism: Beyond "theory of mind." *Cognition, 50,* 115–132.

Gaffney, G. R., Kuperman, S., Tsai, L. Y., and Minchin, S. (1988). Morphological evidence for brainstem involvement in infantile autism. *Biol. Psychiatry, 24,* 578–586.

Gaffney, G. R., Tsai, L. Y., Kuperman, S., and Minchin, S. (1987). Cerebellar structure in autism. *Am. J. Dis. Child., 141,* 1330–1332.

Gao, J. H., Parsons, L. M., Bower, J. M., Xiong, J., Li, J., and Fox, P. T. (1996). Cerebellum implicated in sensory acquisition and discrimination rather than motor control [see comments]. *Science, 272,* 545–547.

Gelehrter, T. D., and Collins, F. S. (1990). *Principles of Medical Genetics.* Baltimore: Williams & Wilkins, p. 3.

George, M. S., Costa, D. C., Kouris, K., Ring, H. A., and Ell, P. J. (1992). Cerebral blood flow abnormalities in adults with infantile autism. *J. Nerv. Ment. Dis., 180,* 413–417.

Gillberg, C., Steffenburg, S., Wahlström, J., Gillberg, I. C., Sjöstedt, A., Martinsson, T., Liedgren, S., and Eeg-Olofsson, O. (1991). Autism associated with marker chromosome. *J. Am. Acad. Child Adolescent Psychiatry, 30,* 489–494.

Green, G., Brennan, L., and Fein, D. (1997). Intensive behavioral intervention for an infant at risk for autism. Paper presented at the Meeting of the Association for Behavior Analysis, Chicago.

Greenough, W. T., Larson, J. R., and Withers, G. S. (1985). Effects of unilateral and bilateral training in a reaching task on dendritic branching of neurons in the rat motor-sensory forelimb cortex. *Behavioral and Neural Biology, 44,* 301–314.

Guerin, P., Lyon, G., Barthelemy, C., Sostak, E., Chevrollier, V., Garreau, B., and Lelord, G. (1996). Neuropathological study of a case of autistic syndrome with severe mental retardation. *Dev. Med. Child Neurol., 38,* 203–211.

Haas, R. H., Townsend, J., Courchesne, E., Lincoln, A. J., Schreibman, L., and Yeung-Courchesne, R. (1996). Neurologic abnormalities in infantile autism. *J. Child Neurol., 11,* 84–92.

Hagerman, R. J. (1996). Biomedical advances in developmental psychology. The case of fragile X syndrome. *Dev. Psychol., 32,* 416–424.

Hagerman, R. J., Hull, C. E., Safanda, J. F., Carpenter, I., Staley, L. W., O'Connor, R. A., Seydel, C., Mazzocco, M. M., Snow, K., Thibodeau, S. N., and et al. (1994). High functioning fragile X males: Demonstration of an unmethylated fully expanded FMR-1 mutation associated with protein expression. *Am. J. Med. Genet., 51,* 298–308.

Harris, N. S., Courchesne, E., Carper, R., Chisum, H., and Egaas, B. (1998). Neuroanatomic contributions to slowed orienting of attention in children with autism. *J. Int. Neuropsychol. Soc., 4,* 47.

Harris, N. S., Courchesne, E., Townsend, J., Carper, R., and Lord, C. (1999). Neuroanatomic contributions to slowed orienting of attention in children with autism. Submitted for publication.

Hashimoto, T., Tayama, M., Murakawa, K., Yoshimoto, T., Miyazaki, M., Harada, M., and Kuroda, Y. (1995). Development of the brainstem and cerebellum in autistic patients. *J. Autism Dev. Disord., 25,* 1–18.

Haznedar, M. M., Buchsbaum, M. S., Metzger, M., Solimando, A., Spiegel-Cohen, J., and

Hollander, E. (1997). Anterior cingulate gyrus volume and glucose metabolism in autistic disorder. *Am. J. Psychiatry, 154,* 1047–1050.

Hobson, R. P., Ouston, J., and Lee, A. (1988). Emotion recognition in autism: Coordinating faces and voices. *Psychol.. Med., 18,* 911–923.

Holttum, J. R., Minshew, N. J., Sanders, R. S., and Phillips, N. E. (1992). Magnetic resonance imaging of the posterior fossa in autism. *Biological Psychiatry, 32,* 1091–1101.

Homanics, G. E., DeLorey, T. M., Firestone, L. L., Quinlan, J. J., Handforth, A., Harrison, N. L., Krasowski, M. D., Rick, C. E., Korpi, E. R., Mäkelä, R., Brilliant, M. H., Hagiwara, N., Ferguson, C., Snyder, K., and Olsen, R. W. (1997). Mice devoid of gamma-aminobutyrate type A receptor beta3 subunit have epilepsy, cleft palate, and hypersensitive behavior. *Proc. Nat. Acad. Sci. U.S.A., 94,* 4143–4148.

Hotof, M., and Bolton, P. (1995). A case of autism associated with partial tetrasomy 15. *J. Autism Dev. Disord., 25,* 41–49.

Hsu, M., Yeung-Courchesne, R., Courchesne, E., and Press, G. A. (1991). Absence of magnetic resonance imaging evidence of pontine abnormality in infantile autism. *Arch. Neurol., 48,* 1160–1163.

Ingram, J. L., Croog, V. J., Tisdale, B., and Rodier, P. M. (1996). Valproic acid treatment in rats reproduces the cerebellar anomalies associated with autism. *Teratology, 53,* 86.

Ito, M. (1984). *The Cerebellum and Neural Control.* New York: Raven Press.

Kandel, E. R., Schwarz, T. M., and Jessel, J. H. (1991). *Principles of Neural Science.* New York: Elsevier.

Kanner, L. (1943). Autistic disturbances of affective contact. *Nerv. Child, 2,* 217–250.

Killackey, H. P. (1990). Neocortical expansion: An attempt toward relating phylogeny and ontogeny. *J. Cog. Neurosci., 2,* 1–17.

Kimura, S., Nakamura, H., Matsumura, K., Morohashi, S., Ueoka, Y., Hasegawa, A., and Yonekura, Y. (1989). [Crossed "cerebral" diaschisis? Seven cases with unilateral cerebellar vascular lesion which showed decreased perfusion in the contralateral cerebral cortex]. *Kaku Igaku, 26,* 1259–1266.

Kleiman, M. D., Neff, S., and Rosman, N. P. (1992). The brain in infantile autism: are posterior fossa structures abnormal? *Neurology, 42,* 753–760.

Koegel, R. L., and Rincover, A. (1976). Some detrimental effects of using extra stimuli to guide responding in autistic and normal children. *J. Abnorm. Child Psychol., 4,* 59–71.

Koegel, R. L., and Wilhelm, H. (1973). Selective responding to the components of multiple visual cues by autistic children. *J. Exp. Child Psychol., 15,* 442–453.

Kolo, D. J., Anderson, L., and Campbell, M. (1980). Sensory preference and overselective responding in autistic children. *J. Autism Dev. Disord., 10,* 259–271.

Laurie, D. J., Wisden, W., and Seeburg, P. H. (1992). The distribution of thirteen GABAA receptor subunit mRNAs in the rat brain. III. Embryonic and postnatal development. *J. Neurosci., 12,* 4151–4172.

Leekam, S., Baron-Cohen, S., Perrett, D., Milders, M., and Brown, S. (1997). Eye-direction detection: A dissociation between geometric and joint attention skills in autism. *Br. J. Dev. Psychol., 15,* 77–95.

Leiner, H. C., Leiner, A. L., and Dow, R. S. (1995). The underestimated cerebellum. *Hum. Brain Mapp., 2,* 244–254.

Lewy, A. L., and Dawson, G. (1992). Social stimulation and joint attention in young autistic children. *J. Abnorm. Child Psychol., 20,* 555–566.

Lisberger, S. G. (1998). Cerebellar LTD: A molecular mechanism of behavioral learning? *Cell, 92,* 701–704.

Logan, C. G., and Grafton, S. T. (1995). Functional anatomy of human eyeblink conditioning determined with regional cerebral glucose metabolism and positron-emission tomography. *Proceedings of the National Academy of Sciences of the United States of America, 92,* 7500–7504.

Lovaas, O. I. (1987). Behavioral treatment and normal educational and intellectual functioning in young autistic children. *J. Consult. Clin. Psychol., 55,* 3–9.

Lovaas, O. I., Schreibman, L., Koegel, R., and Rehm, R. (1971). Selective responding by autistic children to multiple sensory input. *J. Abnorm. Psychol., 77,* 211–222.

Macagno, E. R., Lopresti, V., and Levinthal, C. (1973). Structure and development of neuronal connections in isogeneic organisms: Variations and similarities in the optic system of Daphnia magna. *Proc. Nat. Acad. Sci. U.S.A., 70,* 57–61.

Martin, A., Haxby, J. V., Lalonde, F. M., Wiggs, C. L., and Ungerleider, L. G. (1995). Discrete cortical regions associated with knowledge of color and knowledge of action. *Science, 270,* 102–105.

McDougle, C. J., Naylor, S. T., Cohen, D. J., Volkmar, F. R., Heninger, G. R., and Price, L. H. (1996). A double-blind, placebo-controlled study of fluvoxamine in adults with autistic disorder. *Arch. Gen. Psychiatry, 53,* 1001–1008.

McEvoy, R. E., Rogers, S. J., and Pennington, B. F. (1993). Executive function and social communication deficits in young autistic children. *J. Child Psychol. Psychiatry Allied Disciplines, 34,* 563–578.

McHugh, T. J., Blum, K. I., Tsien, J. Z., Tonegawa, S., and Wilson, M. A. (1996). Impaired hippocampal representation of space in CA1-specific NMDAR1 knockout mice. *Cell, 87,* 1339–1349.

Miall, R. C., Weir, D. J., Wolpert, D. M., and Stein, J. F. (1993). Is the cerebellum a Smith predictor? *J. Motiv. Behav., 25,* 203–216.

Middleton, F. A., and Strick, P. L. (1994). Anatomical evidence for cerebellar and basal ganglia involvement in higher cognitive function. *Science, 266,* 458–461.

Minshew, N. J., Goldstein, G., Dombrowski, S. M., Panchalingam, K., and Pettegrew, J. W. (1993). A preliminary 31P MRS study of autism: Evidence of undersynthesis and increased degradation of brain membranes. *Biol. Psychiatry, 33,* 762–773.

Mitchell, D. E. (1988). The extent of visual recovery from early monocular or binocular visual deprivation in kittens. *J. Physiol., 395,* 639–660.

Modahl, C., Green, L., Fein, D., Morris, M., Waterhouse, L., Feinstein, C., and Levin, H. (1998). Plasma oxytocin levels in autistic children. *Biol. Psychiatry, 43,* 270–277.

Movshon, J. A., and Kiopes, L. (1990). The role of experience in visual development. In J. R. Coleman (ed.): *Development of Sensory Systems in Mammals.* New York: John Wiley & Sons, pp. 155–202.

Müller, R.-A., Behen, M. E., Rothermel, R. D., Chugani, D. C., Muzik, O., Mangner, T. J., and Chugani, H. T. (1999a). Brain mapping of language and auditory perception in high-functioning autistic adults: A PET study. *J. Autism Dev. Disord.* (in press).

Müller, R.-A., Chugani, D. C., Behen, M. E., Rothermel, R. D., Muzik, O., Chakraborty, P. K., and Chugani, H. T. (1999b). Impairment of dentatothalamo cortical pathway in autistic men: Language activation data from PET. *Neurosci. Lett., 245,* 1–4.

Murakami, J. W., Courchesne, E., Press, G. A., Yeung-Courchesne, R., and Hesselink, J. R. (1989). Reduced cerebellar hemisphere size and its relationship to vermal hypoplasia in autism. *Arch. Neurol., 46,* 689–694.

Nadler, L. S., Guirguis, E. R., and Siegel, R. E. (1994). GABAA receptor subunit polypeptides increase in parallel but exhibit distinct distributions in the developing rat cerebellum. *J. Neurobiol., 25,* 1533–1544.

Newman, P. P., and Reza, H. (1979). Functional relationships between the hippocampus and the cerebellum: An electrophysiological study of the cat. *J. Physiol., 287,* 405–426.

O'Leary, D. D. M. (1989). Do cortical areas emerge from a protocortex? *Trends Neurosci., 12,* 400–406.

O'Leary, D. D. (1992). Development of connectional diversity and specificity in the mammalian brain by the pruning of collateral projections. *Curr. Opin. Neurobiol., 2,* 70–77.

Osterling, J., and Dawson, G. (1994). Early recognition of children with autism: A study of first birthday home videotapes. *J. Autism Dev. Disord., 24,* 247–257.

Ozonoff, S. (1995). Executive functions in autism. In E. Schopler and G. B. Mosibov (eds.): *Learning and Cognition in Autism.* New York: Plenum Press, pp. 199–240.

Paulin, M. G. (1993). The role of the cerebellum in motor control and perception. *Brain Behav. Evol., 41,* 39–50.

Pennington, B. F., and Ozonoff, S. (1996). Executive functions and developmental psychopathology. *J. Child Psychol. Psychiatry Allied Disciplines, 37,* 51–87.

Petersen, S. E., Fox, P. T., Posner, M. I., Mintun, M., and Raichle, M. E. (1989). Positron emission tomographic studies of the processing of single words. *Journal of Cognitive Neuroscience, 1,* 153–170.

Pickles, A., Bolton, P., MacDonald, H., Bailey, A., Le Couteur, A., Sim, C. H., and Rutter, M. (1995). Latent-class analysis of recurrence risks for complex phenotypes with selection and measurement error: A twin and family history study of autism. *Am. J. Hum. Genet., 57,* 717–726.

Pierce, K., Glad, K. S., and Schreibman, L. (1997). Social perception in children with autism: An attentional deficit? *J. Autism Dev. Disord., 27,* 265–282.

Pierce, K., and Schreibman, L. (1995). Increasing complex social behaviors in children with autism: Effects of peer-implemented pivotal response training. *J. Appl. Behav. Anal., 28,* 285–295.

Pierce, K., and Schreibman, L. (1997). Multiple peer use of pivotal response training to increase social behaviors of classmates with autism: Results from trained and untrained peers. *J. Appl. Behav. Anal., 30,* 157–160.

Piven, J., and Arndt, S. (1995). The cerebellum and autism. *Neurology, 45*(2), 398–402.

Piven, J., Nehme, E., Simon, J., Barta, P., Pearlson, G., and Folstein, S. E. (1992). Magnetic resonance imaging in autism: Measurement of the cerebellum, pons, and fourth ventricle. *Biol. Psychiatry, 31,* 491–504.

Plomin, R., Owen, M. J., and McGuffin, P. (1994). The genetic basis of complex human behaviors. *Science, 264,* 1733–1739.

Posner, M. I., Walker, J. A., Freidrich, F. A., and Rafal, R. D. (1984). Effects of parietal injury on covert orienting of attention. *Journal of Neuroscience, 4,* 1863–1874.

Quartz, S. R., and Sejnowski, T. J. (1997). The neural basis of cognitive development: A constructivist manifesto. *Behav. Brain Sci., 20,* 537–596.

Raichle, M. E., Fiez, J. A., Videen, T. O., MacLeod, A. M., Pardo, J. V., Fox, P. T., and Petersen, S. E. (1994). Practice-related changes in human brain functional anatomy during nonmotor learning. *Cereb. Cortex, 4,* 8–26.

Raymond, G. V., Bauman, M. L., and Kemper, T. L. (1996). Hippocampus in autism: A Golgi analysis. *Acta Neuropathol., 91,* 117–119.

Raz, N., Torres, I. J., Spencer, W. D., White, K., and Acker, J. D. (1992). Age-related regional differences in cerebellar vermis observed in vivo. *Archives of Neurology, 49,* 412–416.

Reiss, A. L., Aylward, E., Freund, L. S., Joshi, P. K., and Bryan, R. N. (1991). Neuroanatomy of fragile X syndrome: the posterior fossa. *Annals of Neurology, 29,* 26–32.

Reiss, A. L., Freund, L., Plotnick, L., Baumgardner, T., Green, K., Sozer, A. C., Reader, M., Boehm, C., and Denckla, M. B. (1993). The effects of X monosomy on brain development: monozygotic twins discordant for Turner's syndrome. *Annals of Neurology, 34,* 95–107.

Rincover, A., and Ducharme, J. M. (1987). Variables influencing stimulus overselectivity and "tunnel vision" in developmentally delayed children. *Am. J. Ment. Defic., 91,* 422–430.

Ritvo, E. R., Freeman, B. J., Scheibel, A. B., Duong, T., Robinson, H., Guthrie, D., and Ritvo, A. (1986). Lower Purkinje cell counts in the cerebella of four autistic subjects: Initial findings of the UCLA-NSAC Autopsy Research Report. *Am. J. Psychiatry, 143,* 862–866.

Rodier, P. M., Ingram, J. L., Tisdale, B., Nelson, S., and Romano, J. (1996). Embryological origin for autism: Developmental anomalies of the cranial nerve motor nuclei. *J. Comp. Neurol., 370,* 247–261.

Rousseaux, M., and Steinling, M. (1992). Crossed hemispheric diaschisis in unilateral cerebellar lesions. *Stroke, 23,* 511–514.

Rumsey, J. M., Duara, R., Grady, C., Rapoport, J. L., Margolin, R. A., Rapoport, S. I., and Cutler, N. R. (1985). Brain metabolism in autism. Resting cerebral glucose utilization rates as measured with positron emission tomography. *Arch. Gen. Psychiatry, 42,* 448–455.

Saitoh, O., Courchesne, E., Egaas, B., Lincoln, A. J., and Schreibman, L. (1995). Cross sectional area of the posterior hippocampus in autistic patients with cerebellar and corpus callosum abnormalities. *Neurology, 45,* 317–324.

Schain, R. J., and Freedman, D. X. (1961). Studies on 5-hydroxyindole metabolism in autistic and other mentally retarded children. *J. Pediatr., 58,* 315–320.

Schmahmann, J. D. (1997). *The Cerebellum and Cognition.* San Diego: Academic Press.

Schmahmann, J. D., and Sherman, J. C. (1997). Cerebellar cognitive affective syndrome. *Int. Rev. Neurobiol., 41,* 433–440.

Schreibman, L., and Lovaas, O. I. (1973). Overselective response to social stimuli by autistic children. *J. Abnorm. Child Psychol., 1,* 152–168.

Schroer, R. J., Phelan, M. C., Michaelis, R. C., Crawford, E. C., Skinner, S. A., Cuccaro, M., Simensen, R. J., Bishop, J., Skinner, C., Fender, D., and Stevenson, R. E. (1998). Autism and maternally derived aberrations of chromosome 15q. *Am. J. Med. Genet., 76,* 327–336.

Shah, A., and Frith, U. (1983). An islet of ability in autistic children: A research note. *J. Child Psychol. Psychiatry, 24,* 613–620.

Shah, A., and Frith, U. (1993). Why do autistic individuals show superior performance on the block design task? *J. Child Psychol. Psychiatry, 34,* 1351–1364.

Sheinkopf, S. J., and Siegel, B. (1998). Home based behavioral treatment of young children with autism. *J. Autism Dev. Disord., 28,* 15–23.

Singer Harris, N. (1997). *Relationship Between Degree of Neuroanatomic Abnormality and Visual Orienting Deficits in Young Children With Autism.* San Diego: UCSD/SDSU, pp. 1–169.

Sirevaag, A. M., Black, J. E., Shafron, D., Greenough, W. T. (1988). Direct evidence that complex experience increases capillary branching and surface area in visual cortex of young rats. *Brain Research, 471,* 299–304.

Stone, R. L., Aimi, J., Barshop, B. A., Jaeken, J., Van den Berghe, G., Zalkin, H., and Dixon, J. E. (1992). A mutation in adenylosuccinate lyase associated with mental retardation and autistic features. *Nat. Genet., 1,* 59–63.

Stout, J. T., and Caskey, C. T. (1985). HPRT: Gene structure, expression, and mutation. *Annu. Rev. Genet., 19,* 127–148.

Talairach, J., and Tournoux, P. (1998). *Co-planar Stereotaxic Atlas of the Human Brain.* New York: Thieme Medical Publishers.

Townsend, J., and Courchesne, E. (1994). Parietal damage and narrow "spotlight" spatial attention. *J. Cog. Neurosci., 6,* 220–232.

Townsend, J., Courchesne, E., and Egaas, B. (1996a). Slowed orienting of covert visual–spatial attention in autism: Specific deficits associated with cerebellar and parietal abnormality. *Dev. Psychopathol., 8,* 563–584.

Townsend, J., Courchesne, E., Singer-Harris, N., Covington, J., Westerfield, M., Lyden, P., and Press, G. (1999). Cerebellar damage slows orienting of visual attention. Manuscript in submission.

Townsend, J., Harris, N. S., and Courchesne, E. (1996b). Visual attention abnormalities in autism: Delayed orienting to location. *J. Int. Neuropsychol. Soc., 2,* 541–550.

Turner, A. M., and Greenough, W. T. (1985). Differential rearing effects on rat visual cortex synapses. I. Synaptic density and synapses per neuron. *Brain Res., 329,* 195–203.

Verkerk, A. J., Pieretti, M., Sutcliffe, J. S., Fu, Y. H., Kuhl, D. P., Pizzuti, A., Reiner, O., Richards, S., Victoria, M. F., Zhang, F. P., et al. (1991). Identification of a gene (FMR-1) containing a CGG repeat coincident with a breakpoint cluster region exhibiting length variation in fragile X syndrome. *Cell, 65,* 905–914.

Volkmar, R. F., and Greenough, W. T. (1972). Rearing complexity affects branching of dendrites in visual cortex of the rat. *Science, 176,* 1455–1447.

Waterhouse, L., and Fein, D. (1997). Genes tPA, Fyn, and FAK in autism? *J. Autism Dev. Disord., 27,* 220–223.

Waterhouse, L., Fein, D., and Modahl, C. (1996). Neurofunctional mechanisms in autism. *Psychol. Rev., 103,* 457–489.

Williams, R. S., Hauser, S. L., Purpura, D. P., DeLong, G. R., and Swisher, C. N. (1980). Autism and mental retardation: Neuropathologic studies performed in four retarded persons with autistic behavior. *Arch. Neurol., 37,* 749–753.

Williams, R. W., and Herrup, K. (1988). The control of neuron number. *Annu. Rev. Neurosci., 11,* 423–453.

Wisden, W., Laurie, D. J., Monyer, H., and Seeburg, P. H. (1992). The distribution of 13 GABAA receptor subunit mRNAs in the rat brain. I. Telencephalon, diencephalon, mesencephalon. *J. Neurosci., 12,* 1040–1062.

Yeung-Courchesne, R., and Courchesne, E. (1997). From impasse to insight in autism research: From behavioral symptoms to biological explanations. *Dev. Psychopathol., 9,* 389–419.

Yu, S., Pritchard, M., Kremer, E., Lynch, M., Nancarrow, J., Baker, E., Holman, K., Mulley, J. C., Warren, S. T., Schlessinger, D., et al. (1991). Fragile X genotype characterized by an unstable region of DNA. *Science, 252,* 1179–1181.

Zilbovicius, M., Garreau, B., Samson, Y., Remy, P., Barthelemy, C., Syrota, A., and Lelord, G. (1995). Delayed maturation of the frontal cortex in childhood autism. *Am. J. Psychiatry, 152,* 248–252.

IV

INTERVENTIONS

14

Issues in Developing
Effective Interventions

SUSAN H. LANDRY

This chapter deals with the development of effective interventions for children with developmental disorders that are associated with central nervous system (CNS) abnormalities. The disorders emphasized include pervasive developmental disorders (PDD), such as autism, PDD-not otherwise specified (NOS), and Asperger syndrome. Intervention issues in communication and nonverbal learning disorders associated with specific brain abnormalities and acquired insults, including focal brain lesions and cerebellum and midbrain dysmorphologies such as spina bifida, are also discussed. The nature of learning problems associated with these developmental disorders is described in the first section. Because these disorders are the focus of other chapters, learning problems are only briefly described in an attempt to highlight the areas of development that need to be addressed in interventions for children with these developmental disorders. Next, the importance of recent findings in basic science research in guiding the development of intervention models for developmental disorders is discussed. In addition to findings from developmental neurobiology, the chapter highlights the importance of interventions incorporating the powerful influence of caregivers as revealed by the literature on the development of normal children.

The chapter then presents a conceptual framework for early intervention. In this section, a four-step process is outlined: *(1)* delineation of a group of specific developmental deficits to be targeted in an intervention, *(2)* the types of teaching strategies parents use that provide direct support for these developmental deficits, *(3)* the adaptations that parents make across time in relation to the child's changing skills that facilitate better outcomes, and *(4)* a controlled study to verify the effectiveness of intervention techniques for enhancing outcomes. As a contrast to this proposed model, the chapter briefly describes the broad range of interventions currently available for children with PDD-NOS, autism, and other related disorders.

Nature of Disorders

Children with PDD have a broad range of learning problems including deficiencies in verbal and gestural communication, attention, social relatedness, emotional reciprocity, and pretend play (Dawson and Adams, 1984; Green, 1996a; Lord, 1984; Sigman and Capps, 1997; Tager-Flusberg, 1982). These disorders are also associated with deficiencies in attention (Burack et al., 1997; Dawson and Lewy, 1989) and visual–perceptual or sensorimotor integration skills (Smith, 1996). Although children with PDD-NOS and autism may have average intelligence, they always have deficiencies in their language skills, particularly their *use* of spontaneous social language. The social and communication problems associated with PDD require systematic intensive interventions for children to develop basic social language skills such as initiating, greeting, or requesting information. The full range of developmental problems associated with this disorder are described in more detail in Chapters 12–13.

Children with specific CNS abnormalities such as spina bifida meningomyelocele and Dandy-Walker syndrome frequently have problems in the development of fine and gross motor skills, nonverbal cognitive functions, attention, and specific areas of communication, and social functioning. The developmental problems associated with this disorder are described in detail in Chapters 7 and 8. While children with spina bifida meningomyelocele often have relatively average intelligence levels, they frequently have particular difficulties with the identification and pursuit of cognitive and social goals that are appropriate to the specific demands of a task (Dennis and Barnes, 1993; Landry et al., 1994). Their conversational responses have been described as loose and tangential. Although motivated to interact, these children often have difficulty assembling verbal information to provide appropriate responses in quickly changing social interactions (Dennis and Barnes, 1993). They also demonstrate difficulties incorporating contingent feedback into their problem-solving approaches in order to efficiently carry out a task (Fletcher et al., 1996). These problems are important to address in intervention programs because these skills are put to use in most areas of a child's life, including scholastic performance, social interactions, and daily living tasks. Although there is limited information on the early development of children with brain abnormalities such as those associated with spina bifida, the absence of appropriate early interventions for their early motoric, attentional, and oculomotor deficits put these children at even greater risk for learning, social, and behavior problems at later ages.

The Role of Basic Science Research
in the Development of Early Interventions

The development of effective interventions for children with developmental disorders is of critical importance. Recently, there have been major advances in delineating the effects of differential experiences on the structure and function of the developing brain. Some of these important advances are described in earlier chapters of this book (e.g., Chapters 2 and 3). Advances have also been made in relating the central nervous system structure and function of developmental disorders with behavioral manifestations associated with these disorders (see Chapters 7 and 13). In light of these advances, a major challenge is determining how to use these new research findings to guide the development of models of intervention for children with developmental disorders. For example, this research can help us make certain decisions about *the timing* of interventions. There may be *critical periods* in development when children are more receptive to particular types of environmental influences than other periods (Spreen et al., 1995; see Chapter 10). Some of the neuroscience research findings provide important information regarding the plasticity of the young child's developing brain that may allow interventionists to better understand when the CNS is more likely to change in response to specific environmental influences. Intervention models, therefore, need to take into account the specific times when children develop those skills that will be targeted for intervention.

The first few years of life are critically important for the young child's development because of the rapid pace at which the brain develops at this time. It is apparent that the brain undergoes a series of extraordinary changes during these early years, and these changes are determined to a certain extent by the type of environmental input the young child receives (see Chapters 1 and 2). The brain is potentially producing trillions of connections between neurons, many more than it can possibly use. Through a complex "sorting out" process, some of these connections are eliminated, while others form a complex network. In animal models, the quantity and quality of the stimulation the immature animal receives in the early years has an effect on the differentiation and function of these neurons. It is this process that contributes to the great diversity in human development. The quantity and quality of the early input the brain receives play an important role in this "sorting out" process as it influences the ultimate structure and functioning of a child's brain. While we often cannot change what happens to the young child's brain prior to birth, we may be able to change what happens after birth, particularly as knowledge accumulates on how environmental factors influence brain maturation, plasticity, and reorganization of function after insult.

The Parent as the Child's Early Teacher

The parents are a young child's most important teachers during early childhood. Parents' use of particular behaviors or strategies in their interactions with their young children provide support for children to attend and learn normally (Bakeman and Adamson, 1984; Belskey et al., 1980; Bornstein and Tamis-LeMonda, 1989; Bruner, 1977; Kuczynski and Kochanska, 1990; Parpal and Maccoby, 1985; Wertsch, 1979). Some of the different developmental disorders described in other chapters (see Chapters 7, 8, and 12–13) manifest attentional and learning problems in infancy and early childhood. Children with these disorders may have more difficulty learning in interactions with others because of these problems.

For example, very young children with PDD have problems attending to aspects of their environment, particularly in social interactions, when they are required to move their attentional focus in order to share interest in objects or toys with their caretakers (Landry and Loveland, 1989; Sigman et al., 1986). Organizing a motoric or social response is often difficult for these children, particularly when they are required to understand social and nonsocial contingencies. Children with CNS malformations (spina bifida, Dandy-Walker syndrome) also have problems in early childhood shifting their attentional focus and organizing behavioral responses (Dennis et al., 1981; Jennings et al., 1988). Deficits in the ability to regulate and organize behavior in response to changing cognitive and social demands may be one type of early developmental deficiency that a number of developmental disorders have in common.

To understand how to teach these children at young ages to effectively interact with others, we need to develop models that delineate the processes that underlie changes in their attending and organizing skills. Interventions may be most effective if they focus on parenting behaviors that directly target the young child's developmental problems; that is, the interventions must provide specific techniques to support the type of deficits the child is showing. Providing parents with stimulation techniques that directly facilitate the child's ability to attend and respond more appropriately so that learning can occur should enhance the young child's ability to make effective use of his or her experiences for learning. To illustrate, Rovee-Collier (1995) described a conceptual framework for understanding how children's early experiences with their environment work together to facilitate their development. In this process, referred to as *time windows,* children develop networks of associations through their experiences with the environment. These networks are developed by assimilating new information with information in their memory from a prior related experience. Infants and young children develop more efficient memories (i.e., learned skills) when they have had a series of successful early learning experiences that occur while the previous memory is still retained.

Young children with developmental deficiencies may have more difficulty obtaining successful learning experiences on which to build networks of associations. For example, children who have early attention and motor problems may have difficulty learning contingencies through experiences with objects and toys because of problems coordinating their attention and motoric responses. Therefore, the memory of a contingency experience may not be as strong for them as for a normally developing young infant because of less success exploring a toy. Because the strength of associations between old and new experiences may be deficient for these children, they lose the ability to use those older experiences in understanding and learning from the newer experiences; they must re-learn the same lessons over and over rather than building upon earlier experiences. This type of inefficiency in learning suggests that children with developmental problems may be more dependent on parents providing early specialized support. The provision of support that allows them to have successful learning experiences in spite of attentional and organizational delays may establish a more optimal foundation on which later, more complex cognitive and social behaviors are built. If this is the case, understanding the types of techniques that facilitate learning is critically important.

A Conceptual Framework for a Model of Early Intervention

We recently developed an intervention model for a group of children at high degrees of risk for developmental disorders. The focus of this model was on infants who were born prematurely with low birth weights (<1,500 g) and significant medical complications (lung disease, brain hemorrhage) that caused them to be at high risk for problems in cognition, motor, attention, social, and language development. These infants had particular problems in organizing their behavior in response to stimulation in the environment and in attending to stimuli. In the first few years of life, parents often find interactions with preterm very-low-birth-weight (VLBW) infants more difficult because the ways in which the infants signal their needs are often not clear. These infants can easily become overwhelmed by stimulation in their environment, show greater amounts of disorganization and irritability, and have difficulty focusing and orienting their attention.

This intervention model was developed in four steps. We first described the types of early developmental problems these premature infants showed that could potentially interfere with their learning. *Second,* we examined the types of teaching techniques that parents used in interactions with their premature infants and the extent to which certain techniques were successful. *Third,* we examined parent–child interactions longitudinally across the first 3 years of the child's life. This was done to better understand the types of adaptations parents made that achieved faster rates of change in the child's development of cognitive, language, and social skills. *Fourth,* we randomly assigned mothers and their infants to either a parenting intervention that incorporated the information we gained from the first three steps or to a developmental screening program. These four steps are described below in more detail.

Step one

An initial step was to delineate the types of early attentional problems these infants had that would interfere with their ability to learn. A series of studies were conducted to examine early attentional, exploratory, and joint attention skills. In a study of visual attention skills (Landry et al., 1985), the premature infants were divided into high-risk and low-risk groups based on the type and severity of their neonatal medical problems. The high-risk children had complications that included moderate to severe intraventricular hemorrhages with associated hydrocephalus and/or periventricular leukomalacia as well as chronic lung disease. The low-risk children had mild to moderate respiratory problems and/or mild hemorrhages. These two groups were compared with a full-term group with similar sociodemographic variables.

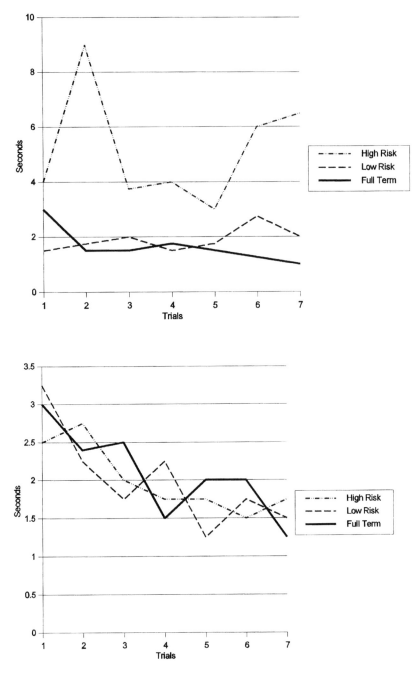

Figure 14-1. *(Top)* Comparison of the mean latencies of the infants in the medically high-risk and low-risk and the full-term groups. The high-risk infants had significantly longer latencies in shifting attention to the blinking light than the other two groups. *(Bottom)* Com-

When examining the infants' ability to move their attention from a blinking light (12 inches to the left of a slide of a simple geometric pattern) to a geometric pattern, we found that the high-risk infants took significantly longer to move their attention to the pattern once the light stopped blinking and the slide went on. Figure 14-1 illustrates the significant differences in the latencies for the high-risk group for orienting their attention compared with the low-risk and full-term groups.

Once the high-risk infants did orient their attention to the geometric pattern, we examined whether they attended to the patterns for similar amounts of time as the other two groups and whether they processed information in similar ways. Results showed that the high-risk infants' processing and dishabituation patterns were quite similar to those of the low-risk and full-term infants' (Figure 14-1). Hence, once they were able to move and orient their attention, the ability to focus and take in information by the high-risk group was not different from the other two groups.

This initial step revealed that early problems in the movement of attentional focus could interfere with high-risk infants' ability to learn from experiences with their environment. Others describe preterm infants as requiring longer periods of focused attention to process information than full-term infants (Rose, 1983) and as requiring longer latencies to organize an exploratory response after focusing on a toy (Ruff, 1986). Because the attentional capacity of infants is critical to their responses in early joint play interactions (Landry, 1995), understanding how to support these early problems is important.

Step two

We then needed to determine whether there were certain behaviors a parent could use to support the high-risk infants' particular problems in moving attentional focus and organizing a response. Hopefully, improved attentional skills would allow them a greater chance of having successful learning experiences. In a study describing the relation of parenting strategies to children's exploratory play responses, we focused on parents' attempts to *maintain* their infants' focus of interest on a toy rather than *redirect* their interest to a different toy than the one they were already attending to (Landry et al., 1996). This strategy was expected to be particularly effective for the high-risk infants because it places fewer demands on their more immature attentional capacity and allows them to use more of their cognitive capacity to process information. The reduction in demands occurs because, when mothers maintain the child's attentional focus, the child is not having to inhibit a response to one stimuli, move attentional focus to another, and then attend and process information about it. In contrast, when mothers attempt to attract children's attention to a different toy than the one they are currently interested in (*redi-*

---

parison of the mean fixation times of infants in the medically high-risk and low-risk and the full-term groups. In spite of the longer latencies to shift attention (top), the high-risk group was comparable with the other groups in showing dishabituation to repeated exposures of a visual stimuli.

recting style), they were expected to be less likely to show the same degree of learning because of decreased attentional and cognitive resources.

We focused on mothers' use of this maintaining versus redirecting style and also looked at whether the verbal content of their maintaining requests made a difference. Specifically, if mothers provided more information about what type of response was expected of the child (i.e., "put the block in the cup") versus comments or orienting statements (i.e., "that's it" or "look at that one"), we hypothesized that the high-risk children would show a higher rate of successful experiences because the technique provided additional support in organizing their responses. We examined sociodemographically comparable groups of premature high-risk, low-risk, and full-term children in toy center play interactions with their mothers.

We found that high-risk children were as likely as low-risk and full-term children to have an increased exploratory response to toys following a maintaining strategy (Fig. 14-2). However, the high-risk infants were significantly less likely than the low-risk infants to increase their exploratory play response when the mothers attempted to redirect their attention to a toy different from the one they were

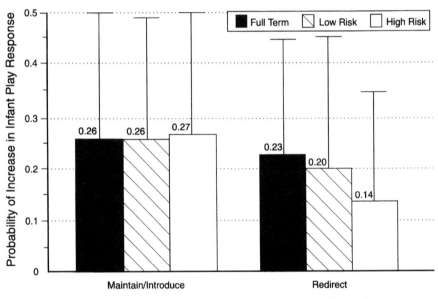

Timing of Maternal Attention-Directing Behaviors

Figure 14-2. Relationship between timing of maternal attention-directing behaviors and increases in mean probabilities of infant exploratory play responses in high-risk, low-risk, and full-term infants. Results show that the high-risk group was significantly less likely to increase the level of exploratory play response than the low-risk and full-term groups when mothers attempted to redirect the infants' attention to a toy other than the one they were attending to. In contrast, when mothers maintained the infants' attention or introduced toys when they were not currently attending to a toy, the high-risk group responded similarly to the other groups in showing an increased response to a toy.

currently interested in. Also, providing more information about specifically what response is expected of the child was most effective when combined with a maintaining strategy rather than a redirecting strategy. Comments, orienting words, and questioning statements were not as effective as the information providing strategies whether they were used with a maintaining or a redirecting approach.

Mothers' sharing of a focus of interest with their infants by maintaining the infants' attention during joint play is thought to be an effective technique in part because the mothers' social behavior in these situations is contingent on and reciprocal to the infants' behavior (for review, see Dunham and Dunham, 1995). In a more recent study with large sample sizes of preterm and full-term children, increased rates of maintaining behaviors early in development predicted faster rates of cognitive, language, and social development across 6 months to 3.5 years of age (Landry et al., 1997). For infants with early developmental problems (e.g., attention and motor delays), a high degree of reciprocity in their interactions with caretakers may be particularly important for optimal learning to occur. These mothers' use of maintaining techniques and avoidance of redirection may also help their children to develop a sense of autonomy in environmental exploration. An important component of exploratory play competence is children's development of a sense that they can master their environment, including their own response to that environment (Lewis and Goldberg, 1969). Because high-risk infants may be particularly dependent on parental involvement in their learning, their mothers may facilitate exploratory mastery by finely tuning their interactions with their infants to avoid undue control (e.g., redirection of attention). Developing intervention techniques that are contingent on the child's behavior and establish a high degree of reciprocity between the child and the interactive partner may be important for a young child with a developmental disorder because they encourage the child to begin to take an active role in learning.

Step three

Because children's development of skills across the first few years of life reflects increasing change rather than stability, the third step in our model development was to determine what types of adaptations in stimulation techniques were effective for promoting continued increases in the development of social and communication skills. This question was addressed by examining the types of parenting strategies that were responsive to the changing abilities of the children in order to describe the influence of these parenting behaviors on the children's changing skills (Landry et al., 1998). We expected that mothers who were able to increase their levels of maintaining across the first 3 years of life would support development of social and language skills. Again, we expected this relation of increased maintaining with faster rates of change in social and communication skills to be stronger for the high-risk children because maintaining strategies target a specific deficit for them (i.e., problems in shifting attentional focus).

Figure 14-3 illustrates that higher levels of maintaining (representing increases in mothers' use of this strategy across this period) were related to greater gains in

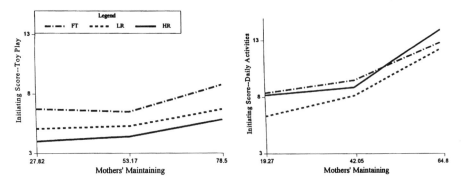

Figure 14-3. Relationship between changes in mothers' maintaining and children's development of initiating for full term (FT), low-risk (LR), and high-risk (HR) groups. The levels of mothers' maintaining relate to the children's average rate of growth in initiating for each of the three risk groups in each context. The midpoint on the x-axis is the grand mean of mothers' maintaining, which is based on maintaining across all times and for all mother–child dyads. Points on either side represent ±1 SD from this grand mean. Results show that increases in mothers' maintaining across the first 3 years of the child's life predict faster rates of social development, particularly in mother–child interactions that occur in the context of daily activities.

social and communication skills. The influence (predictiveness) of maintaining for greater growth in social skills was higher for the high-risk children than for the other two groups. While maintaining has been related to social skills at early time points, the present results demonstrate that increases in the rate at which children develop these skills also depends on caregivers increasing their use of this supportive strategy. The importance of caregivers providing specialized support in interactions with young children (scaffolding) for promoting development extends beyond infancy and has a changing rather than static nature. Moreover, these results suggest that it is not enough for parents to provide specialized stimulation only during early periods in children's development, particularly for children at risk for developmental problems. They also need to adapt to children's changing skills by increasing their support into early childhood. This adaptational process is highlighted by the finding that both premature groups, who had slower rates of social development, responded to higher levels of maintaining to a greater extent than did the full-term children. Moreover, those premature children with greater degrees of biological risk (i.e., high-risk group) showed even greater gains in their development when their mothers adapted by showing further increases in their maintaining strategies. A high degree of directiveness (i.e., telling the child specifically what response is expected) did not result in greater increases in social and communication skills; rather, increases in parents' use of directive strategies were associated with slower rates of development in these skills. Again, this relation was more evident for the high-risk children. Across the first 3 years of the child's life, when parents show higher amounts of direction about what their child should do, they may not promote the development of more active roles in social interactions (Kuczynski et al., 1987). Alternatively, children who have greater difficulty taking active roles may influence their parents to provide more direction. Unfortunately, high amounts of control and structure may also interfere with children developing a willingness to work with others in a cooperative manner. It will be important in future studies to carefully look at the cognitive demands of particular social and communication skills when identifying the types of intervention techniques to target in intervention programs.

Step four

We conducted an experimentally controlled pilot study with random assignment of mothers to either an intervention program or a developmental assessment program (attention control group). In the intervention program, mothers were trained to understand the importance of using maintaining strategies and to include more information about how the child was expected to respond. Mothers also learned to use these strategies in a manner that was responsive to their child's signals and at a pace that allowed the child time to organize a response. The nonintervention mothers received information from developmental screening tests about their child's abilities in various developmental areas.

The intervention targeted mothers' use of *maintaining* rather than *redirecting* strategies. Higher levels of maintaining were expected to enhance the premature infants' development because this strategy places fewer demands on their immature attentional skills, thus allowing them to use their more limited attentional capacity to organize their behavior and process information. We also targeted mothers' *provision of information* about a toy or activity (e.g., demonstrations, verbal directions) in combination with their use of maintaining strategies. Premature infants are more likely to organize an appropriate response when provided with information about the type of response that is expected. In the intervention group, mothers were actively involved in determining what worked with their infants. During the 10 weekly treatment sessions that occurred when the infants were 6–10 months of age, the facilitator and mothers worked together using videotapes of mothers using the targeted behaviors, live modeling, and role playing.

Prior to the start of the intervention, we compared mothers in the two groups on video-taped play, teaching, and feeding interactions with their infants and again several weeks following the completion of the intervention. As Figure 14-4 shows, we found that the intervention mothers had dramatic increases in maintaining and decreases in redirecting compared with the nonintervention mothers. In the intervention group, mothers' maintaining strategies also were less restrictive (i.e., "not that way" or "stop shaking it so hard") and more responsive to the needs of the child (i.e., appropriate pacing, attentive to the infant's signals) and included more information to the child about the type of response that was expected compared with mothers in the control group. The infants in the intervention group (Fig. 14-5), who we expected to show improved development because of changes in their mothers' behavior, showed more initiating and social responsiveness with an ex-

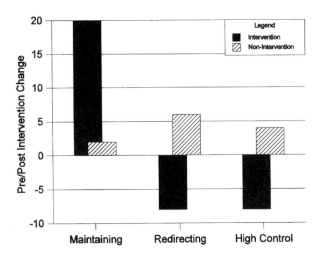

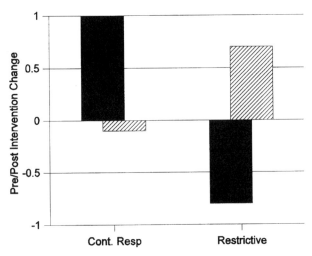

Figure 14-4. Pre- versus postintervention changes in targeted maternal behaviors for the intervention group and the nonintervention group. *(Top)* Mothers in the intervention group demonstrated significantly greater increases in their use of maintaining strategies and decreases in their use of redirecting and high control ("put the ball here") strategies than mothers in the nonintervention group. *(Bottom)* Mothers' use in the intervention group of strategies that were contingently responsive to the child's signals significantly increased while restricting the child's behavior decreased. For mothers in the nonintervention group there were decreases in the use of contingently responsive strategies and increases in restrictiveness.

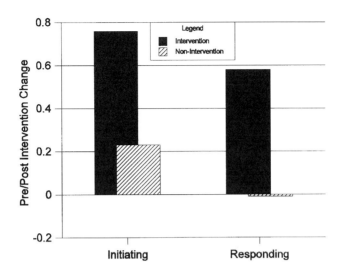

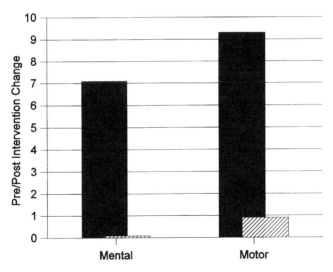

Figure 14-5. Pre- versus postintervention changes in infant behaviors in both intervention and nonintervention groups. *(Top)* Compared with infants in the nonintervention group, infants in the intervention group showed significantly greater increases in social initiating and responding in toy play interactions with an examiner. *(Bottom)* Significantly greater increases in mental and motor scores as measured by the Bayley Scales of Infant Development for infants in the intervention versus the nonintervention group.

aminer from the pre- to post-test evaluations than the nonintervention infants. They also had higher cognitive, language, and information processing scores on standardized measures of development. During learning interactions with their mothers they showed greater decreases in their irritability and disorganization behaviors.

Summary

The results of these studies illustrate an approach to the development of intervention models for infants and children with developmental disorders. We found it useful first to identify the type of developmental deficits shown by a particular "at-risk group" and then to determine what particular interactive behaviors should be targeted to provide specialized support for this deficit. Targeting intervention techniques that directly supported the high-risk premature children's deficiencies was expected to result in increases in these children's ability to take in and process more information from their social and nonsocial learning experiences. This, in turn, was expected to allow them to build the types of networks of associations that ultimately develop into solid memories or skills (Rovee-Collier, 1995).

While it was important to delineate the mechanism by which these strategies were expected to influence outcomes, this step in our model development could not substitute for a controlled study. Our controlled pilot study (step four), therefore, was a necessary step to determine intervention effectiveness.

These studies also show that there are a number of complex issues to address in the development of effective intervention models for young children with developmental disorders. One consideration is an understanding of the importance of delineating the *mechanism* by which an intervention strategy is expected to facilitate or alter the development of a particular skill. We have illustrated that mothers' maintaining strategies (i.e., attention to and support for the child's focus of attention) facilitate medically high-risk infants' social, language, and cognitive development because these strategies place fewer demands on young children's immature attentional skills, thus increasing their attentional and cognitive capacities to process information. Similarly, parents' use of strategies that provide specific information about the type of response expected of the child make it more likely that children with behavioral organization problems will respond in appropriate ways because of the structure inherent in this strategy.

Other types of developmental deficiencies will potentially require different interventions. It will, therefore, be important to engage a similar process for each specific developmental disorder to delineate the child's specific developmental deficiencies and the types of techniques that support these deficiencies, including the adaptations necessary to promote continued increases in skills across time.

Intervention Approaches for Children With PDD

Examination of the current intervention approaches for children with developmental disorders such as PDD-NOS and autism reveals a large variety. The interest in these disorders has resulted in many studies examining the types of problems these children exhibit. However, the results of these descriptive studies have rarely been used directly to guide the development of controlled studies evaluating the effectiveness of interventions for these children. Therefore, questionable treatments have sometimes been developed without a good conceptual or empirical basis.

The current interventions for PDD and autism can be classified into categories of behavioral treatment approaches, special education approaches, sensorimotor therapies, and language-based programs (Smith, 1996). These approaches and available studies examining their effectiveness are described in detail elsewhere (Smith, 1996; Green, 1996b). Descriptions of language programs for children with autism have also been recently published (Prizant et al., 1997; Olley and Reeve, 1997). The following is a brief outline of the range of approaches currently being used for children with the types of problems associated with PDD-NOS and autism.

Behavioral treatment

The behavioral treatment approach, which began in the 1960s with Lovaas' work, breaks autism down into distinct behavior problems and attempts to treat the broad number of problems associated with this disorder (for detailed descriptions of this approach, see Lovaas et al., 1981; Lovaas and Smith, 1988). This approach isolates small units of behavior and, through detailed analysis of each behavior, systematically targets each behavior with a specific treatment approach. These methods differ from other approaches such as sensorimotor therapies or language-based programs that focus on one central problem associated with autism.

Behavioral approaches are based on the premise that children with autism do not learn from typical environments but can learn if instruction is specialized. Programs using behavioral techniques focus on the various deficit areas of this disorder, such as increasing language skills or decreasing aggression, two areas that have been of great interest (Smith, 1996). Behavioral approaches are often designed for each child's individual needs. Although there have been concerns about using behavioral approaches to train language skills (Green, 1996a), behavioral techniques are now often used to target social communication skills. To address concerns about the lack of generalization with behavioral approaches, communications training is often carried out in home, clinic, and community settings because training across social contexts provides more opportunities for generalizing skills to different social situations.

Special education approaches

The TEACCH program (for a detailed history and description, see Schopler, 1997) was formally organized in the early 1970s as a state-mandated program in North Carolina for children with autism and related communication disorders. Three main areas of focus for children in TEACCH include home adjustment, education, and community adaptation. The program uses a comprehensive approach and provides diagnostic assessment, parent training and support, consultation, and professional training. This program is more eclectic than the Lovaas program because it uses a broad variety of techniques, often drawing on both cognitive and behavioral procedures to teach certain skills or to manage disruptive behaviors (Smith, 1996). Their approaches to language training, however, are not typically based on behavioral strategies because behavioral approaches to language training are thought to result in poor generalization (Schopler et al., 1980). There is an emphasis in programs using the TEACCH approach on the use of assessments that incorporate normed instruments and clinical observations of the child across a broad range of outcomes. Through these assessments, developmentally appropriate targets for the intervention as well as prescriptions for instructional approaches are determined. Emphasis is also placed on establishing a warm relationship with clients and their families and to encourage a close parent–professional collaboration.

The TEACCH program and its variations are used throughout the United States in several public school systems in special education programs for children with autism. No experimentally controlled studies have been conducted to evaluate the effectiveness of TEACCH. One study with large numbers of past and present students ($n = 657$), some diagnosed with autism (51%) and the remainder with other communication disorders, was conducted to evaluate outcomes related to various types of involvement with TEACCH (Schopler et al., 1982). Based on 53% of the evaluation questionnaires sent to families that were returned, TEACCH was reported to be helpful to most families, with the highest ratings coming from families with the most program contact.

Sensorimotor and related therapies

There are a number of therapies that use a specific deficit model approach, targeting usually one aspect of the disorder. The effectiveness of these approaches has not been determined. The sensory processing problems that have been described for autistic and PDD individuals have resulted in a therapy known as Sensory Integration Therapy (Ayers, 1972, 1979). This approach is based on observations that children with PDD-NOS and related disorders are unresponsive to sensory input from their environment and was developed to increase children's responsiveness and ability to process and integrate stimulation. Children with sensorimotor deficits are thought to show ritualistic behaviors (rocking, spinning, hand flapping) in order to moderate their arousal levels. Activities such as swinging, spinning, and movement exercises that require balance and motor control are often components of this type of program because they stimulate the vestibular system.

Auditory integration training is a related component of this type of therapy and is based on particular problems some autistic children have with hypersensitivity to certain sounds. An audiogram of each child determines the frequency at which hearing is overly acute and then the child spends numerous hours listening to sounds—sometimes music played through a device that filters out the sounds to which the child is hypersensitive. One random assignment study with small numbers of children showed some beneficial effects of this approach on behavioral and auditory problems (Reilly et al., 1983). There were numerous drawbacks to this study, however, that make the results difficult to interpret.

The facilitated communication approach is based on the observation that autistic children have motor deficits that make it difficult for them to express themselves in spite of adequate intelligence (Bilken, 1993). Therefore, a trained facilitator holds a child's forefinger, wrist, or arm and helps the child to type out messages on a keyboard. This approach has attracted a great deal of publicity because of some of the claims for sudden increases in normal language skills. These claims, however, have never been evaluated in appropriate designs. The few studies that have examined this approach show that it is the facilitator rather than the client who is producing the message (for a more complete description of this approach, see Smith, 1996).

Specific language interventions

Natural language paradigms (Koegel et al., 1987), including incidental teaching approaches (Hart and Risley, 1975), were developed to enhance generalization of language beyond what is thought to occur from standard behavioral approaches. These approaches are used to get elaborated language by waiting for the child to initiate conversation or make some vocal or verbal sound and then to respond in ways that encourage more language or vocalizations from the child. Children are taught language skills with the use of everyday stimuli (e.g., common objects and toys) in naturally occurring situations. Therapists set up language-promoting activities by encouraging curiosity in the child. Modeling is often used to encourage verbal behavior, and an emphasis is placed on using less structured contexts (i.e., a school walk) and generalization to new contexts. The programs involving peers in incidental teaching strategies are described in more recent research as encouraging the development of conversational skills for children with autism with their peers in normal school and play situations. Better generalization is thought to occur in these approaches because the treatment situation is set up more like an everyday life situation. Few empirical studies have been done to examine the effectiveness of these programs. In many cases, they are used to supplement standard Lovaas-based behavioral approaches.

Summary

There are few controlled studies evaluating the effectiveness of the various treatment or intervention approaches available for children with PDD-NOS and autism. Of the studies that have been conducted, the results suggest that interventions that use behavioral techniques and target the child's deficient behaviors with systematic and skillfully implemented approaches by dedicated staff achieve the best outcomes. In addition, programs that are intensive and provide high levels of structure are thought to be effective for children with this disorder. In Rutter and Bartak's comparison (1973) of three different models for classroom teaching for autistic children, those classrooms offering the most structure and teaching time were the most effective. A consensus also exists that intervention needs to be implemented as early as possible, particularly within the first 3 years of life, with parental involvement and school and community focus (Green, 1996b). Programs also need to be modified and adapted as the child develops new skills. While there is consensus that intensity of treatment is important, there is little agreement on how to determine the appropriate level of intensity. For example, Lovaas and colleagues (1981) suggest that autistic children need to receive as much treatment as possible in their programs, at least in the initial phases; treatment is approximately 30–40 hours per week in this approach. Other approaches involve the child in treatment for considerably shorter periods of time. The paucity of good information from controlled studies concerning the effectiveness of existing treatment approaches demonstrates a need for future research in this area. Without such research, children with severe developmental disorders will continue to receive treatments without the benefit of appropriate controlled studies evaluating their effectiveness on outcomes. In the next section a number of important issues related to evaluating treatment effectiveness are described.

Considerations for Future Intervention Studies

It is important that future intervention study designs take into account the many complexities inherent in this type of research. Researchers need to clearly delineate the mechanisms by which the treatment is expected to influence the child's behavior. However, understanding the mechanism underlying the intervention's expected effectiveness is not sufficient for evaluating outcomes. Future intervention studies also need to use controlled designs with large sample sizes to adequately examine the numerous factors that could contribute to individual differences in long-term outcomes. Careful attention needs to be paid to the selection of the children who are included in these studies. For example, in intervention studies for children with diagnoses within the PDD/autism spectrum, inclusion criteria need to be clearly specified and based on well-established approaches to diagnosis. Studies that delineate diagnostic subgroups within the PDD/autism or other developmental disorders may provide useful information on the type of developmental profile (i.e., child's level of functioning across a number of skill areas) that is most strongly affected by a particular intervention approach. Currently, there is limited information concerning the differential effectiveness of programs in relation to children's type and severity of problems.

In relation to this, important questions remain to be addressed such as how much intervention intensity is necessary to produce a good outcome. Is it necessary that the intervention be one on one, or can the same effect be achieved with one interventionist and small groups of children? This, of course, may vary depending on the developmental needs of the child. To date, little is known regarding the effectiveness of particular interventions in relation to co-morbid deficits frequently associated with particular developmental disorders. Although high intensity and individualized programs may be effective, if similar effects can be achieved with less costly approaches, more children are likely to be impacted (Lyon and Moats, 1997).

Programs with multiple components need to evaluate what components are producing what effects and for what type of child. Operational definitions need to be provided for the targeted behaviors in intervention programs so that all behaviors of interest can be directly observed and measured. In evaluating the effectiveness of an intervention, a broad range of skills should be measured to evaluate how comprehensive a particular program is in effecting change in the child's outcome. In addition to standardized measures of cognition, language, motor, and academic skills, emphasis needs to be placed on additional areas of functioning such as skills that demonstrate social competence (i.e., social interactions with peers, ability to effectively negotiate, and friendships), adaptive behaviors in home and community settings, and flexibility in problem-solving situations.

An important factor in evaluating the effectiveness of an intervention, particularly with children, is accounting for the change over time in a particular developmental process. To date, few intervention studies for children with developmental disabilities have examined the process of change in children's abilities across time in terms of the specific treatment and contextual factors that impact change. In addition to the specific treatment program a child receives, factors such as the parental level of involvement and compliance, the child's experiences with siblings and exposure to a range of social activities, as well as the availability of extended family may be important in understanding individual differences in outcomes within a treatment group. Greater family support and more opportunities to use the newly learned communication skills may influence faster rates of increases in children's skill attainment. While it is critically important to standardize the amount of training provided to each parent in the treatment group, parents may vary greatly in their level of expertise in using the techniques; this variability may provide important information concerning treatment effectiveness. Similarly, intervention outcomes may be affected by differences across the clinicians providing the program. Variability in the training and experience levels of clinicians and teachers affect children's response to the treatment.

Understanding the factors that influence changes in children's skills will require longitudinal methodologies and careful measurement of a broad range of treatment and contextual factors that are selected because of sound rationales regarding their potential importance (Applebaum and McCall, 1983). Our recent research examining the influence of changes in parental behaviors on children's rates of increased skill development (Landry et al., 1998) demonstrates the importance of attending to the process of change in both the children and their caregivers. In this study, mothers who adapted their input appropriately to their children's changing competencies influenced greater change in the children's skill development.

While this adaptational process between parents and their developing children is quite complex, there are effective statistical methods that allow for examination of associations between patterns of change in caregivers' and children's behaviors (Willet, 1989). Hierarchical linear modeling is one of several methods that allows for modeling the rate of growth in skill development for individual participants and the direct examination of potential predictors of these growth curves (Bryk and Raudenbush, 1987). The use of this type of statistical approach in intervention research has the potential to account for multiple causes of change in children's behavior. To date, few studies use available growth curve modeling methodologies to examine the way in which various treatment and contextual factors influence rates and patterns of change in children with developmental disorders. Growth modeling methods are appealing because of their flexibility and their ability to describe how multiple factors predict different patterns of development from assessments collected over time (for detailed descriptions, see Burchinal and Applebaum, 1991; Rogosa and Willet, 1985). Researchers gain flexibility with this approach because each child's growth can be modeled even if measurement points differ somewhat across subjects (Wohlwill, 1970). The same flexibility in the use of different measurement points is not possible with more traditional repeated measures analysis of variance.

While growth curve modeling has not been used to evaluate treatment effectiveness for children with significant developmental disorders, Lyon and Moats (1997) describe its effective application in recent reading intervention research (Foorman et al., 1998; Francis et al., 1996; Torgesen et al., 1998). Through the use of growth modeling analysis, these researchers have delineated a deficit rather than a developmental lag as characteristic of a reading disability (Francis et al., 1996); they also delineated the range and importance of individual differences among reading disabled children with respect to treatment outcomes (Foorman et al., 1998; Torgesen et al., 1998).

With respect to intervention research for children with significant developmental disorders, growth curve approaches could provide information on differences across subtypes of a particular disorder in terms of patterns of change in children's response to a specific treatment. Longitudinal designs using hierarchical linear modeling approaches can reveal more about the influence of the timing of a particular treatment and how treatments need to be modified and adapted to the child's changing competencies. Treatment and contextual correlates or predictors of individual differences in children's responses to treatment can be delineated so that families and clinicians can better determine what conditions are necessary for a child to benefit from a particular treatment approach. As intervention studies adopt designs that allow for examination of the high degree of complexity inherent in this research area, intervention models can be developed that more closely match the treatment stimuli with the type of input the brain needs in order to change. With longitudinal designs, complex statistical methodologies, and the use of relevant information from basic science research, intervention models can optimize opportunities to significantly alter the developing brains of children with developmental disorders.

References

Studies described in this chapter were supported by NIH grants HD23800 and HD25128.

Applebaum, M. I., and McCall, R. B. (1983). Design and analysis in developmental psychology. In P. Mussen (ed.): *Handbook of Child Psychology,* vol. 1. New York: Wiley, pp. 415–476.

Ayers, A. J. (1972). *Sensory Integration and Learning Disorders.* Los Angeles: Western Psychological Association.

Ayers, A. J. (1979). *Sensory Integration and the Child.* Los Angeles: Western Psychological Association.

Bakeman, R., and Adamson, L. (1984). Coordinating attention to people and objects in mother–infant and peer–infant interaction. *Child Dev., 55,* 1278–1289.

Belsky, J., Goode, M. K., and Most, R. K. (1980). Maternal stimulation and infant exploratory competence: Cross-sectional, correlational, and experimental analyses. *Child Dev., 51,* 1163–1178.

Biklen, C. (1993). *Communication Unbound: How Facilitated Communication Is Challenging Traditional Views of Ability/Disability.* New York: Teachers College.

Bornstein, M., and Tamis-LeMonda, C. S. (1989). Maternal responsiveness and cognitive development in children. In M. H. Bornstein (ed.): *Maternal Responsiveness: Characteristics and Consequences.* San Francisco: Jossey-Bass, pp. 49–61.

Bruner, J. (1977). Early social interaction and language acquisition. In H. R. Schaffer (ed.): *Studies in Mother–Infant Interaction.* New York: Academic Press, pp. 271–289.

Bryk, A. S., and Raudenbush, S. W. (1987). Application of hierarchical models to assessing change. *Psychol. Bull., 101,* 147–158.

Burack, J. A., Enns, J. T., Stauder, J. E. A., Mottron, L., and Randolph, B. (1997). Attention and autism: Behavioral and electrophysiological evidence. In D. J. Cohen and F. R. Volkmar (eds.): *Handbook of Autism and Pervasive Developmental Disorders.* New York: John Wiley & Sons, pp. 226–247.

Burchinal, M., and Applebaum, M. I. (1991). Estimating individual developmental functions: Methods and their assumptions. *Child Dev., 62,* 23–43.

Dawson, G., and Adams, A. (1984). Imitation and social responsiveness in autistic children. *J. Abnorm. Child Psychol., 12,* 209–225.

Dawson, G., and Lewy, A. (1989). Arousal, attention, and the socioemotional impairments of individuals with autism. In G. Dawson (ed.): *Autism: Nature, Diagnosis, and Treatment.* New York: Guilford Press, pp. 49–74.

Dennis, M., and Barnes, M. A. (1993). Oral discourse after early-onset hydrocephalus: Linguistic ambiguity, figurative language, speech acts, and script-based inferences. *J. Pediatr. Psychol., 18,* 639–652.

Dennis, M., Fitz, C. R., Netley, C. T., Sugar, J., Harwood-Nash, D. C., Hendrick, E. B., Hoffman, H. J., and Humphreys, R. P. (1981). The intelligence of hydrocephalic children. *Arch. Neurol., 38,* 607–615.

Dunham, P. J., and Dunham, F. (1995). Optimal social structures and adaptive infant development. In C. Moore and P. J. Dunham (eds.): *Joint Attention: Its Origins and Role in Development.* Hillsdale, NJ: Lawrence Erlbaum Associates, Inc., pp. 159–188.

Fletcher, J. M., Brookshire, B. L., Landry, S. H., Bohan, T. P., Davidson, K. C., Francis, D. J., Levin, H. S., Brandt, M. E., Kramer, L. A., and Morris, R. D. (1996). Attentional skills and executive functions in children with early hydrocephalus. *Dev. Neuropsychol., 12,* 53–76.

Foorman, B. R., Francis, D. J., Fletcher, J. M., Schatschneider, C., and Mehta, P. (1998). The role of instruction in learning to read: Preventing reading failure in at-risk children. *J. Ed. Psychol., 90,* 37–58.

Francis, D. J., Shaywitz, S. E., Steubing, K., Shaywitz, B. A., and Fletcher, J. M. (1996). Developmental lag vs. deficit models of reading: A longitudinal, individual growth curve analysis. *J. Educ. Psychol., 88,* 3–17.

Green, G. (1996a). Evaluating claims about treatments for autism. In C. Maurice (ed.): *Behavioral Intervention for Young Children With Autism.* Austin, TX: Pro-Ed, Inc., pp. 15–27.

Green, G. (1996b). Early behavioral intervention for autism. In C. Maurice (ed.): *Behavioral Intervention for Young Children with Autism.* Austin, TX: Pro-Ed, Inc., pp. 29–44.

Hart, B. M., and Risley, T. R. (1975). Incidental teaching of language in the preschool. *J. Appl. Behav. Anal., 8,* 411–420.

Jennings, K. D., Connors, R. E., and Stegman, C. E. (1988). Does a physical handicap alter the development of mastery motivation during the preschool years? *J. Am. Acad. Child Adolescent Psychiatry, 27,* 312–327.

Koegel, R. L., O'Dell, M. C., and Koegel, L. K. (1987). A natural language teaching paradigm for nonverbal autistic children. *J. Autism and Developmental Disorders, 17,* 187–199.

Kuczynski, L., and Kochanska, G. (1990). Development of children's noncompliance strategies: From toddlerhood to age 5. *Dev. Psychol., 26,* 398–408.

Kuczynski, L., Kochanska, G., Radke-Yarrow, M., and Girnius-Brown, O. (1987). A developmental interpretation of young children's noncompliance. *Developmental Psychology, 23,* 799–806.

Landry, S. H. (1995). The development of joint attention in preterm infants. Effects of maternal attention-directing behaviors. In C. Moore and P. Dunham (eds.): *Joint Attention: Its Origins and Role in Development.* Hillsdale, NJ: Erlbaum Assoc., pp. 223–250.

Landry, S. H., Garner, P. W., Swank, P. R., and Baldwin, C. D. (1996). Effects of maternal scaffolding during joint toy play with preterm and full-term infants. *Merrill-Palmer Q., 42,* 1–23.

Landry, S. H., Jordan, T., and Fletcher, J. M. (1994). Developmental outcomes for children with spina bifida and hydrocephalus. In M. B. Tramontana and S. R. Hopper (eds.): *Advances in Child Neuropsychology,* vol. 2. New York: Springer-Verlag, pp. 85–117.

Landry, S. H., Leslie, N., Fletcher, J. M., and Francis, D. J. (1985). Effects of intraventricular hemorrhage on visual attention in very premature infants. *Infant Behav. Dev., 8,* 309–322.

Landry, S. H., and Loveland, K. (1989). The effects of social context on the functional communication skills of autistic children. *J. Autism Dev. Disord., 19,* 283–299.

Landry, S. H., Smith, K. E., Miller-Loncar, C. L., and Swank, P. R. (1997). Predicting cognitive—linguistic and social growth curves from early maternal behaviors in children at varying degrees of biologic risk. *Dev. Psychol., 33,* 1–14.

Landry, S. H., Smith, K. E., Miller-Loncar, C. L., and Swank, P. R. (1998). The relation of change in maternal interactive styles with infants' developing social competence across the first three years of life. *Child Dev., 69,* 105–123.

Lewis, M., and Goldberg, S. (1969). Perceptual—cognitive development in infancy: A generalized expectancy model as a function of mother–infant interaction. *Merrill-Palmer Q., 15,* 81–100.

Lord, C. (1984). Development of peer relations in children with autism. In F. Morrison, C. Lord, and D. Keating (eds.): *Applied Developmental Psychology,* vol. 1. New York: Academic Press, pp. 166–230.

Lovaas, O. I., Ackerman, A., Alexander, D., Firestone, P., Perkins, M., Young, D. B., Carr, E. G., and Newsom, C. (1981). *Teaching Developmentally Disabled Children: The ME Book.* Austin, TX: Pro-Ed, Inc.

Lovaas, O. I., and Smith, T. (1988). Intensive behavioral treatment for young autistic children. In B. B. Lahey and A. E. Kazdin (eds.): *Advances in Clinical Child Psychology* vol. 11. New York: Plenum, pp. 285–324.

Lyon, G. R., and Moats, L. C. (1997). Critical conceptual and methodological considerations in reading intervention research. *J. Learning Disabil., 30,* 578–588.

Olley, J. G., and Reeve, C. E. (1997). Issues of curriculum and classroom structure. In D. J. Cohen and F. R. Volkmar (eds.): *Handbook of Autism and Pervasive Developmental Disorders.* New York: John Wiley & Sons, Inc., pp. 484–511.

Parpal, M., and Maccoby, E. E. (1985). Maternal responsiveness and subsequent child compliance. *Child Dev., 56,* 1326–1334.

Prizant, B. M., Schuler, A. L., Wethersky, A., and Rydell, P. (1997). Enhancing language and communication development: Language approaches. In D. J. Cohen and F. R. Volkmar (eds.): *Handbook of Autism and Pervasive Developmental Disorders.* New York: John Wiley & Sons, Inc., pp. 572–605.

Reilly, C., Nelson, D. L., and Bunday, A. C. (1983). Sensorimotor versus fine motor activities in eliciting vocalizations in autistic children. *Occup. Ther. J. Res., 3,* 199–211.

Rogosa, D. R., and Willitt, J. B. (1985). Understanding correlates of change by modeling individual differences in growth. *Psychometrics, 50,* 203–228.

Rose, S. A. (1983). Differential rates of visual information processing full-term and preterm infants. *Child Dev., 54,* 1189–1198.

Rovee-Collier, C. (1995). Time windows in cognitive development. *Dev. Psychol., 31,* 147–169.

Ruff, H. A. (1986). The measurement of attention in high-risk infants. In P. Vietze and H. G. Vaughan (eds.): *Early Identification of Infants At Risk for Mental Retardation.* New York: Grune & Stratton, pp. 282–296.

Rutter, M., and Bartak, L. (1973). Special educational treatment of autistic children: A comparative study. II. Follow-up findings and implications for services. *Journal of Child Psychology and Psychiatry, 14,* 241–270.

Schopler, E. (1997). Implementation of TEACCH philosophy. In D. J. Cohen and F. R. Volkmar (eds.): *Handbook of Autism and Pervasive Developmental Disorders.* New York: John Wiley & Sons, Inc., pp. 767–792.

Schopler, E., Mesibov, G. B., and Baker, A. (1982). Evaluation of treatment for autistic children and their parenting. *J. Am. Acad. Child Psychiatry, 21,* 262–267.

Schopler, E., Reichler, R. J., and Lansing, M. (1980). *Individualized Assessment and Treatment for Autistic and Developmentally Disabled Children, vol. 2, Teaching Strategies for Parents and Professionals.* Austin, TX: Pro-Ed, Inc.

Sigman, M., and Capps, L. (1997). *Children With Autism: A Developmental Perspective.* Cambridge, MA: Harvard University Press.

Sigman, M., Mundy, P., Sherman, T., and Ungerer, J. (1986). Social interactions of autistic, mentally retarded and normal children and their caregivers. *J. Child Psychol. Psychiatry Allied Disciplines, 27,* 647–656.

Smith, T. (1996). Are other treatments effective? In C. Maurice (ed.): *Behavioral Intervention for Young Children With Autism.* Austin, TX: Pro-Ed, Inc., pp. 45–59.

Spreen, O., Risser, A. H., and Edgell, D. (1995). *Developmental Neuropsychology.* New York: Oxford University Press.

Tager-Flusberg, H. (1982). Pragmatic development and its implications for social interaction in autistic children. In D. Park (ed.): *Proceedings of the International Symposium for Research in Autism.* Washington, DC: National Society for Autistic Children, pp. 103–108.

Torgesen, J. K., Wagner, R. K., Rashotte, C. A., Alexander, A. W., and Conway, T. (1997). Preventive and remedial interventions for children with severe reading disabilities. *Learning Disabil. Multidisciplinary J., 8,* 51–62.

Wertsch, J. V. (1979). From social interaction to higher psychological processes. *Hum. Dev., 22,* 1–22.

Willett, J. B. (1989). Some results on reliability for the longitudinal measurement of change: Implications for the design of studies in individual growth. *Educ. Psychol. Measure., 49,* 587–602.

Wohlwill, J. F. (1970). The age variable in psychological research. *Psychol. Rev., 77,* 49–64.

15

Pervasive Developmental Disorders: Listening Training and Language Abilities

MICHAEL M. MERZENICH, GABRIELLE SAUNDERS,
WILLIAM M. JENKINS, STEVEN MILLER,
BRET PETERSON, AND PAULA TALLAL

By definition, children diagnosed with pervasive developmental disorders (PDD, autistic [PDD-A]; pervasive developmental disorder–not otherwise specified [PDD-NOS]) have severe language impairments. Some scientists have argued that their especially severe early receptive language difficulties, resulting in the predominance of a thinking-in-pictures rather than a thinking-in-words cognition, are at the core of their complex panoply of neurobehavioral deficits (e.g., Rutter, 1974; Tager-Flusberg, 1993, 1996). Others have argued that language difficulties are one of many parallel and substantially independent deficits or "principal factors" that can have widely variable expressions in this population (e.g., Siegel et al., 1989; Eaves et al., 1994; Sevin et al., 1995; Hameury et al., 1995; Waterhouse et al., 1996a,b; Rapin, 1997).

Twin studies have shown that nearly all monozygotes of children with PDD-A and PDD-NOS have language impairments, but that the language (and other neurobehavioral) deficits of the identical twin are commonly of a different severity and can be expressed in a moderate form (Lainhart and Piven, 1995; Le Couteur et al., 1996). It has long been argued that children can also develop PDD-like symptoms, including a correspondingly severe language impairment from a variety of other inherited and postnatal neurological causes, such as intrauterine rubella, tuberous sclerosis, herpes simplex encephalitis, phenylketonuria, or fragile-X syndrome (for review, see Rapin, 1997). While these children may comprise only a small fraction of individuals identified as "autistic" (Bailey et al., 1993, 1995), they raise a very important question: What do these inherited and disease-induced conditions have in common that could result in such similar expressions of very severe language impairment? Moreover, how do the language impairments of children with PDDs relate to the often milder language impairments of their siblings or monozygotic twins—or to the neurological origins and expressions of language deficits in children with less severe impairments, in general? Are the language impairments of children with PDDs on a neurological continuum with those of children with specific language impairments (SLIs)? Can similar remedial training strategies be expected to ameliorate speech and language usage in both populations? This current study is a part of an extended series of experiments that are designed to address these important questions.

Neurologically Based Remediation of Phonological Processing, Language Reception, Comprehension, and Expression in Language Impaired Children

A new methodology has been developed for ameliorating the fundamental signal reception problems that underlie milder forms of language learning impairments (Tallal et al., 1995, 1999; Merzenich et al., 1996, 1998). There is increasing evidence that children with SLIs have different language learning progressions across the first year of life (Benasich and Tallal, 1996) that result in their processing aural speech inputs in an alternative way (see Tallal and Piercy, 1974, 1975; Tallal et al., 1993, 1999; Merzenich et al., 1993, 1999; Merzenich and Jenkins, 1995; Wright et al., 1997). Over 50% of infants with a family history of SLI do not develop the normal ability to make accurate fine-grained acoustic distinctions over the first 6 months of postnatal life (Benasich and Tallal, 1996; Spitz et al., 1997). Specifically, they integrate representations of complex acoustic inputs, including speech, over longer than normal processing times, resulting in relatively coarse-grained spectrotemporal signal resolution and subsequently delayed language development.

Studies of the brain plasticity underlying learning in monkeys and humans have led to the discovery that the accuracy with which rapidly successive and rapidly changing inputs are represented and processed by the cerebral cortex is subject to powerful behavioral training–induced plasticity (for reviews, see Merzenich and Jenkins, 1995; Merzenich and DeCharms, 1996; Merzenich et al., 1998, 1999). The principles of the neuroscience of complex signal learning derived in these basic experiments have been applied by us to children with SLI who have special problems at just these skills. Training exercises disguised as "computer games" were created *(1)* to drive progressive improvements in the fundamental complex-acoustic-signal reception abilities of children with SLI; *(2)* to generalize training gains to the wider contextual conditions that apply for the accurate reception of aural speech; and *(3)* in parallel, to train children at graduated exercises designed to drive improvements in their grammatical and syntactical abilities.

In each of these exercises, training stimuli were synthetically altered to initially disambiguate them for the child with receptive impairments. To reduce successive signal masking interferences and to thereby facilitate signal distinction and learning in children with SLI, brief and rapidly changing sound components of complex acoustic stimuli including speech were initially *(1)* prolonged in time, *(2)* differentially amplified, and *(3)* separated apart in time from one another. Through adaptive training exercises based on the neuroscience of the brain plasticity underlying complex signal learning and on well-established principles of experimental psychology (see Merzenich and Jenkins, 1995; Tallal et al., 1996; Merzenich et al., 1996, 1998, 1999), children were then trained to make accurate distinctions about and to accurately receive progressively more rapidly successive or more rapidly changing (for speech, progressively more natural) inputs. The end points of all seven listening exercises was a normal ability to distinguish and identify rapidly changing and rapidly successive acoustic events, including the phonological parts of speech—and thereby to achieve more accurate speech reception and language usage abilities.

The majority of children with SLIs who have participated in our studies have been successfully trained by these computer-guided procedures to achieve more normal fine-grained, fast successive signal reception abilities that were successfully generalized to the multiple contextual conditions of speech (Tallal et al., 1996, 1997, 1999; Merzenich et al., 1996, 1998, 1999; Miller et al., 1997). Furthermore, most of these 5–12-year-old children with SLIs who have completed the training program demonstrated significant improvements in their speech and language abilities based on comparisons between pre- and post-training standardized language assessments (Tallal et al., 1996, 1999; Miller et al., 1997; Merzenich et al., 1998, 1999).

Application of The Training Procedures to PDD Children

Rationale

It has been argued that children with PDDs, like children with SLIs, have language deficits that are characterized by a compromised ability to decode the rapid acoustic stimuli that characterize speech (e.g., see Ramberg et al., 1996; Rapin, 1996, 1997; Rapin and Dunn, 1997). As noted above, the training tools that have been very successfully applied to children with SLIs were designed specifically to overcome just such deficits. Moreover, it was reasoned that because children with PDDs often have siblings and even identical twins who are more mildly language impaired, and because previous studies have shown that computer-based training had a positive impact on the language abilities of a group of child with SLIs, gains with our adaptive training program might also be achieved in children with PDD. On those bases, this novel training method was applied to 29 children with PDD (10 PDD-A, 19 PDD-NOS) as part of a >400-child field trial of the efficacy of this training program, which we called *Fast ForWord*.

Training exercises

Circus Sequence. In Circus Sequence, the first of seven hierarchical exercises, the child was trained to identify and reconstruct the sequences of presentation of rapidly successive pairs of frequency glides. The durations of frequency-modulated (FM) stimuli ranged from 80 to 20 msec in six steps; interstimulus intervals ranged from 500 ms to 0 msec in 45 steps in difficulty. The FM sweep rate was maintained constant at 16 dB/octave. The two stimuli in each pair extended across the identical frequency range. The child received any one of four glide pairs (up–up, up–down, down–up, down–down) and was required to represent the stimulus presentation order by a button press sequence. In this and in all following computer-based exercises, the child performed an observing response (a "button press" with the computer mouse) to initiate a trial. The child listened to the successive stimuli on headphones and then responded with the computer mouse.

In all seven exercises, the child received feedback about correct and incorrect responses by *(1)* a progress indicator; *(2)* accumulating points on a point counter; and *(3)* sounds and lights. In all games, a brief reward animation and "bonus points" were obtained whenever the child got a fixed number of answers correct. The child worked at all exercises in a token economy based on the accumulation of points earned in these training exercises. The numbers of tokens obtained at the end of each training session were designed to reflect the child's game-play intensity and effort.

In this and in the following two exercises, a new stimulus set was loaded into the game whenever the child reached a performance asympote signaled by a preset number of hit–miss crossovers.

Stimulus sets in this game were adjusted in a 3-up, 1-down adaptive training schedule that was designed to ensure that the child always got about 80% of trials correct. As noted above, variable parameters included stimulus duration and interstimulus interval. Stimulus sweeps were delivered in three frequency ranges: 0.5–1.0 kHz, 1.0–2.0 kHz, and 2.0–4.0 kHz.

The objective of this game was to develop a more normal ability to identify brief, rapidly changing and rapidly successive acoustic stimuli that fall within the same frequency-processing channels of hearing and to generalize these fast signal receptive abilities across the frequency range required for the accurate reception of rapid acoustic transitions in speech. FM sweep rates of these stimuli paralleled those that apply for consonant–vowel (CV) transitions in normal English.

Phoneme Identification. A second exercise was designed to train the child to identify confusable CV stimuli. In this two-alternative forced-choice task, the child's observing response triggered the aural presentation of a target CV or vowel–consonant–vowel (VCV). Two characters in the "game" then vocalized the two contrasting syllabic (or bisyllabic) stimuli in random sequence. The child's task was to identify the character that produced the target sound.

Adaptive stimulus variables included the formant transition duration (in six steps) and the differential intensity (in seven steps) of the frequency transitions (and of other fast acoustic components) of these synthetic CVs or VCVs, as well as the time intervals between stimuli in the pair (from 500 to 10 msec in 13 graded steps). Specific contrasts used in the game included /ba/ versus /da/; /be/ versus /de/; /bi/ versus /di/; /va/ versus /fa/; and /aba/ versus /ada/. These specific synthetically produced contrasts were chosen because they are subject to relatively strong successive signal interference effects in children with SLIs and because (to support training generalization) they covered a reasonably broad spectrotemporal stimulus range.

Old McDonald's Flying Farm. This signal discrimination-based, limited-hold reaction-time task was used to train the child to make distinctions between synthetic speech sounds that differed by a single temporal acoustic parameter, that is, either by voice onset time or fricative-vowel time separation. The child's observing response required the "capture" of a beeping animal by a computer mouse click-and-hold that resulted in the animal producing a control CV at a regular rate. Following a random number of presentations of this control CV, a target CV was presented, followed by an additional control CV. The child's task was to signal the presentation of the target CV by a mouse button release. The reaction time window for "hits" in the "game" was 1,000 msec from the time of stimulus onset. Variables included the component durations and inter-event intervals of these synthetic CV contrasts critical for categorically distinguishing them, as well as the interstimulus intervals between CVs, which stepped from 1,000 to 300 msec. Stimuli were again varied in difficulty across these continua along a 3-up:1-down staircase. Specific contrasts in the game were /shu/ versus /chu/, /do/ versus /to/; /gi/ versus /ki/; /si/ versus /sti/; and /ge/ versus /ke/.

Phonic Match. The fourth exercise in the Fast ForWord training program was designed to provide generalization training for many contextual conditions in which fine spectrotemporal distinctions have to be made in normal speech reception. The stimuli were 48 CVCs and CVs, with the training list biased to emphasize the most commonly occuring syllables that present strong, between-element acoustic masking interferences. This exercise was an acoustic stimulus matching "game" played on a 2×2, 3×3, or 4×4 grid game board. The child's task was to match squares that evoked the same sounds. A correct match was signalled by "removing" the correctly matched panels and by a point accumulator and a sound. A graphic indicator signalled the accumulated number of matching attempts. When the child completed a grid, bonus points were awarded in inverse relationship to the number of attempts that had been taken to complete sound stimulus matching on the "game" board. The child was given a limited number of matching attempts per board, set as the number required for board completion if the child adopted an optimal strategy based on the ability to remember the previous two sounds. If the child required fewer match attempts to complete a board, additional points were awarded.

The stimuli used in this exercise were natural speech items that were modified using a speech processing algorithm in which the speech was prolonged in time (by 1.5×, 1.25×, 1.0×) and in which rapidly changing and brief acoustic elements in the acoustic stream were differentially amplified in decending steps from +20 dB. The processing algorithm that was employed to generate these stimuli has been described in detail elsewhere (Nagarajan et al., 1998).

In training, the child progressed from maximally processed speech (1.5× expansion; +20 dB differential amplification) on all game boards in four graded steps to normal (unprocessed) speech (the fifth difficulty level). The speech processing level was advanced when the child consistently cleared 4 × 4 game boards with a pre-set minimum number of match attempts. With that attempt number, we were assured that the child reliably distinguished each of the presented speech sounds and that the children were able to accurately and consistently recall the previous two sounds.

Phonic Word. This single-word reception/picture pointing exercise was designed to provide the child with practice at making correct phonetic distinctions between sounds presented in word contexts. Forty-seven word contrast pairs were applied in these exercises, with pictures representing target and foil initial or final consonant sounds. Again, acoustically modified speech stimuli were used for training (Nagarajan et al., 1998). As in the previously described game, the child advanced through four levels of temporally extended and/or fast-element-amplified speech to a fifth natural speech level. In this and in the following two exercises, the speech processing difficulty level advanced one step toward the normal when the child achieved a 90% performance level on a complete stimulus set.

Block Commander. This language comprehension exercise was designed to train children to comprehend commands of increasing length and grammatical complexity. In the task, related to the progressive Token Test for Children, the child received instructions to point to or to move colored geometric shapes on a game board. Verbal comands progressed through six levels of increasing instruction length and complexity. Again, the child moved across five speech processing levels culminating in natural speech, as outlined above.

Language Comprehension Builder. The objective of this "game" was to adaptively train a child to make age-appropriate grammatical distinctions in a sentence context. In this language comprehension/grammatical training exercise adapted from the CYCLE assessment battery (Curtiss and Yamada, unpublished data), the children heard a spoken sentence. Their task was to point to one of two to four pictures that correctly depicted the sentence. The incorrect foil pictures were carefully designed and tested to ensure that correct responses could be made based on vocabulary that required explicit understanding of the grammatical rule being trained. Sentences varied in terms of their grammatical or syntactical structure and complexity. The child progressed through 40 grammatical tasks encompassing the range of grammatical ability that is appropriate for a normal 8-year-old. Again, five levels of speech processing were applied in training.

Response Monitoring; Training Program Administration. Each of the training exercises provided a measurement of a child's ability at each "game" on every training day. All relevant information about their responses and performance times were recorded trial by trial during "game" play. At the end of Fast ForWord training sessions, this information was uploaded via the Internet to a central database, where it was analyzed, graphed, and then sent back to the supervising clinician over the Internet. The objective of this approach was to provide assistance to the clinician in guiding each child's training program. The database automatically documented daily performance progress at multiple levels of detail. It alerted the professional supervising the training whether children had compliance problems, had difficulties playing a particular "game" by the rules, were not advancing at a particular exercise, or had successfully accomplished different specific acoustic or language listening skills represented by specific dimensions of "game" play.

Experimental design

The primary data reported in this study originate from a subset of children diagnosed with PDD who took part in a large field trial of Fast ForWord (see Merzenich et al., 1998; Tallal et al., 1999). Subjects were diagnosed with PDD on the basis of standard DSM-IV criteria by a neurologist, psychiatrist, or psychologist. The clinicians involved in the field trial were each interviewed to confirm the current validity of the PDD diagnoses. Several children for whom a diagnosis of PDD was uncertain were omitted from these analyses. Their inclusion in this sample would not affect any of its conclusions.

Twenty-nine children with PDD completed Fast ForWord training. Ten were classified as PPD-A and 19 as PDD-NOS. Their mean age was 7.95 years (SD, 2.25; range, 5.00–13.74); 8 were girls, and 21 were boys. Children with PDD worked at the seven exercises described above for an average total of 55 training hours achieved over an average training period of 31 training days.

We also report data comparing these 29 children with PDD with the 219 other SLI children trained in this large field trial of Fast ForWord. These other SLI children were diagnosed with a variety of disorders including one or more of a language-based learning disorder; a receptive, expressive, or mixed communication disorder; a central auditory processing disorder; and any of the above along with a co-morbid attention deficit disorder. The mean ages of these children was 8.48 years (SD, 1.98; range, 4.25–13.53); 61 were girls, and 158 were boys. The mean age of children with PDD did not differ from that of the other children in this field trials ($t = 1.33$, $p = 0.19$), nor did the proportion of boys to girls differ for the two groups ($c^2 = 0.001$, $p = 0.98$).

Language training of children with PDD was supervised by 16 clinicians working independently at speech pathology clinics distributed across the United States (see Acknowledgments). Speech reception, language comprehension, and comprehensive language batteries were administered to each child before and after Fast ForWord training. The independent clinicians participating in this field trial were specifically instructed to apply whatever standardized speech and language testing battery they normally used in their assessment of the language abilities of PDD children. Different clinicians applied different measures. Here, we report data derived from all speech reception or language tests that were used to assess pre- versus post-training abilities of at least five children with PDD trained with Fast For-Word in this field trial.

Results: Positive Changes in Acoustic Signal Reception, Language Comprehension, and Expression Resulted From Fast ForWord Training

The accurate reception of sounds in words is a common deficit of children with SLI and PDD (e.g., Liberman et al., 1974; Bird et al., 1995; Ramberg et al., 1996; Rapin and Dunn, 1997; Rapin, 1997; for review, see Leonard, 1998). This is a principal skill that was trained by Fast ForWord. Marked performance improvements were recorded in standarized measures of this fundamental ability after training in 14 children with PDD to whom the Goldman-Fristoe-Woodcock (GFW) Test of Auditory Discrimination–Quiet (Fig. 15-1) was administered. In this test, the child points to one of four pictures representing an aurally presented word. The other three pictures represent confusable words that differ by an initial or final consonant sound. In these trained children with PDD, z-scores advanced by an average of 1.65; that is, performances improved with training on average by 1.65 standard deviations. For the 11 children who were given the GFW–Noise (simulating speech reception in a classroom noise environment), scores improved by an average of 2.0 SD (Fig. 15-1 and Table 15-1).

At the initiation of training, 57% (8) of these children fell within the 1st percentile in performance at these tests. After training, several of these children advanced to above the normal mean (i.e., above the 50th percentile). Repeated measures ANOVA showed a significant main effect of pre- versus post-training change ($F = 22.2, p < 0.001$), with no differences between quiet and noise test gains ($F = 1.0$, n.s.). There were no differences in the gains made by children with PDD-A versus PDD-NOS children ($F = 0.2$, n.s.; Table 15-2). The average post-training scores moved to near the normal median performance for both tests—and for both PDD groups—after training (Fig. 15-1).

In our large trial, the children with PDDs had lower post-training scores than did children with SLIs without a PDD diagnosis (Fig. 15-2). At the same time, changes in performances achieved by children with PDDs were not significantly different from the changes in performances achieved by the rest of our trained population, who were predominantly less severely language impaired (e.g., GFW-Quiet, PDD versus non-PDD, $F = 1.1$, n.s.; GFW-Noise, $F = 0.8$, n.s.; Token Test, $F = 1.3$, n.s.; TOLD/CELF Listening Quotients, $F = 1.8$, n.s.; TOLD/CELF speaking quotients, $F = 1.4$, n.s.; Table 15-1 and Fig. 15-2).

Another hallmark of the child with PDD is a fundamental difficulty in accurately receiving and acting on verbal instructions. With the improved accuracy in

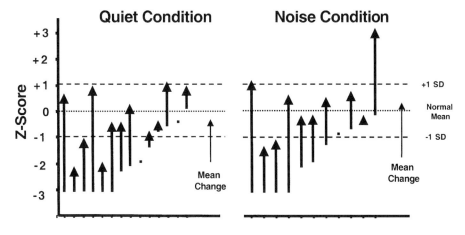

Cases Ordered by Pre-Training Score

Figure 15-1. z-Scores obtained for children tested on the Goldman-Fristoe-Woodcock Test of Auditory Discriminination, administered before and after Fast ForWord training. Quiet condition, $n = 14$; Noise condition, $n = 11$. Cases are ordered by pre-training scores, with children with PDDs with the lowest pre-training performance abilities displayed at the left for each condition. Each arrow represents the test scores of an individual child: the bottom of the arrow indicates the pre-training score; the tip of the arrowhead indicates the post-training score. Group mean performances are shown by the lighter arrows. The dotted lines mark the normal population mean; dashed lines mark performance levels that are 1 SD above or below the normal U.S. population mean.

their reception of speech sounds demonstrated above, it was not surprising that most (not all) of these severely impaired children made major gains on overall speech intelligibility measures. For example, on the Token Test for Children, in which a child has to receive, remember, and carry out verbal instructions of variable length and complexity, the performance of children with PDD advanced by an average of 1.6 SD ($n = 29$; $t = 7.0$, $p < 0.0005$; see Fig. 15-3). Average gains were identical for children with PDD-A and PDD-NOS.

Eleven of these children completed age-appropriate versions of the Clinical Evaluation of Language Function (CELF) language battery before and after training. Eight completed an age-appropriate version of the Test of Language Development (TOLD). These two assessment batteries are commonly used to evaluate the language skills of children in the United States.

The PDD children here showed significant pre-training versus post-training gains for all of the quotients obtained with both language batteries except the "phonology quotient" on the TOLD, for which only five children were assessed (Table 15-1 and Fig. 15-4). Those highly significant score advances are noteworthy, given the relatively small numbers involved.

Table 15-1. Means, standard deviations and results of *t*-tests comparing pre- and post-test *z*-scores on language measures for all children with PDD

Test Measure	Number of Cases	Pre-Test		Post-Test		*t*-value	*p* < (Pre- vs. Post-Test
		Mean	SD	Mean	SD		
Token Test							
Total age-standardized score	29	−3.11	2.09	−1.52	1.82	−7.0	0.0005
GFW Test of Auditory Discrimination							
Quiet subscale	14	−2.00	1.18	−0.35	2.11	−4.8	0.0005
Noise subscale	11	−1.82	1.16	0.18	1.25	−5.1	0.0005
TOLD (P:2 and 1:2 combined)							
Spoken language quotient	8	−1.90	1.00	−1.04	1.17	−3.6	0.008
Listening quotient	8	−1.92	0.91	−1.1	0.81	−3.3	0.014
Speaking quotient	8	−1.88	1.15	−0.89	1.45	−3.3	0.013
Semantics quotient	8	−1.65	0.63	−0.92	0.95	−3.1	0.018
Syntax quotient	8	−1.93	0.93	−1.08	1.28	−3.0	0.021
Phonology quotient	5	−1.20	1.56	−0.64	1.37	−1.9	0.135
CELF (Preschool and −3 combined)							
Receptive language quotient	11	−2.19	0.69	−0.87	0.95	−5.2	0.0005
Expressive language quotient	10	−2.36	0.92	−1.31	1.24	−7.0	0.0005

Table 15-2. Means, standard deviations (SD; in parentheses) and results of *t*-tests comparing changes in score for children with PDD-Autism versus PDD–NOS

Test Measure	Mean Change in *z*-Score (SD)		*t*-value and *p* (PDD-A vs. PDD–NOS)
	PDD-autism	PDD–NOS	
Token Test			
Total age-standardized score	1.58 (0.82)	1.61 (1.41)	0.1 n.s.
	n = 10	*n* = 19	
GFW Test of Auditory Discrimination			
Quiet subscale	1.44 (1.14)	1.77 (1.41)	0.4 ns.
	n = 5	*n* = 9	
Noise subscale	1.86 (1.23)	2.12 (1.46)	0.3 ns.
	n = 5	*n* = 6	
CELF (Preschool and −3 combined)			
Receptive language quotient	1.6 (1.15)	1.09 (0.47)	1.0 ns.
	n = 5	*n* = 6	
Expressive language quotient	1.01 (0.63)	1.08 (0.32)	0.2 ns.
	n = 5	*n* = 5	

It is important to note that expressive as well as receptive language quotients advanced in trained children. The *z*-scores for receptive language quotients on the CELF advanced by an average of 1.3. The *z*-scores for expressive language quotients on the CELF advanced by an average of 1.1 (Table 15-1). For children diagnosed as PDD-A, the average receptive and expressive language quotient gains were 1.6 and 1.0, respectively (Table 15-2). For children diagnosed as PDD-NOS, they were 1.1 and 1.1, respectively. Repeated measures ANOVA showed a significant main effect of pre- versus post-training change for receptive and expressive CELF language quotients ($F = 30.2, p < 0.002$). No differences in changes in receptive versus expressive quotients ($F = 0.6$, n.s.) or for the different PDD groups ($F = 0.3$, n.s.) were recorded.

For the eight children with PDDs given the TOLD battery (Fig. 15-4), the speaking quotient advanced by 1.0 SD (Table 15-1).

Taking the CELF- and TOLD-tested children together, ANOVA showed significant effects of pre- versus post-training change for both the receptive/listening quotient and the speaking/expressive quotients ($F = 19.7, 0.0005$) but not for a comparison between them ($F = 0.1$, n.s.).

Overall Language Benefits for Trained Children

These positive score changes represented significant advances in the language abilities of many, but not all, children trained with Fast ForWord. For example, on

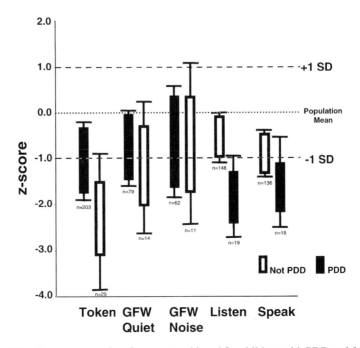

Figure 15-2. Comparisons of performances achieved for children with PDD and for other trained children with language impairments. The numbers of each population group are shown with each bar. The bottom of each bar represents the mean pre-training score for the tests shown on the abscissa. The top of each bar represents the mean post-training score. Standard errors for the pre-training and post-training data are indicated at the ends of each bar.

GFW-Quiet tests administered before training, children with PDD had initial phonetic reception performance abilities that placed most of them within the lowest percentiles of children of the same age in the American population. After training, on the average, the children with PDD in this study performed within the normal range—at about the 45th percentile for U.S. children of the same age. In GFW-Noise tests simulating phonetic reception abilities in a noisy environment, the performance of the majority of trained children was at the third percentile or below before traning. After training, children advanced, on the average, to above the normal mean for children of the same age in the American population. The GFW-Noise condition is important because it reflects speech reception abilities in the noise environment of the average school.

Advances on language comprehension abilities measured by the Token Test were more limited, even though children were trained in Fast ForWord at a closely related task. Twelve trained children did not achieve post-training scores that advanced to within 1 SD of the normal mean performance level. Nonetheless, the performance of all but five of those children advanced toward the normal performance level by at least 1 SD, which represented a substantial test score advance. The remaining 17 children all advanced from <1 SD below the normal mean into the normal performance range. Six of these children achieved post-training scores that reached or exceeded the normal mean performance level for children of the same age.

Of 19 children administered CELF or TOLD language batteries, 12 (68%) advanced from impaired levels (<1 SD below the normal mean for children of the same age) into the normal range for receptive language abilities. After training, the performances of two of those children scored above the normal mean. The scores of four children with PDDs changed little on any post-training versus pre-training measure that was applied.

Expressive language abilities changed only modestly for 5 of the 17 children administered a full complement of TOLD or CELF expressive language battery tests before and after training. Scores of 10 children with PDDs advanced by more than 1 SD. Seven of 18 tested children (39%) advanced from an "impaired" level group into the normal range. After training, the expressive language quotients of five children with PDDs was very near to or exceeded the normal median.

Note that the least impaired and the most questionably PDD child (from the perspective of language impairment) advanced little on both expressive and receptive language measures, while another relatively language-capable child with PDD advanced from just below or just within the low-normal performance range

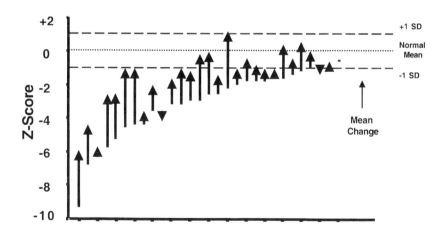

Cases Ordered by Pre-Training Score

Figure 15-3. *z*-Score changes for 29 children with PDDs who were administered the Token Test for Children before and after Fast ForWord training. Cases are ordered by pre-training scores at this task. The bottom of each arrow is the pre-training score; the arrowhead tip is the post-training score. See Figure 15-1 and text for further details.

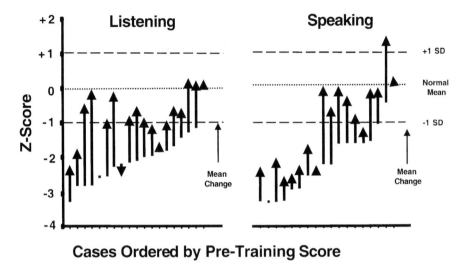

Cases Ordered by Pre-Training Score

Figure 15-4. *(Left) z*-Score changes for 19 children for whom receptive language quotients (CELF battery) and listening quotients (TOLD battery) were defined before and after training. *(Right)* Expressive language quotients (CELF) and speaking quotients (TOLD). Cases are ordered by pre-training scores. Each arrow represents performances defined before (base of arrow) and after (tip of arrowhead) training for an individual child.

to an above-normal ability at both receptive and expressive language abilities that brought him up to the 85th and 99th percentiles in these language performance measures, respectively.

Twenty-five of these 29 children advanced by ≥1 SD on at least one of the test measures derived after training; 17 of the 29 children advanced by more than 2 SD on at least one test measure; seven children advanced by more than 3 SD on at least one test measure; and more than half (15 of 29) of the children with PDD trained with Fast ForWord advanced by at least 1 SD on *every one* of up to six test measures. Because the Fast ForWord training exercises focussed on developing better listening skills, it had been expected that receptive language skills would improve more than expressive skills. That was not the case. In fact, it is striking that the benefits of this training were measured for nearly *all* aspects of language ability in these children with PDDs. These across-the-board performance gains mirror a broad sweep of positive test changes obtained in generally more mildly language impaired populations (Tallal et al., 1996, 1999; Miller et al., 1998; Merzenich et al., 1998).

We have argued that this wide-ranging improvement in perceptual, cognitive, and expressive skills in children with less severe SLIs might be explained by the fact that their training has improved the accuracy with which they receive incoming speech (see Tallal et al., 1996, 1998; Merzenich et al., 1998, 1999). This hypothesis, supported by very large test score advances in simple tests of phonetic reception fidelity, suggests that with a sharp improvement in complex acoustic signal (speech) input salience, *all* measures of perceptual, short-term memory–related, and cognitive abilities employing aurally received speech also advance (see Merzenich et al. [1998b] for an explanation of these effects expressed in neurological terms). Similarly, those abilities of speech production that operate with newly refined neurological representations and with newly refined sensory feedback are improved in parallel. These across-the-board improvements in higher functions after positive advances in basic processing precision are not unprecedented. For example, visual perception, cognition, and visuomotor skils are all broadly and rapidly improved in children with visual impairments once their defective visual reception is corrected, that is, with corrective lenses.

Some Precautions

Training effects are usually positive, but trained children still have language impairments

It should be emphasized that only 13 of 19 trained PDD children who were administered CELF or TOLD language batteries in this trial (68%) achieved receptive or listening language battery quotients that moved from the "impaired" range into the "normal" range after training. Moreover, in a simple test of language comprehension, the Token Test for Children, only 16 of 29 children (55%) advanced from <1 SD below the normal mean into the range within 1 SD of normal. All but five of those children only advanced as far as the "low-normal" domain.

At the same time, most of these children—and, indeed, most other trained children—achieved substantial score advances in the direction of normal. At the same time the majority of these chldren continued to require additional speech and language services.

The trained population was a selected one

It should be noted that this population was specially selected: *(1)* Eleven other PDD children initiated training, but because of behavioral problems did not complete it. *(2)* An unknown number of other children with PDD-A and PDD-NOS were excluded by therapists from participating in this trial because they could not undergo reliable standardized language asessments pre-training or were judged not to have the behavioral or conceptual competencies that the professional judged to be required for completing it.

Some selectivity may also apply for the tests chosen for administration to different children in this limited series. In interpreting these findings, it should *not* be assumed that test results would be identical had all children been administered any one of these tests.

The specific bases of training-induced gains in language abilities in this special population are not well understood

Positive changes in the receptive abilities of children were tracked through the course of game play in Fast ForWord training. It is reasonable to believe that these measured improvements in acoustic (and speech) signal resolution contributed to the advance of language scores following training. At the same time, there are other important facets of this intensive acoustic signal/aural language training that also undoubtedly contribute to the often-dramatic positive changes in language behaviors. It drills children in attention, working memory, and response rate processing skills. It intensively trains children in syntactic and grammatic skills. Our understanding of the fundamental receptive, attentive, memory, cognitive, and pragmatic/behavioral aspects of the language-related deficits of these children is still incomplete. Given both this small sample and the limited assessments of language-related (and other neurobehavioral) abilities of these children, any proportional attribution of the gains of training to different specific aspects of this training regime must await further study.

Training-induced changes in language abilities were paralleled by changes in real-world language abilities in some children, but mismatches were recorded

Therapists reported that training-based gains in language abilities were paralleled by obvious changes in pragmatics and fluency in many—but clearly not in all—of these trained children with PDDs. Moreover, therapists' reports of "real-world" outcomes indicated that there were several notable mis-matches between measured speech and language gains and gains in practical language usage. For example, in two of the children in whom no statistically significant advances in speech reception or language abilities were recorded through standardized testing, the therapists noted unequivocally positive, *major* changes in communicative competencies and behaviors. The relationship of positive changes in language abilities to other psychological indices that characterize the autistic spectrum remains undocumented.

These initial findings should be viewed as preliminary

Further studies are clearly required to derive a more quantitatively ascertained PDD Fast ForWord training-response sample. Although all children in this study were medically disgnosed as PDD, no quantitative data based on standized diagnostic measures beyond these basic speech and language measures has been considered in this interpretation of these findings. Comparisons with a more completely documented sample and with well-matched control samples need to be undertaken to more fully interpret the findings of this preliminary study. A larger experimental study designed to address many of the questions raised by this en-couraging preliminary survey has now been initiated.

Discussion: Some Conclusions; Remaining Questions

PDD-Autism and PDD-NOS are marked by symptoms that combine the signature deficits of severe or profound language learning impairments with parallel, severe sensori-perceptual, cognitive, and social behavioral deficits (for review, see Rapin, 1997; Waterhouse et al., 1996b). The very positive gains in language abilities achieved in these short-term, intensive training studies raise important questions about this population.

What accounts for the apparently stronger penetration of inherited deficit(s) in the severely impaired child with PDD versus a more moderately language (and commonly in parallel, psychologically) impaired sibling or twin? We know that children with SLIs who inherit their language problems have a dif-ferent language learning progression in early childhood (Benasich and Tallal, 1996). Through that progression, they do not develop the normal ability to ac-curately distinguish the rapidly successive and rapidly changing spectrotempo-ral fine structures of speech. Are the language impairments expressed in the autistic spectrum disorder simply a more severe form of what is essentially the same defective language learning progression, or are there other contributing neurological factors that augment their often especially severe language learn-ing problems? Do special behavioral or experiential factors contribute to these striking differences in genetic expression? Does the progressive deterioration between the first and second year of postnatal development of language de-scribed in patient histories as occuring in about one third of children in the PDD spectrum (see Rapin, 1997) manifest a different—or a second—language-de-grading process or event that results in the differentiation of the PDD child from the SLI child? The current study shows that whatever the differences or com-malities that apply to language learning deficits in children with PDDs versus children with SLIs, Fast ForWord training was equally effective in driving im-provements in their language abilities. No significant differences in the magni-tudes of performance gains achieved with training were recorded for *any* of a series of applied speech reception or language usage measures in children with PDD versus children with language impairment attributed to other (non-PDD) diagnoses.

Given the broad sweep of changes in perceptual, cognitive, and communica-tive skills recorded in this study, and given the movement of some children's abil-ities into the normal range with Fast ForWord training, can relatively normal lan-guage performances be achieved by the more extended training of this population? There is no indication that most children with PDD in this trial—which involved an average total of only 55 hours of training—reached any hard and fast speech reception/language performance ceiling. New training tools are now being developed that should facilitate the extension of training through another training period to determine whether still higher rapidly achieved performance gains can be obtained in them.

Given an effective treatment of these fundamental aural signal reception problems and the reduction of the language-based isolation of these children, to what extent could the other complex perceptual, cognitive, metacognitive, and emotional problems that mark the PDD spectrum disorder be altered or ameliorated? Individual case studies now indicate that there can be major parallel positive behavioral impacts of this training in some children in this small PDD population sample. A new investigation has been initiated to more specifically define the possible, extended impacts of this intensive language training on other aspects of the autistic behavioral spectrum.

What aspects of a complex disability like PDD-A or PDD-NOS *cannot* be ameliorated or altered by the achievement of more normal acoustic/speech reception and language abilities? What other intensive training tools might be brought to bear to ameliorate other complex deficits that characterize these children? A principal-factors analytic approach can now be applied to differentially define important positive impacts of this intensive training. Such an approach should help determine how training might be further elaborated to provide even greater amelioration of the complex panoply of deficits that limit the potential achievements of children with PDDs.

Finally, what could account for the apparent failure to drive any positive advances in language abilities in a small percentage of these trained children?

The answer to this important question strikes at the heart of our understanding of the true nature of the origins of the language and nonlanguage impairments that characterize the PDD spectrum of disorders. These training results open the door to many potential studies that hold the prospect of still further improving the capacities and potentials of children with PDDs.

References

The authors thank the therapists who supervised the training of children with PDDs in this trial: Dr. Gail Bedi, Learning and Development Center, New York, NY; Mary Ann Ceriotti, San Francisco Hearing and Speech Center, San Francisco, CA; Dr. Martha Burns, Evanston, IL; Jane Gould-Caulfield, Scottish Rite Language Clinic, Oakland, CA; Sabra Gelfond, National Speech/Language Therapy Center, Bethesda, MD; Dr. Nancy Polow, Suburban Speech Center, South Orange, NJ; Julie Burgess-Dennis, Talk, Learn, Communicate, Seattle, WA; Ann Osterling, Ann Osterling Therapy Associates, Savoy, IL; Dr. Vicki Simms, Mann Center, Los Angeles, CA; Andrea Jobe, Stanbridge Academy, Santa Clara, CA; Dr. Marlene Rissman, Children's Hospital, San Diego, CA; Judith LeDuc, Chicago, IL; Dr. Christine Weber-Fox, Mills Peninsula Hospital, San Mateo, CA; Karen Grites, Children's Health Council, Palo Alto, CA; Jeri Weinstein, Beth Israel Medical Center, New York, NY; and Dr. Alan Wachtel, Family Health Associates, New York, NY.

The Fast ForWord training program was produced by Scientific Learning Corporation in Berkeley, CA, and provided to participating therapists and families without charge. The independent therapists who participated in this trial were not reimbursed by Scientific Learning Corporation for their participation. For further information about the Fast ForWord program, see www.FastForWord.com.

Bailey, A., Bolton, P., Butler, L., Le Couteur, A., Murphy, M., Scott, S., Webb, T., and Rutter, M. (1993). Prevalence of the fragile X anomaly amongst autistic twins and singletons. *J. Child Psychol. Psychiatry, 34,* 673–686.

Bailey, A., LeCouteur, A., Gottesman, I., Bolton, P., Simonoff, E., Yuzda, E., and Rutter, M. (1995). Autism as a strongly genetic disorder: Evidence from a British twin study. *Psychol. Med., 25,* 63–77.

Bailey, A., Phillips, W., and Rutter, M. (1996). Autism: Towards an integration of clinical, genetic, neuropsychological and neurobiological perspectives. *J. Child Psychol. Psychiatry, 37,* 89–126.

Benasich, A. A., and Tallal, P. (1996). Auditory temporal processing thresholds, habituation, and recognition memory over the first year. *Infant Behav. Dev., 19,* 339–357.

Bird, J., Bishop, D. V., and Freeman, N. H. (1995). Phonological awareness and literacy development in children with expressive phonological impairments. *J. Speech Hear. Res., 38,* 446–462.

Bishop, D. V. M. (1992). The underlying nature of specific language impairment. *J. Child Psychol. Psychiatry, 33,* 3–66.

Eaves, L. C., Ho, H. H., and Eaves, D. M. (1994). Subtypes of autism by cluster analysis. *J. Autism Dev. Dis., 24,* 3–22.

Hameurey, L., Roux, S., Barthelemy, C., Adrien, J. L., Desombre, H., Sauvage, D., Garreau, B., and Lelord, G. (1995). Quantified multidimensional assessment of autism and other pervasive developmental disorders. Application for bioclinical research. *Eur. Child Adolesc. Psychiatry, 4,* 123–135.

Lainhart, J. E., and Piven, J. (1995). Diagnosis, treatment and neurobiology of autism in children. *Curr. Opin. Pediatr., 7,* 392–400.

Le Couteur, A., Bailey, A., Goode, S., Pickles, A., Robertson, S., Gottesman, I., and Rutter, M. (1996). A broader phenotype of autism: The clinical spectrum in twins. *J. Child Psychol. Psychiatry, 37,* 785–801.

Leonard, L. (1998). *Children with Language Impairment.* Cambridge, MA: MIT Press.

Liberman, I., Shankweiler, D., Fischer, F. W., and Carter, B. (1974). Explicit syllable and phoneme segmentation in the young child. *J. Exp. Child Psychol., 18,* 201–212.

Merzenich, M. M., and De Charms, R. F. (1996). Neural representations, experience and change. In Rollinus and P. Churchlord (eds.): *The Mind–Brain Continuum.* Boston: MIT Press, pp. 61–81.

Merzenich, M. M., and Jenkins, W. M. (1995). Cortical plasticity, learning and learning dysfunction. In B. Julesz and I. Kovacs (eds.): *Maturational Windows and Adult Cortical Plasticity.* New York: Addison-Wesley, pp. 247–272.

Merzenich, M., Jenkins, W., Johnston, P. S., Schreiner, C., Miller, S. L., and Tallal, P. (1996). Temporal processing deficits of language-learning impaired children ameliorated by training. *Science, 271,* 77–80.

Merzenich, M. M., Miller, S., Jenkins, W., Sauners, G., Protopapas, A., Peterson, B., and Tallal, P. (1998). Amelioration of the acoustic reception and speech reception deficits underlying language-based learning impairments. In C. V. Euler, (ed.): *Basic Neural Mechanisms in Cognition and Language.* Amsterdam: Elsevier, pp. 144–172.

Merzenich, M. M., Schreiner, C., Jenkins, W. M., and Wang, X. (1993). Neural mechanisms underlying temporal integration, segmentation and input sequence representation: some implications for the origin of learning disabilities. *Ann. N.Y. Acad. Sci., 682,* 1–22.

Merzenich, M. M., Tallal, P., Peterson, B., Miller, S. L., and Jenkins, W. M. (1999). Some neurological principles relevant to the origins of—and the cortical plasticity based remediation of—language learning impairments. In J. Grafman (ed.): *Neuroplasticity: Building a Bridge From the Laboratory to the Clinic.* Amsterdam: Elsevier (in press).

Miller, S. L., Merzenich, M. M., Saunders, G. H., Jenkins, W. M., and Tallal, P. (1997). Improvements in language abilities with training of children with both attentional and language impairments. Soc. Neurosci. Abstr., 23, 490.

Nagarajan, S. S., Wang, X., Merzenich, M. M., Schreiner, C. E., Johnston, P., Jenkins, W. M., Miller, S. M., and Tallal, P. (1998). Speech modification algorithms used for training language learning impaired children. *IEEE Trans. Rehabil. Eng.*, 6, 257–268.

Ramberg, C., Ehlers, S., Nyden, A., Johansson, M., and Gillberg, C. (1996). Language and pragmatic functions in school-age children on the autism spectrum. *Eur. J. Dis. Commun.*, 31, 387–413.

Rapin, I. (1996). Practitioner review: Developmental language disorders: A clinical update. *J. Child Psychol. Psychiatry*, 37, 643–655.

Rapin, I. (1997). Autism. *N. Eng. J. Med.*, 337, 97–104.

Rapin, I., and Dunn, M. (1997). Language diorders in children with autism. *Semin. Pediatr. Neurol.*, 4, 36–92.

Rutter, M. (1974). The development of infantile autism. *Psychol. Med.*, 4, 147–163.

Sevin, J. A., Matson, J. L., Coe, D., Love, S. R., Matese, M. J., and Benavidez, D. A. (1995). Empirically derived subtypes of pervasive developmental disorrders: A cluster analystic study. *J. Autism Dev. Dis.*, 25, 541–578.

Siegel, B., Vukicevic, J., Elliott, G., and Kraemer, H. (1989). The use of signal detection theory to assess DSM-IIIR criteria for autistic disorder. *J. Am. Acad. Child Psychiatry*, 28, 542–548.

Spitz, R., Tallal, P., Flax, J., Benasich, A. (1997). Look who's talking: a prospective study of familial transmission of language impairments. *J. Speech. Lang. Hear. Res.*, 40, 990–1010.

Tager-Flusberg, H. (1993). What language reveals about the understanding of other minds in children with autism. In S. Baron-Cohen, H. Tager-Flusberg, and D. J. Cohen (eds.): *Understanding Other Minds.* New York: Oxford University Press, pp. 138–157.

Tager-Flusberg, H. (1996). Brief report: Current theory and research on language and communication in autism. *J. Autism Dev. Dis.*, 26, 169–172.

Tallal, P., Merzenich, M. M., Miller, S., and Jenkins, W. M. (1999). Language learning impairments: Integrating basic science, technology and remediation. *Exp. Brain Res.*, (in press).

Tallal, P., Miller, S. L., Bedi, G., Byma, G., Wang, X., Nagarajan, S. S., Schreiner, C., Jenkins, W. M., and Merzenich, M. M. (1996). Language comprehension in language-learning impaired children improved with acoustically modified speech. *Science*, 271, 81–84.

Tallal, P., Miller, S., and Fitch, R. H. (1993). Neurobiological basis of speech: A case for the preeminence of temporal processing. *Ann. N.Y. Acad. Sci.*, 682, 27–47.

Tallal, P., and Piercy, M. (1974). Developmental aphasia: Rate of auditory processing and selective impairment of consonant perception. Neuropsychologia, 12, 83–93.

Tallal, P., and Piercy, M. (1975). Developmental aphasia: The perception of brief vowels and extended stop consonants. *Neuropsychologia, 13*, 69–74.

Tallal, P., Saunders, G. H., Miller, S., Jenkins, W. M., Protopapas, A., and Merzenich, M. M. (1997). Rapid training-driven improvement in language ability in autistic and PDD-NOS children. *Soc. Neurosci. Abstr., 23*, 490.

Waterhouse, L., Fein, D., and Modahl, C. (1996a). Neurofunctional mechanisms in autism. *Psychol. Rev., 103*, 457–489.

Waterhouse, L., Morris, R., Allen, D., Dunn, M., Fein, D., Feinstein, C., Rapin, I., and Wing, L. (1996b). Diagnosis and classification in autism. *J. Autism Dev. Dis., 26,* 59–86.

Wright, B. A., Lombardino, L. J., King, W. M., Puranik, C.S., Leonard, C. M., and Merzenich, M. M. (1997). Deficits in auditory temporal and spectral processing in language-impaired children. *Nature, 387,* 176–178.

V

CONCLUSIONS

16

Development, Learning, and Neuroplasticity: Where We Are Now

BENNETT A. SHAYWITZ

As a scientist who knew little about neural plasticity before being cajoled by the editors into writing a commentary and, as a result, having to carefully listen to 2 days of extraordinary presentations, the resulting volume can be considered a crash course in neural plasticity. What strikes this novice is not only the great range of studies that comprise plasticity but the extraordinary progress in the field. Though the volume has been divided into four sections, in fact we can consider two general domains of plasticity: animal models and studies in children.

Parts I and II, comprising Chapters 1–6, consider animal models of plasticity; those of us who study children view such studies with envy for they allow a different level of knowledge than is possible in human studies. Chapters 1–3 emphasize the similarities between those mechanisms involved in learning and those involved in shaping the developing nervous system. Though it comes as the second chapter, historically the studies of Mark Rosenzweig and his colleagues were among the first studies of environmental factors in plasticity. Rosenzweig provides a personal account of how he and his colleagues came to this work; they were trying to explain individual differences in performance in rats. As a student of Hebb in 1947, Rosenzweig related how Hebb was amused that he (Hebb) was credited with the Hebbian plasticity hypothesis of cell assemblies, which is the idea of increases in synaptic strength between neurons that fire together. In fact, Hebb's hypothesis resembled formulations by William James in the latter part of the nineteenth century. Rosenzweig used acetylcholinesterase as a marker of neuronal activity and initially studied rats trained on a progressive series of tasks. The logistics of the training led him to turn to environmental changes, particularly how the rats were housed. His studies compared rats reared in enriched conditions (large groups of 10–12 animals per cage with a variety of stimulus objects), standard conditions (three animals per cage), and impoverished conditions (single animal per cage). Not only did he find increases in acetylcholinesterase, he also found that neocortical weight was increased in those rats in the enriched condition, providing the first evidence that enrichment of the environment could lead to structural changes in brain. Later studies, this time using chicks, provided evidence that the enriched experience was related to neurochemical events, particularly protein synthesis. Central to these observations was that "experience caused changes in specific cortical regions and not undifferentiated growth of brain." (See Chapter 2 of this volume.) Rosenzweig nicely addresses the issue of whether the neural mechanisms of learning and development are the same. Quoting Marcus, he notes that the critical examination of this question will come from studies that examine whether the same process is required for both neuronal development and synaptic plasticity; such studies have not yet been performed.

Philip Nelson and Roger Davenport review their work in Chapter 1, which focuses on synapse elimination at the neuromuscular junction. The phenomenon they are investigating is this: Within several weeks after birth, synapse elimination reduces the initial polyneuronal innervation of individual muscle fibers to mononeuronal innervation. The authors have developed a tissue culture preparation designed to analyze this phenomenon that they call *activity-dependent synapse reduction.* They use an *in vitro* preparation of neurons and muscle dissociated from fetal and neonatal mice and placed into a three-compartment chamber so that axons from two separate populations of cholinergic neurons converge on and innervate a common population of muscle cells. Using this elegant model system, Nelson and Davenport have begun to dissect the mechanisms involved in synapse elimination. Their results suggest that chronic electrical stimulation initiates synapse elimination and that this process involves a cascade of chemically mediated events, involving, for example, the thrombin receptor. More generally, these events may involve the actions of protein kinase C. What is still not clear is now chemically mediated synapse elimination can so precisely affect one synapse while sparing its immediate neighbor; future studies are directed at just this question.

In Chapter 3, William Greenough and his associates review those studies examining the effects of postnatal experience on the structure of the developing and adult brain. They note that the basic organization of the mammalian nervous system is impervious to experience, presumably to protect the organism from minor perturbations during development. In contrast, some species have found it advantageous to adapt their brains to their environment or to incorporate information from the environment, the process of experience-dependent neural plasticity. Greenough et al. use the complex or "enriched" environment paradigm similar to that developed by Rosenzweig, which manipulates differences in the complexity of the environment to examine the mechanisms of synapse formation and elimination in the rat. Rats reared in enriched environments have larger dendritic fields with a greater number of synapses per neuron than rats reared individually. Furthermore, cerebellar cortex from rats raised in environmentally complex conditions demonstrate increases in the number of synapses, capillary volume, and glia. These changes appear related to learning, not simply to aggregate neuronal activity reflecting increases in motor activity. More recent studies using preparations of synaptoneurosomes from these animals indicate that the increase in synapses reflects increases in protein synthesis, perhaps involving increases in receptors. Greenough et al. have extended their studies to try to relate plasticity in animals to a developmental disorder, specifically fragile-X syndrome. Their findings suggest that the fragile-X mental retardation protein found in this syndrome might be necessary for the normal developmental process of synapse maturation and elimination. Greenough et al. have also shown that mice with knockout of the fragile-X gene have immature dendritic spines and failure of synaptic elimination processes. They have also used intensive experiential therapy in an animal model of fetal alcohol syndrome.

In the second part of the chapters on animal models (Chapters 4–6), three investigators review their work examining the mechanisms of reorganization in the central nervous system. In the first chapter of this section (Chapter 4), Craig Bailey discusses the structural changes underlying long-term memory. Bailey studies the gill-and-siphon withdrawal reflex of the marine mollusc *Aplysia californica.* This reflex can be modified by nonassociative learning, specifically habituation and sensitization. Bailey focuses on the monosynaptic connection between mechanoreceptor sensory neurons and their associated motor neuron. Using intracellular labeling techniques combined with serial sections, he was able to compare synapses from control and behaviorally modified animals. He found that long-term memory is accompanied by structural modifications of the synapse, specifically alterations in focal regions of membrane specialization of the synapse as well as in the total number of presynaptic varicosities per sensory neuron. These changes can also be affected by cAMP activated by serotonin. More recent studies suggest that at the molecular level synaptic reorganization involves cell adhesion molecules, particularly isoforms of the immunoglobulin-related cell adhesion molecule named apCAM. Bailey suggests that the serotonin modulates apCAMs resulting in membrane remodeling at the synapse, a process that may represent the first morphological step underlying long-term facilitation.

Asaf Keller in Chapter 5 reviews issues related to the development and plasticity of local circuits in the motor cortex. The focus of his work is understanding the mechanisms by which cortical representations of movement patterns are modified by behavioral experience, both during development and in mature animals. He shows that an innocuous manipulation that affects sensorimotor activity—whisker clipping—results in dramatic but reversible changes in these cortical representations. These changes are thought to be generated by changes in synaptic interactions mediated by intracortical circuits. Using anatomical, electrophysiological, and functional imaging approaches, Keller shows that these interactions are highly specific in that they preferentially link cells located within representations related to the same movement patterns. He also shows that the efficacy of these interactions is influenced by inhibitory processes. Furthermore, a long-lasting increase in the efficacy of these interactions (long-term potentiation) can be produced by repetitive stimulation. These findings support the role of local circuits in shaping movement representation maps in the motor cortex.

Bertram Payne (Chapter 6) studies lesions of the visual cortex, comparing the effects of lesions in the immature visual cortex in the kitten with similar lesions in the mature cat. His studies reveal global rewiring of the visual system with repercussions throughout the neural circuitry of vision (retina, thalamus, midbrain, and extrastriate cortex). As a result of lesions in the primary visual cortex, he finds regressive effects in some regions (i.e., specific death of neurons), while in other regions there is evidence of expansion of specific pathways. In still other regions, there is neural compensation reflected as increased neural traffic. These studies suggest that, given the widespread effects of lesions, multiple therapeutic strategies might need to be adopted to attenuate the effects of the system wide lesion.

Part III, the longest section, examines the issues of neuroplasticity within the framework of human neurodevelopmental disorders. In the first of this group of chapters, Hannay, Fletcher, and Brandt (Chapter 7) exploit magnetic resonance imaging to examine the corpus callosum as a model for brain plasticity. The Houston group studies defects of the corpus callosum in children with congenital brain malformations; the most common of these are children who were born with spina bifida meningomyelocele, most of whom experience a combination of defects associated with partial agenesis of the corpus callosum and/or hypoplasia of the corpus callosum as well as abnormalities of the cerebellum and midbrain. These children are compared with children with aqueductal stenosis, a congenital disorder leading to hydrocephalus and often partial agenesis and hypoplasia of the corpus callosum, but with a normal cerebellum. Another group are children with Dandy-Walker syndrome, also associated with defects of the corpus callosum and partial to complete agenesis of the cerebellar vermis. Children with these abnormalities share common neurobehavioral deficits, particularly difficulties with motor coordination and spatial cognition. Hannay, Fletcher, and Brandt set out to explore the neural mechanisms underlying these cognitive deficits. They consider three possibilities that might affect motor and spatial function: *(1)* general effects of hydrocephalus on thinning the posterior regions of the cerebral cortex; *(2)* abnormalities of the cerebellum (common in spina bifida and Dandy-Walker syndrome but not aqueductal stenosis; *(3)* abnormalities of the corpus callosum accounting for some of the deficits. Good evidence by Hannay, Fletcher, and Brandt strongly implicates the third possibility, that is, that the motor and spatial deficits are related to the integrity of the corpus callosum. In more recent studies they have begun to explore the neural reorganization that takes place in hydrocephalic children with abnormalities of the corpus callosum using auditory, visual, and somatosensory laterality tasks to test these hypotheses more directly.

Maureen Dennis and her associates (Chapter 8) are interested in age-based functional plasticity in children with congenital malformations of the cerebellum and midbrain. In contrast to older views of the cerebellum's role in coordination of motor movements, more contemporary views consider that, in addition, the cerebellum plays a role in the temporal integration of discrete motor movements and in cognitive function (e.g., language, learning, and skill acquisition). To determine the structure–function relationships, Dennis and her associates study children with congenital malformations of the cerebellum of the same type studied by Hannay and colleagues, as well as acquired disorders of the cerebellum. Data from both groups of subjects suggest an apparent absence of age-based functional plasticity in motor tasks and in tasks addressing cognitive timing. In contrast to the cerebral cortex, age-based functional plasticity does not appear to be the rule in cerebellar lesions in children.

Barry Gordon and his associates (Chapter 9) examine the recovery of reading impairments in adults undergoing surgery for epilepsy, tumors, or arteriovenous malformations. Because these investigators were able to evaluate their patients prior to and during surgery, and at early and later times following surgery, they were able to follow the course of recovery after a surgical-induced focal brain lesion. They focus on four subjects who developed impairments in reading following resections of the left inferior temporal region (in three of four) and left lateral occipital cortex. All subjects recovered to nearly their baseline. A number of possible mechanisms could explain this recovery, including residual neural tissue. They point out that only about 10%–20% of neural tissue is necessary for adequate functioning to occur; even this small amount of residual tissue may be capable of achieving near-normal function. Extrapolating to a developmental disorder (autism), they suggest that very targeted training may be more effective than currently available therapies.

In surely one of the most provocative chapters in this volume, Elizabeth Bates (Chapter 10) reviews her findings of language development in children with early injuries (within the first 6 months of life) to one side of the brain. In a series of studies she and her collaborators have reported that such children "usually acquire language abilities within the normal or low-normal range, with little evidence for effects of lesion side or lesion site." But rather than simply reviewing her previous data, Bates discusses the implications of her findings "for the nature and origins of language localization in the adult, providing an account of how this neural system might emerge across the course of development." Bates proposes what she refers to as "the emergentist perspective" of language development (Elman et al., 1996), a view at odds with a modular and instinctual (innate) view of language development espoused by, for example, Fodor (1993) and Pinker (1994). In Bates' view "there has to be something special about the human brain that makes language possible, but that 'something' may involve highly distributed mechanisms that serve many other functions."

Dorothy Aram (Chapter 11) examined the effects of unilateral brain lesions on language development in a population of children similar to those studied by Bates, addressing the question of the degree of early specialization versus plasticity of the brain for language. Her studies focused on behavioral plasticity and inferred the neural plasticity from the behavioral data. Over a 14-year period she recruited 25 children with left lateralized lesions and 15 children with right lateralized lesions. Remarkably, at follow up few significant deficits were noted on either cognitive or language testing. To be sure, Aram found mild deficits in left-lesioned children on spoken syntax, syntactic comprehension, lexical development and retrieval, and mathematics; right-lesioned subjects tended to exhibit mild deficits in intelligence, attention, and lexical development. Yet on a battery of tests assessing phonological analysis, decoding, reading comprehension, and spelling, the majority of subjects did well. Nor did the age at which the lesion occurred produce any predictable effect on language and learning. Lesions involving the left subcortical structures were associated with the most persistent and pronounced residual deficits. Aram concludes that children with unilateral brain injury tend to have a relatively good prognosis.

Marian Sigman and Norman Kim (Chapter 12) describe continuity and change in the symptoms of a severe developmental disability, autism. Sigman has followed 51 autistic children longitudinally and describes stability or change in their tested intelligence and in a number of other cognitive and behavioral domains. Over an 8–9-year period there was little change in IQ scores for the children with autism in contrast to children with Down syndrome, whose IQ dropped 20 points in this period of time. Of particular interest was the findings that "the most hopeful result of this investigation was that a surprising number of children with autism who tested in the mentally retarded range at intake had scores above that range at follow up some 8–9 years latter." Thus, about half the children with autism showed increases in intelligence, and about 25% of children with autism who had scored in the mentally retarded range 8–9 years before now scored in the borderline to average range with just one child showing a comparable decline in IQ. Such findings lead the authors to conclude that "plasticity is possible in the life course of individuals with autism."

In the final chapter in this section Eric Courchesne, Rachel Yeung-Courchesne, and Karen Pierce (Chapter 13) examine the biological and behavioral heterogeneity in autism. Courchesne and colleagues have provided something extremely important in this chapter, a new way of thinking about the biological substrates of autism. They theorize that it is just those biological mechanisms, pleiotropy and epigenesis, "that are designed to create efficiency and adaptive neuroplasticity during development [which] simultaneously and inevitably open the door to many different possible developmental outcomes." Pleiotropy, a mechanism for genetic coding efficiency, represents the phenomenon whereby a single gene is responsible for multiple actions in many different kinds of cells at different times. While this is indeed efficient, it also means that mutations in a single gene's code may cause multiple problems in multiple cells. Epigenesis refers to the incredibly large number of influences, both internal and external to the organism, that shape the development of the brain. Adapting an argument made by Quartz and Sejowski, epigenesis means that the developing nervous system is designed to be perturbable. Courchesne et al. hypothesize that these mechanisms may occur in autism. Thus, in the initial sections of their chapter they marshall an impressive array of data (incorporating behavioral, anatomical, and brain morphometric and functional imaging studies), much of it from their own laboratory, that suggests that an insult during the early stages of gestation, perhaps around the fifth fetal week, affecting the cerebellar vermis and its connections with other brain structures may be involved in autism.

In Part IV, the final two chapters focus on interventions for children with developmental disabilities, a natural extension of the animal and the human studies of plasticity. In the first part of Chapter 14, Susan Landry reviews her experience with intervention for very-low-birth-weight infants. These children are at great risk for developing disorders affecting attention, motor functions, and language. Results from a pilot study suggest that structured interventions directed toward maternal behaviors, such as teaching the mother to orient infants toward stimuli, may be an important component of any therapeutic program. The second portion of the chapter, a critical review of interventions for children with pervasive developmental disorders, is particularly informative. She notes that one of the most popular and widely used intervention programs (TEACCH) has never been assessed in controlled studies. Clearly, longitudinal studies combined with new techniques, such as growth curve modeling, may be helpful in better assessment of interventions. Future interventions must be tested with experimental designs that incorporate good sample sizes, longitudinal methodology, careful attention to diagnostic criteria, and outcomes that assess a broad range of skills.

In Chapter 15, Michael Merzenich and his colleagues describe a language-based intervention in children with pervasive developmental disorder. What is so interesting here is that Merzenich, one of the pioneers in the study of neural plasticity (see Buonomano and Merzenich, 1998) has developed an intervention for children based on his work on neural plasticity in animal models. The intervention, the computer-based program Fast ForWord, resulted in improvement of at least 1 SD in at least one of the tests in 25 of 29 children with pervasive developmental disorders, and 17 of 29 children advanced by at least 2 SD on at least one of the tests. The obvious next step is to build on these impressive results from an open trial to test the intervention in a randomized clinical trial.

Future Directions: Functional Imaging

Some of the most interesting and significant questions that begin to be touched on by the contributors to this volume relate to efforts to begin to understand those mechanisms influencing brain development and brain plasticity in human disorders of higher cognitive function. As an optimist I am intrigued by Mark Rosenzweig's quote by the historian of psychology Edwin Boring: "The truth about how the brain functions may eventually yield to a technique that comes from some new field remote from either physiology or psychology. Genius waits on insight, but insight may wait on the discovery of new concrete factual knowledge" (Boring, 1950, p. 4). Perhaps functional imaging, a family of techniques that comes from physics and engineering, may be the lever that allows us such insights, particularly in studies of plasticity in cognitive processes that are uniquely human, such as language and reading.

Functional imaging, the ability to measure brain function during performance of a cognitive task, became possible in the early 1980s. For the first time, rather than being limited to examining the brain in an autopsy specimen, or measuring the size of brain regions using static morphometric indices based on computed tomography or magnetic resonance imaging, scientists were able to think of studying brain metabolism while individuals were performing specific cognitive tasks.

When an individual is asked to perform a discrete cognitive task, that task places processing demands on particular neural systems in the brain. To meet those demands requires activation of neural systems in particular brain regions and those changes in neural activity are, in turn, reflected by changes in brain metabolic activity (e.g., changes in cerebral blood flow or changes in cerebral utilization of metabolic substrates such as glucose); it is possible to measure those changes in metabolic activity in specific brain regions while subjects are engaged in cognitive tasks.

The first studies of this kind used xenon 133 to measure cerebral blood flow, but more recent studies use positron emission tomography (PET). In practice PET requires intraarterial or intravenous administration of a radioactive isotope to the subject so that cerebral blood flow or cerebral utilization of glucose can be determined while the subject is performing the task. Positron-emitting isotopes of nuclei of biological interest have very short biological half-lives and are synthesized in a cyclotron immediately prior to the testing, a factor that mandates that the time course of the experiment conform to the short half-life of the radioisotope. Although much has been learned about language using PET technology, PET uses short-lived radioisotopes, requires a cyclotron and associated team of technicians, and suffers from relatively poor spatial and temporal resolution and sensitivity. Particularly when considering studies in children, the invasive nature of the procedure and radiation exposure as well as the logistics of generating short-lived isotopes limits the utility of PET.

Functional Magnetic Resonance Imaging (fMRI) promises to surpass other methods for its ability to map the individual brain's response to specific cognitive stimuli. Because it is noninvasive and safe, it can be used to repeatedly study humans, including children and neonates, without risk. In principle, the signal used to construct MRI images changes, by a small amount (typically 1%–5%), in regions that are activated by a stimulus or task. The increase in signal results from the combined effects of increases in the tissue blood flow, volume, and oxygenation, though the precise contributions of each of these is still somewhat uncertain. At least in some conditions, the increase in activation produced a flow increase locally that introduces oxygenated blood to a degree that is greater than the increased metabolic demands, with the result that the tissue oxygen tension increases and the venous blood becomes more oxygenated. The significance of this is that the intravascular magnetic susceptibility then more closely matches the surrounding tissue than when the vessels contain deoxyhemoglobin. In the deoxygenated state, the heme group in blood produces a significant paramagnetism that disturbs the homogeneity of the magnetic field in the environment of the vasculature, whereas in oxygenated blood the disturbance is much smaller. This in turn means that the magnetic field experienced by tissue water in the close vicinity of activated volumes is more uniform.

The signal used to construct MR images is derived from the nuclear magnetization produced mainly by tissue water protons. This magnetization can be tipped away from its equilibrium alignment in the direction of an applied external field using radiofrequency pulses, and the resultant signal decays at a measurable rate.

The decay rate is slower, and the MR signal therefore stronger, when the magnetic field is uniform. Thus, MR image intensity increases when deoxygenated blood is replaced by oxygenated blood.

A variety of methods can be used to record the changes that occur. One preferred approach makes use of so-called ultrafast imaging, such as echo planar imaging (EPI), in which complete images are acquired in times substantially shorter than a second. EPI can provide images at a rate fast enough to capture the time course of the hemodynamic response to neural activation and to permit a wide variety of imaging paradigms over large volumes of the brain.

Because fMRI allows repeated scans of the same subject, it is ideal for studying brain plasticity. Experiments can be planned to examine the plasticity of, for example, expressive language in individuals with aphasias as a result of strokes. Tasks engaging language systems can be repeated on the same subject over a period of weeks, months, or even years, and observations can determine activation in specific brain regions that change over time. It is also ideal for studying the effects of an intervention on brain organization in developmental disorders such as developmental dyslexia (Shaywitz et al., 1998).

In collaboration with Benita Blachman at Syracuse University, our research group is using fMRI to study the effects of reading instruction on brain organization in dyslexic children. The project involves, first, the identification of children with dyslexia; fMRI is used to assess brain organization at baseline, 1 year after an intensive phonemically based reading program, and 1 year after the intervention program has finished. We hope to see changes in brain organization that parallel (or perhaps precede) improvement in reading performance. Comparisons of responders and nonresponders may be particularly illuminating.

Conclusions

Despite the wide variation in specific subject matter, the chapters in this volume embody several general themes. The first is that those mechanisms serving to influence the development of the brain are similar to and may be the same as those influencing plasticity. The obvious message from this information is that understanding the mechanisms that influence brain development will help us to understand the mechanisms that affect plasticity. Another general theme is the recognition that mechanisms that have evolved to create efficiency (Courchesne) and experience-dependent adaptive neuroplasticity (Greenough), critical in understanding plasticity, are the same mechanisms that may go awry and result in significant and profound developmental disorders, such as autism. Third, the complementary nature of basic/clinical and animal/human studies is clearly apparent. These studies operate in worlds that overlap and where the relationships are reciprocal—not in isolated chambers of the laboratory and clinic. Finally, treatment is on the horizon. Research on early brain disorders is progressing and to the point where treatment and, equally importantly, prevention will be possible. New treatment and prevention methods will have strong research foundations. The next step, to follow Landry, will be to fully evaluate the efficiency of interventions using well-controlled designs.

What is clear from this volume is the extraordinary program that has been made in understanding neural plasticity and how elucidation of the mechanisms serving plasticity may help to unravel the causes of some of the most disabling developmental disorders in children. The good news is that scientists have identified the questions to address and have developed a range of experimental models both in animals and in humans. The challenge as we enter the twenty-first century is how best to exploit the great progress that has already been made to understand, treat and, yes, perhaps prevent some of these pernicious developmental disorders.

References

Portions of this commentary appeared in Shaywitz, B. A., Shaywitz, S. E., Pugh, K. R., Skudlarski, P., Fulbright, R. K., Constable, R. T., Bronen, R. A., Fletcher, J. M., Liberman, A. M., Shankweiler, D. P., Katz, L., Lacadie, C., Marchione, K., and Gore, J. C. (1996). The functional organization of brain for reading and reading disability (dyslexia). *Neuroscientist, 2,* 245–255, with permission.

Boring, E. G. (1950). *A History of Experimental Psychology.* New York: Appleton-Century-Crofts.

Buonomano, D. V., and Merzenich, M. M. (1998). Cortical plasticity: From synapses to maps. *Ann. Rev. Neurosci., 21,* 149–186.

Elman, J. L., Bates, E. A., Johnson, M. H., Karmiloff-Smith, A., Parisi, D., and Plunkett, K. (1996). *Rethinking Innateness: A Connectionist Perspective on Development.* Cambridge, MA: MIT Press.

Foder, J. M. (1983). *The Modularity of Mind: An Essay on Faculty Psychology.* Cambridge, MA: MIT Press.

Pinker, S. (1994). *The Language Instinct: How the Mind Creates Language.* New York: William Morrow.

Shaywitz, S. E., Shaywitz, B. A., Pugh, K. R., Fulbright, R. K., Constable, R. T., Mencl, W. E., Shankweiler, D. P., Liberman, A. M., Skudlarski, P., Fletcher, J. M., Katz, L., Marchione, K. E., Lacadie, C., Gatenby, C., and Gore, J. C. (1998). Functional disruption in the organization of the brain for reading in dyslexia. *Proc. Natl. Acad. Sci. U.S.A., 95,* 2636–2641.

Index

children
IQ, 217–218, 257–259, 267
language, grammatical development, 219–220, 244, 260–261
language, lexical development, 262
left versus right hemisphere damage, 219–221, 231–232, 262, 269–271, 393–394
limb growth, 256–257
outcomes, academic, 263, 265, 268–269
outcomes, language, 225–229, 244–246, 260–262
outcomes, visuospatial, 226
hemispheric reorganization, 269–270
event-related potentials, 269–270
strokes, 255–256
Forgetting, reduction in synapses in, 82
Fragile X syndrome, 51, 53, 311, 317, 322, 365, 391
mental retardation protein (FMRP) 51, 54, 60–61, 391

γ-aminobutyric acid (GABA) 103, 107
Gene activation, 82–84, 91
Growth factors, 82–83, 87

Habituation, 391
Hebb synapse, 10–11, 17, 27, 107
Hemispherectomy, language recovery of, 229–232
Holoprosencephaly, 157
Hydrocephalus, 157–162, 181, 184–185, 392

IQ, 278–280, 287, 342, 394
children, autism, 278–280
children, focal lesions, 217–218, 246, 257–259, 264–265
discrepancies, 257
stability of scores, in autism, 278–279
stability of scores, in early brain injury, 258–259
reliability, 278
Interhemispheric transmission time (ITT), 154–155, 163–165
Intervention and Training
autism and PDD, 325–328, 330, 354–359, 371–379, 395
complex symbolic functions, 210

Fast ForWord, 367–372, 374–378
limitations of, 379–382, 395
fetal alcohol syndrome, 61–63
neural mechanisms, 210
Intracortical microstimulation technique (ICMS), 98, 100–101, 103, 106

Kainate/α-amino-3-hydroxy-5-methyl-ioxyzole-4 propionic acid (AMPA) glutamate receptors, 101

Language
in autism, 281–283, 342, 365
emergentist view, 235–241, 393
focal lesions, and, 219–220, 231, 244, 261–262, 269–271, 393–394
innate predetermination, 214–215, 230, 233–238, 244, 247, 393
lateralization, 215, 219–220, 246
left temporal cortex, role of, 247
and phrenology, 214, 233–235, 239–242, 247
right hemisphere, role of, 243–245, 264, 271
specific language disorders, 366, 371
Laterality task, tachistoscopic, 163
Learning
and development, 34–37, 73, 77, 90–92, 389–390
and synapse formation, 55–56, 59, 73
Long-term depression (LTD), 12, 107
Long-term facilitation, 83–84, 391
Long-term potentiation, (LTP), 10–12, 91, 107, 391

MacArthur Communicative Development Inventory, 227
Machado-Joseph disease, 180
Marinesco-Sjogren syndrome, 180
Mathematics and early focal lesions, 263, 266
Mean Length of Utterance, 227, 260–261
Medulloblastoma, 181–182, 187–190
Memory, long-term trace, 89–90
and development, 91
formation, neurochemical cascades during, 32–33
Mitogen-activated protein kinase (MAPK), 88